Oral Health Practice for Dental Hygienists

Oral Health Practice for Dental Hygienists

Edited by Patrick Hall

hayle
medical

New York

Hayle Medical,
750 Third Avenue, 9th Floor,
New York, NY 10017, USA

Visit us on the World Wide Web at:
www.haylemedical.com

This book contains information obtained from authentic and highly regarded sources. Copyright for all individual chapters remain with the respective authors as indicated. All chapters are published with permission under the Creative Commons Attribution License or equivalent. A wide variety of references are listed. Permission and sources are indicated; for detailed attributions, please refer to the permissions page and list of contributors. Reasonable efforts have been made to publish reliable data and information, but the authors, editors and publisher cannot assume any responsibility for the validity of all materials or the consequences of their use.

ISBN: 978-1-63241-564-6

Trademark Notice: Registered trademark of products or corporate names are used only for explanation and identification without intent to infringe.

Cataloging-in-Publication Data

Oral health practice for dental hygienists / edited by Patrick Hall.
  p. cm.
Includes bibliographical references and index.
ISBN 978-1-63241-564-6
1. Dental hygiene. 2. Mouth--Care and hygiene. 3. Dental care.
4. Dental public health. 5. Dentistry. 6. Oral medicine. I. Hall, Patrick.
RK60.5 .O73 2019
617.602 33--dc23

Table of Contents

Preface VII

Chapter 1 **Denture and Overdenture Complications**.. 1
Elena Preoteasa, Cristina Teodora Preoteasa, Laura Iosif,
Catalina Murariu Magureanu and Marina Imre

Chapter 2 **Ultrasonic Instrumentation**.. 34
Ana Isabel García-Kass, Juan Antonio García-Núñez
and Victoriano Serrano-Cuenca

Chapter 3 **Panoramic Radiography — Diagnosis of Relevant Structures that
Might Compromise Oral and General Health of the Patient**...................... 55
Ticiana Sidorenko de Oliveira Capote, Marcela de Almeida Gonçalves,
Andrea Gonçalves and Marcelo Gonçalves

Chapter 4 **Improving Antimicrobial Activity of Dental Restorative Materials** 85
J. M. F. A. Fernandes, V. A. Menezes, A. J. R. Albuquerque,
M. A. C. Oliveira, K. M. S. Meira, R. A. Menezes Júnior
and F. C. Sampaio

Chapter 5 **Evidence-Based Control of Oral Malodor**.. 103
Nao Suzuki, Masahiro Yoneda and Takao Hirofuji

Chapter 6 **Oral Fluid Biomarkers in Smoking Periodontitis Patients
and Systemic Inflammation** 119
Anna Maria Heikkinen, Päivi Mäntylä, Jussi Leppilahti,
Nilminie Rathnayake, Jukka Meurman and Timo Sorsa

Chapter 7 **Herbal Dentifrices for Children**.. 138
Marisa Alves Nogueira Diaz, Isabela de Oliveira Carvalho
and Gaspar Diaz

Chapter 8 **Assorted Errands in Prevention of Children's Oral Diseases
and Conditions** 162
H. S. Mbawala, F. M. Machibya and F. K. Kahabuka

Chapter 9 **Comparative School Dental Sealant Program to Alleviate Dental
Caries Problem — Thai versus International Perspective** 184
Sukanya Tianviwat

Permissions

List of Contributors

Index

Preface

This book has been a concerted effort by a group of academicians, researchers and scientists, who have contributed their research works for the realization of the book. This book has materialized in the wake of emerging advancements and innovations in this field. Therefore, the need of the hour was to compile all the required researches and disseminate the knowledge to a broad spectrum of people comprising of students, researchers and specialists of the field.

The practice of maintaining hygiene of the mouth is known as oral hygiene. It is required to be carried out on a regular basis to prevent dental diseases and bad breath. Tooth decay and periodontitis are two of the most common types of dental and gum diseases. Routine dental treatment includes dental filling, tooth extraction, scaling and root planing, and root canal. Teeth cleaning is an important part of oral hygiene. It includes the removal of dental plaque from teeth in order to prevent gum diseases, deposits of tartar and cavities. This book is a compilation of chapters that discuss the most vital concepts and emerging trends in the field of oral health practice. Some of the diverse topics covered in it address the varied branches that fall under this category. The extensive content of this book provides the readers with a thorough understanding of the subject.

At the end of the preface, I would like to thank the authors for their brilliant chapters and the publisher for guiding us all-through the making of the book till its final stage. Also, I would like to thank my family for providing the support and encouragement throughout my academic career and research projects.

Editor

Denture and Overdenture Complications

Elena Preoteasa, Cristina Teodora Preoteasa,
Laura Iosif, Catalina Murariu Magureanu and
Marina Imre

1. Introduction

Dentures and overdentures, the most frequently used treatment options for the complete edentulism, can have local and systemic complications. For their prevention, treatment and reduction of their negative impact, it is necessary to understand their etiological context and to know their particularities of manifestation. Considering the relatively high rate of some complications of denture and overdenture treatment, knowing them is essential for ensuring a treatment that corresponds to the medical standards of care and patients' needs and expectations.

2. Context of denture and overdenture complications

All medical treatments should be approached with a holistic perspective in mind, due to the fact that there are numerous factors which, through interacting each other, have an impact on the final medical outcome. Understanding the problem and its realistic possible approaches, but also considering its treatment limitations and performing an analysis that evaluates the medium and long-term prognosis ensures the highest premises for obtaining a good result.

The previous also applies to the treatment of edentulism using dentures or overdentures. Some of the key aspects that might help understand better the denture and overdenture complications, as they define the etiological context, are mentioned in Table 1.

	General medical and social factors	Medical and social perception of edentulism
		Demographics of edentulism
	Denture and overdenture treatment factors	Treatment difficulty
		Treatment options overview
		Maintenance therapy
Context		Technical and biomechanical considerations
		Previous dental treatments
	Edentulous patient factors	Oral health status
		Systemic health status and medication use
		Age
		Health risk factors
		Patient need and preferences

Table 1. Context of denture and overdenture complications – key factors

2.1. Medical and social perception of edentulism

Edentulism is defined as the loss of all permanent teeth. Tooth loss is an outcome of a complex interaction between disease entities (e.g., caries and periodontal disease) and non-disease entities (e.g. economy, oral healthcare system, access to dental services, dental awareness, cultural tradition, education) [1]. Continuing exposure to risk factors after onset of edentulism (e.g., poor oral hygiene, smoking, deficient dental treatment) can have an etiological role in the occurrence of complication.

Edentulism is a chronic, severe, irreversible medical condition and is described as the final marker of disease burden for oral health [2,3]. It is common for elderly people, but it is not regarded any more as an inevitable phenomenon that comes with age [4].

Edentulism has several deleterious consequences on oral health (e.g., residual ridge resorption, impaired masticatory function, trouble speaking), general health (deficient nutritional status, increased risk for certain systemic diseases), mental and social well-being (dissatisfaction with appearance, avoidance of social contacts) and on quality of life [1,2,4]. The previous have impact on prosthetic treatment to be performed.

Thus, the current perception on edentulism is as non-fatal sequelae of diseases and injuries, which still represents a tremendous global health care burden [5,6]. It can be considered a physical impairment, because important body parts have been lost, a disability, because it associates functional limitations or a handicap, as it sometimes limits or prevents normal life or work activities [1,2,7-9].

Considering the impact and demographics of the edentulism, the health care barriers that older people face, the Active Ageing approach of the World Health Organization (keeping older people socially engaged and productive), intensive measures and new regulations regarding caring for the elderly population are needed. Consequently, implementation of gerodontology, as a new dental specialty, may be appropriate [10].

2.2. Demographics of edentulism

According to the current reports and predictions, edentulism is and will continue to represent a common disease for the elderly people segment.

There is a tendency for reduction of the edentulism prevalence, through the reduction of tooth loss. Thus, in the United States in the period of 1999-2004, the prevalence of tooth retention in seniors (65 years and older) significantly increased from 17.9 teeth to 18.9 teeth and the prevalence of edentulism significantly decreased from approximately 34% to 27% [11]. This phenomenon can be justified through the progress made in the dental field, the emphasis on prevention measures, improved access to dental care services and mass education for approaching a healthy behavior [4]. But, despite these efforts, complete edentulism continues to have a high prevalence, aspect associated mainly to the aging population phenomenon through growth of the life expectancy and thus the number of elderly people and the number of edentulous patients [12,13].

Estimates show that edentulism is found in 2.3% of the world's population regardless of age, respectively in 7-69% of adult populations internationally [5,14]. Considerably high disparities are noted between different countries, different regions, due to the important impact of the socio-economical and behavioral factors.

The prognoses show that edentulism is decreasing, but most probably will continue to be a condition with a significant prevalence, especially in elderly's people, which is estimated to be a growing category in the global population [15]. Douglas estimates that in the United States the population with one or two edentulous jaws will increase from 34 million in 1991 to 38 million in 2020 [1,12]. Felton considers that most probably the necessity for complete denture therapy will not disappear over the next 4 or 5 decades, and the economic conditions may even lead to a growing need [1,6].

2.3. Treatment difficulty

Edentulism is generally regarded as a clinical condition with a high degree of treatment difficulty, often being hard to achieve optimal functional parameters. The complexity of the edentulous condition derives from the extensive oral changes, both anatomical and functional, that sometimes require preprosthetic surgical intervention in order to optimize the biomechanical conditions, which are superimposed on general alterations (related to age, systemic disease, and psychosocial status). In order to support the differentiation of cases according to their treatment difficulty degree, the ACP (American College of Prosthodontists) has put together the Prosthodontic Diagnostic Index (PDI) Classification System for the complete edentulism [16]. Higher complexity of edentulism condition increase the risk of treatment complication (e.g., in cases with severe ridge resorption ill-fitting dentures are more frequently noticed), and complications can also contribute to increasing the degree of treatment difficulty (e.g., wearing unstable dentures accelerate the ridge resorption rate).

2.4. Treatment options overview

Complete denture used to be the only treatment option for the complete edentulism. Nowadays, this is still the most frequently used treatment option, but there can be seen a growing trend towards using implant prosthetic restorations fixed or removable. Each treatment option has the risk of specific complications, dependent on their manufacturing particularities and bio-mechanical features.

Dentures can have both local and systemic complications, such as gingival hyperplasia, denture stomatitis, loss of denture retention, fracture of the denture and functional impairment, mastication deficiencies having a negative impact on the nutritional status. Some patients cannot tolerate the dentures, aspect that can be connected to psychological factors, to patients' needs and expectations, but also to age, oral conditions, denture deficiencies and doctor-patient relationship.

Root supported overdentures, with or without attachment systems, have the advantage of improved retention and stability, with a positive impact on the oral functions and the accommodation with the future dentures. Their possible complications include the ones of the conventional dentures and, additionally, some modifications of the supporting teeth or the attachment system used.

Prosthetic implant restorations, either fixed or a removable, are alternatives that provide an improved functional integration and better treatment outcome, but are more complex and require preprosthetic interventions, with additional biological, financial and time costs. Using these treatment options involves the risk for additional complications, with regards to the higher complexity of the treatment –e.g., treatment plan related, surgical complications, technical complications.

2.5. Maintenance therapy

Maintenance is very important for the longevity of the treatment, having a positive impact in reducing the frequency and severity of its complications. Both type of procedures, those performed in the dental office, by the dentist and at home, by the patient, are relevant in this respect.

Periodical check-ups are essential, considering that there are some complications with a high prevalence rate both for dentures and implant overdentures (e.g., loss of denture stability due to progressive ridge resorption, denture adjustments and relinings, clip activations) [17]. Additionally, the edentulous patients are often elderly patients, and face access barriers to dental care services, in relation to aspects like lack of finances or transportation difficulties [18,19]. Due to this, it is recommended to keep in mind the possible complications and to take the appropriate preventive measures to limit them at the time the treatment is being planned and performed.

Informing and instructing the patient on how to take proper care of the oral care and prosthetic restorations are important aspects, since complications can be tightly related to this (e.g., the lack of appropriate cleaning of the denture, teeth or implants is associated with a higher risk for denture stomatitis, tooth or implant loss). Since we are frequently dealing with elderly people, who have less manual dexterity, it is recommended to choose simpler treatment option (e.g., if applicable, 2-implant overdentures are more appropriate than 4-implant overdenture [20].

2.6. Technical and biomechanical considerations

According to the current level of knowledge, treatment with dentures or implant/root overdentures must consider the risk for developing complications in relation to the technical and biomechanical features (e.g., design, attachment components, materials).

There are different types of design for dentures and overdentures, with different possible complications. Thus, using narrow-diameter implants associates a higher risk of implant fracture. Considering the occlusal scheme, there is evidence that patients prefer dentures with lingualized occlusion [21]. Metal or non-metal (glass and polyethylene fibers) inserts are recommended for denture base reinforcement when there is a high risk of denture fracture or when there are more than 2 teeth or implants supporting the denture [22].

Material used for denture/overdenture fabrication associates the risk of developing complications in relation to their physico-chemical properties and their biocompatibility. For example, polymethylmethacrylate (PMMA), the material mostly used for manufacturing of dentures or overdentures, through its features (porosity, increased wettability, low mechanical strength, monomer release after curing) facilitates the occurrence of complications such as microbial or contact denture stomatitis, fracture of the dentures, artificial teeth discoloration and wear [23].

2.7. Previous dental treatments

A key element in order to achieve a predictable outcome is the analysis of the previous dental and prosthetic treatments, by connecting patient's subjective complaints with prosthetic restoration's objective deficiencies. This gives important information that could be used for decision making in establishing the particularities of the future prosthetic treatment. For example, complete denture intolerance can be linked to personality traits, to objective patient's features that enhance the occurrence of functional deficiencies, or to some objective faults of the dentures. Differentiating between these three situations is the basis for selecting the optimal treatment option, with the possibility to prevent the complications that occurred in the past.

2.8. Oral health status

The complete edentulism cannot be regarded simply as the loss of teeth. It is accompanied by massive, progressive changes of the oral structures and functional alterations, which associates a high degree of treatment difficulty and the occurrence of specific complications. Impact of edentulism on oral health is mainly manifested in 3 directions: modifier of normal physiology; risk factor for impaired mastication; determinant of oral health [2]. Amongst the sequelae of treatment with complete dentures, as the most commonly used treatment option, there can be mentioned residual ridge resorption, mucosal reactions, burning mouth syndrome, denture stomatitis [24].

Considering the severe changes of the oral status in edentulous patients, the increasing elderly population and the relatively frequent barriers to oral health care of older people (e.g., financial hardship, transportation difficulties), Petersen et al. makes a series of recommendations among which are the incorporation of age related oral health concerns into the promotion of general health, that could ease the development of oral health care for older people [25].

2.9. Systemic health status and medication use

Between oral health and general health there are numerous interactions, that sometimes materializes as local or systemic complications.

The impact of complete edentulism on the general health status is manifested as an increased risk of conditions, such as nutritional deficiencies, inflammatory changes of the gastric mucosa, peptic or duodenal ulcers, obesity, noninsulin-dependent diabetes mellitus, hypertension, heart failure, ischemic heart disease, stroke, aortic valve sclerosis, chronic kidney disease, sleep-disordered breathing, including obstructive sleep apnea [2]. Additionally, functional limitations, mental and social well-being alterations that negatively impact the quality of life are more common in edentulous patients.

The impact of general health status and the medication used on the oral health of the edentulous patient is partially manifested through the occurrence of complications. Nutritional deficiencies increase the risk of occurrence of denture stomatitis, traumatic ulcer and burning mouth syndrome [25]. Patient's personality and psychological well-being influences treatment satisfaction and tolerance [10]. Decreased manual dexterity has a negative impact on care and maintenance of dentures/overdentures, which leads to negative effects on oral and systemic health [14].

2.10. Age

Patient's age is an important aspect to consider when planning the prosthetic treatment, being linked to particularities of oral and general health status, to specific needs and expectation towards the prosthetic rehabilitation, to particular medical approaches in order to ensure a good long-term prognosis. Prosthetic treatment of the edentulous patient should take into account the current situation, but also the most probable evolution and, if present, the inherent complications (e.g., preventive measures to reduce alveolar ridge resorption are recommended).

Young-elderly edentulous patients generally have more favorable clinical conditions for prosthetic rehabilitation, a better general health status, a faster adaptation to removable prosthesis if chosen and the ability to perform most accurately the necessary the maintenance procedures. They have higher expectations regarding the esthetics and functionality of the prosthetic rehabilitation and don't easily accept the removable treatment options.

Old-elderly edentulous patients generally register an increased treatment difficulty, as a consequence of numerous factors interacting. In previous ill-fitting complete denture wearers there is a severe ridge resorption [26,27]. The prevalence of co-morbidities is increased, such as physical or mental health problems that have a negative impact on oral health, systemic health, functioning and behavior. Most of the times the elderly people are not regular users of dental services since they overcome physical and psychological access treatment barriers (e.g., the cost of dental care services, transportation problems, doctor's attitudes-lack of responsiveness to patient's concerns, the lack of perceived need for care, fear), which are more significant for the functionally dependent elderly then for the independent elderly [28-30]. They have treatment expectations that target first the rehabilitation of the masticatory function, and second the esthetics. They usually prefer more simple medical procedures, that include limited surgical interventions and that demand easy maintenance procedures. The older completely edentulous patients show a more frequent rate of denture intolerance, probably due to less adaptability to new situations.

Demographic changes, namely population ageing and decreasing prevalence of tooth loss, have impact on the edentulous patient profile. There is an increasing of the age when edentulism occurs, aspects that associates an increased treatment difficulty. Considering the latter, additional measures are necessary to ensure adequate oral health for older edentulous patients e.g., access to and financing for dental services, an adequately trained workforce to provide dental care and appropriate education to edentulous individuals [30].

2.11. Health risk factors

Health risk factors should be assessed since they can explain some of the case particularities and may have a negative impact on the treatment outcome. Among them, there can be mentioned behavioral risk factors (e.g. tobacco and alcohol consumption, obesity related to physical activity and diet), social risk factors (e.g., socio-economical status, social networks and social support, occupational factors, social inequalities), inadequate disease screening practices, exposure to increased stress [31]. Their role is proven both as a cause of complete edentulism and also as a factor that impacts the treatment outcome, being risk factors for some complications.

2.12. Patient need and preferences

Health care decisions require integrating the patient's individual preferences and values, according to the ethical principle of respecting the patient's autonomy [32]. A good relation and communication between doctor and patient offers the best premises for reaching a consensus regarding the medical decision, with a positive effect on the treatment outcome.

Patient preferences are related to numerous variables, e.g., age, social status, personality type, education. Acknowledging them may be difficult, especially in elderly patients, sometimes in relation to objective reasons, as physical changes that affect the communication (e.g., loss of hearing or visual acuity). Additional efforts should be made in order to understand the patient's health needs and preferences, since they can have important consequences, such as rejection of the prosthetic treatment or even avoiding addressing for medical treatment.

3. Classification of denture and overdenture complications

The classification of denture and overdenture complications can enhance practitioner's understanding of them, with a positive effect on their management and prognosis.

Denture and overdenture complications can be classified considering their etiology, according to risk factor's nature and mechanism of action, as described in table 2, or in regarded to some descriptive criteria, as presented in table 3.

Classification of denture and overdenture complications, considering their etiology

---

A. According to the nature of the risk factor

Host or patient related factors
- *edentulism-related*, e.g., ridge resorption, impaired mastication;
- *oral health-related*, excluding the conditions linked to edentulism, e.g., reduced salivary flow increases the risk for denture stomatitis and denture intolerance;
- *systemic health-related*, including medication use, e.g., diabetes mellitus is a risk factor for denture stomatitis; the bisphosphonate treatment is a risk factor for osteonecrosis;
- *patient's behavior and other characteristics-related*, like income and social status, education, physical environment, e.g., poor financial status limits the access to dental treatment;

Dental treatment related factors
- *removable dental prosthesis-related*, considering the manufacturing accuracy, technical features and materials used, e.g., overextended dentures causes traumatic ulcers or hyperplasia; artificial teeth wear is linked to mastication deficiencies; allergic reactions to polymethylmethacrylate (PMMA);
- *teeth or dental implants-related*, e.g., periodontal disease of supporting roots causes denture instability; implant overdentures have additional surgical complications like nerve injury; treatment failure may appear consequently to tooth or dental implant loss;
- *attachment system-related*, e.g., ill-fitting overdenture due to loosening or loss of the matrix;

Dentist's intervention related factors [33]
- *inherent complications*, in which dentist's role is irrelevant, e.g., allergic reaction to polymethylmethacrylate (PMMA), when patients' history is inconclusive;
- *passive intervention*, as improper conduct regarding early signs of disease, e.g., implant loss due to excessive denture pressure or due to ignored early signs of peri-implantitis;
- *wrongful judgment*, as errors in conceiving and conducting the treatment, e.g., improper implant location or number; incorrect registration of maxillomandibular relationship, as an increased vertical dimension of occlusion.

B. According to the mechanism of action of the risk factor

Susceptibility factors increase the chance of complications occurrence, e.g., implant failure is frequenter in smokers and diseases like diabetes;

Initiation factors directly initiate the complication, e.g., overextended dentures cause traumatic lesions of the oral mucosa;

Progression factors cause worsening of a preexistent condition, e.g., ill-fitting dentures increase the rate of alveolar ridge resorption.

Table 2. Classifications of denture and overdenture complications, considering their etiology

Descriptive classification of denture and overdenture complications

A. According to localization

Host

- *oral*, e.g., oral soft and hard tissue complications, functional alterations; remaining teeth complications in case of root overdentures as caries, periodontal disease, root fracture;

- *facial*, e.g., aged prognathic appearance;

- *systemic*, e.g., malnutrition, gastro-intestinal disorders;

Dental restoration

- *removable dental prosthesis*, e.g., denture/overdenture fracture; retention loss; aging of the material, teeth wear

- *dental implants*, that are classified according to Berglundh et al. [34] as biological complications (functional disturbances that affect the tissues supporting the implant, e.g., peri-implantitis) or technical complications (mechanical damage of the implant, implant components and suprastructures)

- *attachment system*, e.g., loosening, loss, damage

B. According to modification type

Anatomical changes, e.g., alveolar ridge resorption; decrease of the muscular mass;

Functional changes, e.g., mastication or phonation deficiencies, protruded mandibular position;

Pathological changes, e.g., traumatic ulcers, atrophic stomatitis, candidiasis.

C. According to severity

Light – few clinical signs, whose treatment is simple, requires reduced costs in terms of biological, financial and clinical time and has a good prognosis, e.g., loosening of attachment system; ulcerations or irritations related to surplus material on denture's base;

Moderate – functional alterations are associated and treatment requires medium costs, e.g., denture base fracture; loss of stability and need for relining; artificial tooth wear;

Severe – associates important functional alterations, can lead to treatment failure, addressing them imply high costs, e.g., damage of inferior alveolar nerve, denture intolerance.

D. According to the moment of occurrence

During the preprosthetic procedures, e.g., pain during the surgical procedures for frenum plastia or reshaping of exostosis;

While manufacturing the removable prostheses, e.g., discomfort due to vomiting reflex;

During the surgical phase of implant placement, according to Misch & Wang [35] being encountered treatment plan-related complications (e.g., wrong angulation or improper implant location), anatomy-related complications (e.g., nerve injury, bleeding, cortical plate perforation, sinus membrane complication), procedure-related complications (e.g., mechanical complications, lack of primary stability, ingestion and aspiration) and others (e.g., iatrogenic damage and human error);

Immediately after inserting the denture/overdenture, e.g., traumatic ulcers;

During maintenance, e.g., root or implant complications, retention loss

Table 3. Classifications of denture and overdenture complications, considering descriptive criteria

4. Main complications of denture and overdenture

Some of the most common complications of the completely edentulous patient, treated by dentures or implant/root overdentures will be presented. Aspects related to their etiology, clinical features and management will be covered.

4.1. Alveolar ridge resorption

The residual ridge derives from the alveolar process after tooth loss. It registers the most significant changes and it supports the highest pressures during the worn of dentures or implant-retained overdentures. The ridge resorption is manifested as a continuous, cumulative and irreversible process, visible as the decrease of the quantity and quality of the bone [36].

Etiology. The ridge resorption is inherent after tooth loss and during denture wearing. It is a cronic plurifactorial condition as a joint result of physical, physiological and pathological factors.

The process of postextractive bone restructuring, after tooth loss, has variable rate and pattern, in relation to general physiological and pathological factors (age, menopause, systemic alterations), local factors (the edentulism and its cause, features of the jaws – volume, density). Also, the rate of bone resorption (the quantity of bone lost in a time period) varies in relation to the moment of tooth loss-it is maximum immediately after it in the first month, high in the first year after the tooth loss and decreases consequently. The pattern of bone resorption registers topographic differences – as for the maxilla and the mandible, for the anterior and posterior regions and in relation to anatomical features. The resorption is maximum at the top of the ridge and is lower at the base of the ridge, in the biostatical areas (maxillary tuberosity, retromolar pad), at the ligaments' insertion site (frenum) and in the region of the hard palate. The ridge resorption occurs from the top to the basis, and is centripetal in the maxilla and centrifugal in the mandible. The pattern of ridge resorption varies according to the anatomical features and the size of the jaws, e.g., in class II skeletal patients, brachicephals, with mandibular micrognathism the resorption is more severe in the mandible, and in class III skeletal patients, dolicocephals, with mandibular macrognathism the resorption is more severe in the maxilla. Also, ridge resorption is more pronounced in women (probably linked to smaller jaws and lower bone density, related to postmenopause osteoporosis), in patients who lost their teeth due to periodontal disease and in those with high occlusal forces (natural teeth as antagonists, bruxism). Systemic conditions, particularly diabetes mellitus and other metabolic disorders, can accelerate the rhythm of ridge resorption.

The dentures accelerate the rate of ridge resorption, mainly through the pressure exercised by them on the support structures during oral functions. The severity of ridge resorption is connected to the parameters of functional and parafunctional forces of occlusion and to biomechanical aspects related to the prosthesis-the support and stability of the denture, the positioning of artificial teeth, type of occlusion, antagonists (teeth, implants, edentulous), and correctness of the registration of maxillomandibular relationship. The support surface for occlusal forces is reduced in edentulous patients, compared to the dentulous ones, and through progressive ridge resorption, both in high and width, consequently the support surface decreases even more. The magnitude of occlusal forces are generally lower in the edentulous patients, but there are variations related to age, sex, parafunctions as bruxism, stress level, food consistency preferences, and also the correctness of prosthetic rehabilitation. Increased duration of occlusion contacts, as a risk factor for ridge resorption, is related to bruxism, ill-fitting dentures, unstable occlusion and increased vertical dimension of occlusion. Compared to maxillary edentulism, mandibular edentulism has greater risk of registering more severe ridge resorption, due to the decreased denture support surface and related higher magnitude of pressure beared. Also, denture wearing associates the risk of specific complications that favor the occurrence of an accelerated rate of ridge resorption, such as inflammatory lesions of the oral mucosa (e.g., denture stomatitis). Due to these factors, it is considered that ridge resorption is in tight relation with the period of wearing the dentures, but is also influenced by the quality of the treatment.

Clinical features. Ridge resorption is characterized by changes of the morphology of the alveolar ridges and of maxillomandibular relationship, with consequences on the prosthetic treatment and its outcome with time.

Ridge resorption implies a decrease in bone volume, as ridges' height (assessed as reduced, medium and severe resorption), ridge's width (assessed as wide, medium or thin "knife edge ridge") and ridge's surface layout (normal or abnormal morphology, with exostosis). The characteristics of the alveolar ridge influence treatment conduct and have impact on its outcome, e.g., severe ridge resorption (Figure 1) is more frequently associated with denture instability and reduced denture tolerance, difficulties in mounting the artificial teeth and esthetic deficiencies.

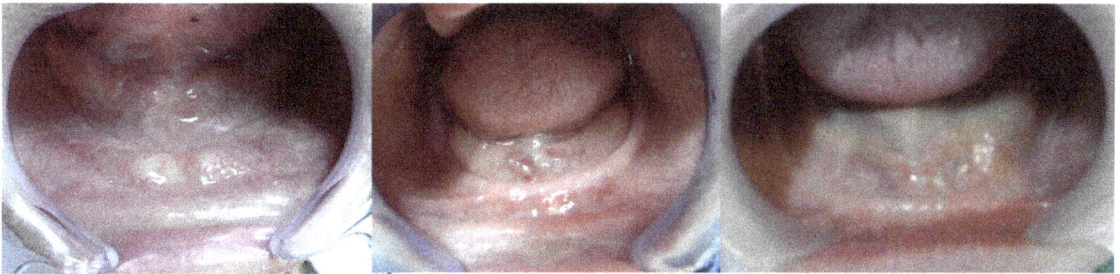

Figure 1. Severe ridge resorption, in long-term denture wearers

Associated to ridge resorption particular aspects of the maxillomandibular relationship can be noticed, as lack of parallelism between the ridges direction and anterior or/and posterior inverse ridge relationship (Figure 2). According to their skeletal jaw relations and in relation with the different patterns of jaws resorption, class III skeletal patients have the tendency to register an inverse ridge relationship, and class II skeletal patients an apparently normal relationship.

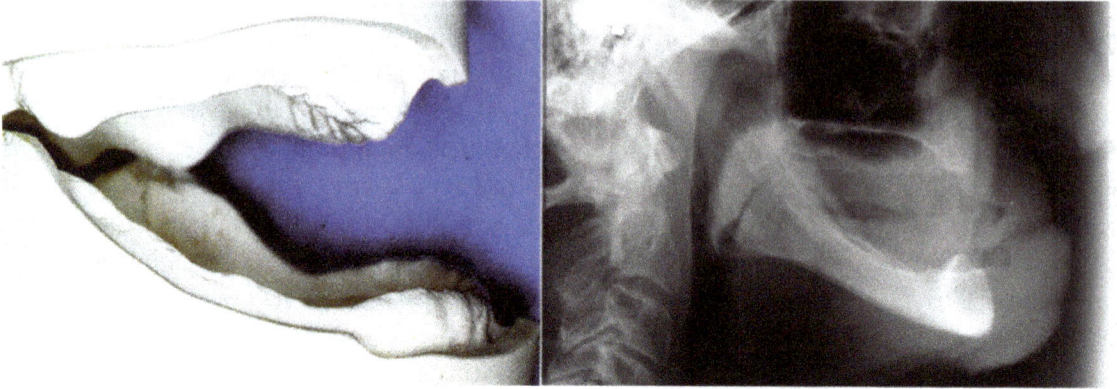

Figure 2. Inverse ridge relationship, related to skeletal class III and the pattern of bone resorption (centripetal in the maxilla and centrifugal in the mandible)

Through resorption and replacement of the bone with fibrous tissue, a floating ridge, usually named "flabby ridge" is noticed. This aspect is most commonly observed in the edentulous anterior maxilla, being related to the excessive pressure of the mandibular anterior teeth (Combination Syndrome). Flabby ridge can also be seen in other places, like maxillary tuberosity or retromolar pad, being linked to instability of the denture or excessive occlusal trauma.

Severe mandibular ridge resorption is accompanied by reduction of the area of the fixed mucosa, difficulties in acknowledgement of the extension of the denture base (due to the sublingual gland herniation through the mylohyoid muscle and modifications of the muscle and ligaments' insertion sites, which can get close to the ridge crest) and pain as a result of dental pressure in the mental foramen area and nerve exposure.

Denture wearing associates inherent ridge resorption, manifested as the occurrence of denture instability. Consequently, clinical procedures as relining or rebasing are required for readjustment of the dentures, in order to correspond to patient's need and to prevent worsening of the edentulous condition.

Management. The ridge resorption, due to its impact on the prosthetic treatment, is the first criteria for the classification of treatment difficulty level according to the Prosthodontic Diagnostic Index (PDI) for complete edentulism of ACP [16]. Thereby, a detailed analysis of the severity of ridge resorption and associated clinical signs is essential in the treatment planning. Useful data can be gained through clinical examination, analysis of the old dentures (when available, they are essential) and evaluation on panoramic and cephalometric radiographs. Computed tomography provides information that are most valuable when implant prosthetic restorations are used, as implant overdentures, especially in complex cases as those with severe ridge resorption or flabby ridge.

In edentulous patients, considering the irreversible and progressive character of bone resorption, preventive interventions should be taken towards reduction of resorption rate and its complications. In this respect, addressing the risk factors and correct management of the supporting tissue should be a priority. In order to limit the bone resorption it is recommended to preserve the tooth roots, to use dental implants, to realize immediate prosthetic rehabilitation, especially in cases with tooth lost due to periodontal disease since this conduct favors a more reduced guided bone resorption. Correctness of dentures manufacturing is essential and it should rely on the principles of retention, stability and support, with proper maintenance and on time replacement. Implant overdentures can be used both as a preventive solution, in order to reduce the bone resorption, and as a curative solution, for solving the cases with severe ridge resorption where conventional dentures did not succeed or were not tolerated.

Severe ridge resorption associates decreased denture stability, which is associated with complications such as pain, lesions of the mucosa, reduced denture tolerance, that need to be addressed. The surgical preprosthetic interventions (bone augmentation, frenectomy, excision of hyperplasic lesions, as in figure 3) and non-surgical interventions (tissue conditioning, antifungal medication, improvement of the nutrition) are preparative treatments that aim achieving better conditions for prosthetic rehabilitation. Taking into account edentulous patient's profile (aged, with systemic co-morbidities), stress related to the fear of surgical interventions and healing parameters (as time needed or remaining scar tissues), the non-surgical or less invasive surgical interventions are preferred. Soft lining materials are indicated since they facilitate the uniformly distribution of the functional stress and can reposition the abused tissues.

The prosthetic treatment of the edentulous patient can be performed using conventional or implant restorations, fixed or removable, with or without preprosthetic interventions, according to the clinical case's particularities and patient's needs. Treatment requirements include accurate physiological impression of the oral structures, correct registration of maxillomandibular relationship and teeth mounting and selection of appropriate occlusal scheme, in order to ensure dentures' stability and esthetic and functional rehabilitation.

Accurate establishment of the peripheral extension of the denture base, considering also the pressures supported by the denture-bearing area, is extremely important, being directly relate to denture's retention, stability and tolerance. In this respect, the correct 2-phase impression technique (primary and custom tray impression) is essential. In edentulous patients with severe ridge resorption, additional adjunctive procedures may be required as tissue conditioning, supplementary functional impressions or usage of neutral zone impression technique. In displaceable or "flabby ridges", the selective pressure impression technique (e.g., using a custom tray with a window opening over the mobile tissue) is more recommended, being at equal importance to other aspects as stable posterior occlusion. Thin mandibular "knife edge ridges", that are accompanied by pain related to denture pressure, needs special treatment conduct, with usage of soft liners, a selective pressure impression technique, preprosthetic surgery (some disagree because ridge reduction implies loss of potential stabilizing zone) and dental implants.

Registration of maxillomandibular relationship is essential for the treatment success. It implies establishing the functional vertical dimension of occlusion, in accordance with minimum speaking space and the freeway space, and respecting the coincidence of maximal intercuspal position and centric relation. The most recommended occlusal schemes for removable prosthesis are the lingualized occlusion, for the bimaxillary complete edentulous patient, in

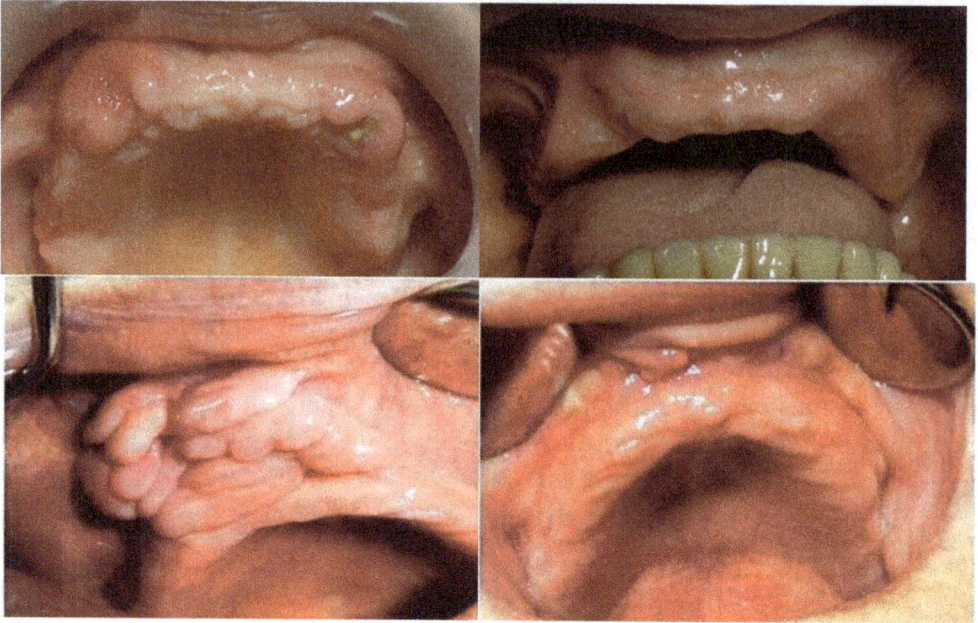

Figure 3. Preprosthetic surgical interventions for excision of hyperplastic lesions

skeletal class II patients or in severe mandibular ridge resorption or the linear occlusion, for mandibular overdentures, in patients with combination syndrome or skeletal class III pattern and severe maxillary ridge resorption.

Mandibular conventional dentures register frequently retention and stability deficiencies, mainly related to ridge resorption. These can be addressed through usage of implant prosthetic restorations, fixed or removable. There are multiple treatment options when considering usage of dental implants, as removable prosthesis (conventional or narrow dental implant overdenture, with different attachment systems as bars, ball, Locator) or fixed restorations (All an four, Fast & Fixed, conventional fixed implant restorations). Current perspective identifies 2 implant overdentures as the minimum standard for mandibular edentulism taking into account performance, patient satisfaction, cost and clinical time [37]. Selecting between them require acknowledgement of case futures and patient's need and preferences. For example, fixed restorations have better treatment outcome, but have limited usage due to aspects like cost and higher complexity of the interventions required (e.g., sometimes surgical procedures as bone augmentation or sinus lift cannot be avoided).

4.2. Traumatic ulcers

Traumatic ulcers are small, painful mucosal lesions that most commonly develop in the first days after insertion of a new denture [38].

Etiology. Traumatic ulcers are caused by dentures with overextended margins, unbalanced occlusion, small excess of material or related to some conditions of the denture bearing area, like exostosis or tori. Ill-fitting dentures can lead to soft tissue irritation or ulceration due to excessive movement of denture. Additional to the mechanical trauma, ulcers can appear due to chemical or thermal insults.

Clinical features. The painful mucosal ulcerations are tender, have a yellowish floor and red margins, with no hardening or thickening of mouth tissues. The irregularly shaped lesions are usually localized in the buccal and lingual sulcus, are covered by a grey necrotic membrane and surrounded by an inflammatory halo. It looks as a hyperemic area, covered or not with fibrin deposits..

Management. Traumatic ulcers usually heal fast, in about a week, after removal of the cause. Usually, denture base and occlusion adjustments are made. Additionally, benzamine hydro-chloride 0.15% mouthwash or spray, to provide symptomatic relief, and chlorhexidine gluconate 0.2% mouthwash for oral rinses and soaking the dentures overnight, to prevent and treat infection, can be recommended [39]. Traumatic ulcer decreased in frequency as the length of denture use increased and occurred more frequently during the first 5 years of denture use [40]. Traumatic ulcers must be differentiated from squamous carcinoma, bacterial, fungal and viral diseases, and other oral mucosal diseases, through their clinical aspect, evolution, lack of response to treatment [39]. Patients with an ulcer of over three weeks' duration should be referred for biopsy or other investigations to exclude malignancy or other serious conditions such as chronic infections.

4.3. Denture related hyperplasia

Denture related hyperplasia is an enlargement of the oral mucosa, appeared in relation to the denture base. There are two main types of denture related hyperplasia, namely denture-related fibrous hyperplasia (epulis fissuratum) and inflammatory papillary hyperplasia.

Etiology. Denture-related fibrous hyperplasia occurs as a reaction to low-grade continuous chronic trauma induced by denture flanges, which have thin sharp edges. Other risk factors are ill-fitting unstable dentures, increased vertical dimension of occlusion and parafunctional habits [41]. Inflammatory papillary hyperplasia occurs in relation to wearing the denture continuously, poor oral and denture hygiene, severe ridge resorption, unstable dentures, smoking, age-related changes and some systemic conditions [42]. Denture related hyperplasia is more common in elderly due to oral mucosa changes and their decreased immune response to infection.

Clinical features. Denture-related fibrous hyperplasia appears as a reactive mucosal enlargement, corresponding to the denture flange, which is more common in the maxillary buccal sulcus. The pedunculated, sessile or nodular formations, single or multiple can be red, hyperemic or light pink, usually being asymptomatic. Microbial colonization can occur, most common being Candida species.

In inflammatory papillary hyperplasia the hard palatal mucosa has an erythematous aspect, with a pebbly or papillary surface [42]. According to its severity, we can see forms with limited localization or that cover the entire hard palatal mucosa. The previously described two types of denture related hyperplasia can be observed in figure 4.

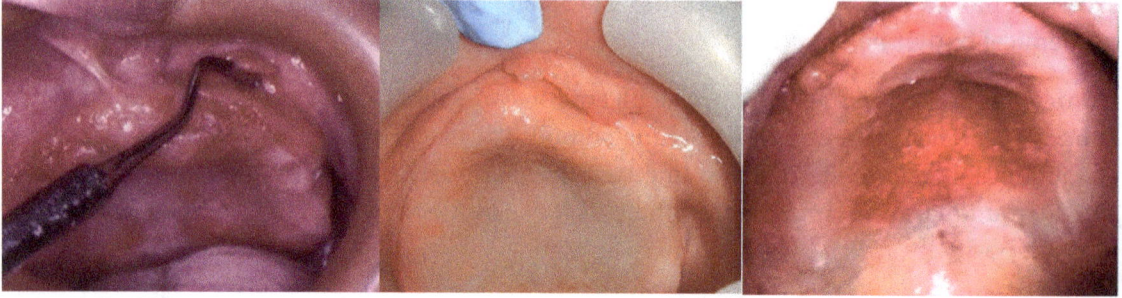

Figure 4. Denture related hyperplasia

Management. Denture-related fibrous hyperplasia usually diminishes considerably, almost entirely, after removal of the cause, correcting the denture flanges. Sometimes minor surgery is required.

The treatment of inflammatory papillary hyperplasia requires removal of the denture at night, improvement of the oral hygiene and denture hygiene. Antifungal therapy, surgical excision of the hyperplastic tissues and renewal of the denture can be recommended in some cases [42].

4.4. Denture stomatitis

Denture stomatitis is a chronic infectious inflammatory disease of the oral mucosa that is in direct contact with the base of the removable prosthesis, either conventional or implant-supported.

Etiology. It has a multifactorial etiology, it is primary related to denture wearing, but the dominant etiological factor is the microbial one-frequently fungal infection with Candida albicans and other sub-strains, but also bacteria such as Staphylococcus and Streptococcus species being identified [43]. Additionally, there are local and systemic and behavioral risk factors.

Acrylic dentures produce ecological changes that facilitate the accumulation of bacteria and yeasts and thus commensal organism may become pathogenic, denture stomatitis being considered an opportunistic infection [44]. A higher prevalence is noticed in cases with poor denture hygiene with denture plaque accumulation, continuous wear of the dentures (including at night) and in ill-fitting dentures. Other risk factors for denture stomatitis are related to the material characteristics, as their changes in time that favor plaque accumulation and microbial colonization (soft linings materials through their fast deterioration and difficulties of achieving proper hygiene; hard acrylic materials through their increased porosity that occurs in time) or as determining hypersensitivity reactions.

Host related risk factors for denture stomatitis include local factors (reduced salivary flow rate, low salivary pH, poor oral hygiene), general factors (physiological such as age, sex, nutritional status and associated medication) which act towards decreasing the resistance and defense mechanisms of the oral mucosa. The prevalence of denture stomatitis is higher among elderly denture users, women, smokers, alcohol consumers, vitamin A deficiency, diabetes and immune deficiency [44-47]. Changes in the salivary flow rate may be signs of a systemic disease, as in Sjögren or Mikulicz syndromes, or associated to medication use, as diuretics, antihypertensive, antipsychotic, anxiolytic, analgesic, anti-inflammatory, antihistaminic drugs. Also, incorrect antibiotic therapy, without fungal protection and broad spectrum antibiotics are seen as risk factors.

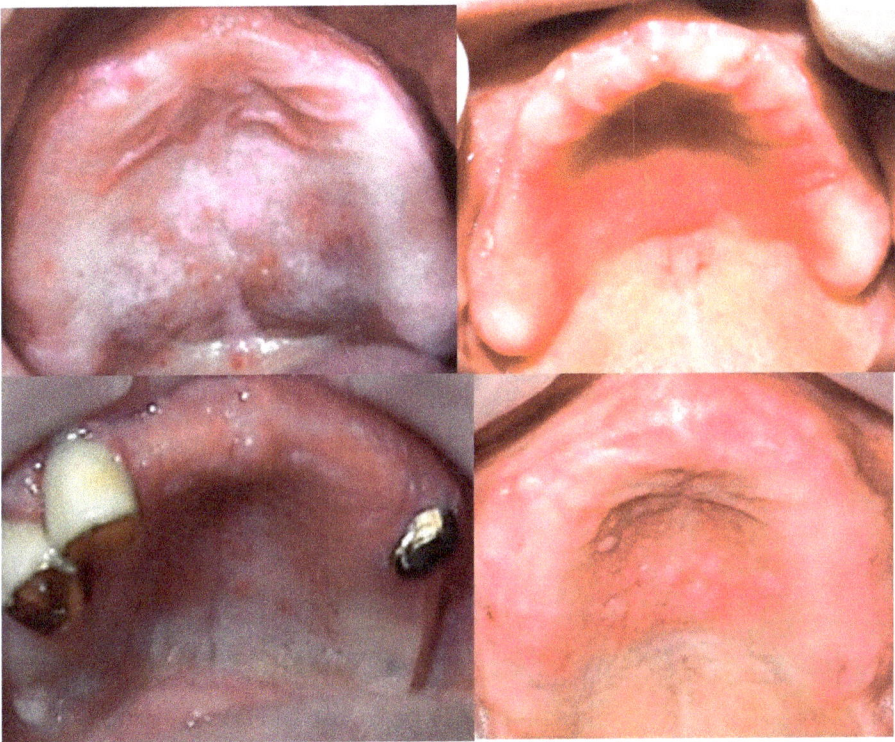

Figure 5. Denture stomatitis – clinical aspect

Clinical features. Denture stomatitis (Figure 5) is characterized by usually asymptomatic inflammatory lesions, with erythema and edema that are found in the denture bearing area, more frequently in the maxilla [44]. The reference classification for denture stomatitis is the one suggested by Newton in 1962, based exclusively on clinical criteria, including 3 types, namely type I (pin-point hyperemic lesions, as a localized simple inflammation), type II (diffuse erythema of the mucosa contacting the denture, as a generalized simple inflammation), and type III: (granular surface, as an inflammatory papillary hyperplasia) [43]. Denture stomatitis can be accompanied by other soft tissue lesions as angular cheilitis, median rhomboid glossitis or candidal leukoplakia.

Management. Considering the relatively high prevalence of denture stomatitis and its relapses, a preventive approach is recommended, by making the patient aware of this disease in order to motivate them to adopt the proper oral and denture hygiene methods, to remove the denture over nighttime and adopt a healthy life-style (quitting smoking, proper nutrition). Since most of the times the condition has no clinical signs, it is recommended to perform a routine basis screening for denture stomatitis. Additional tests may be useful, such as micro-biological exam and thermography –Figure 6 [14,43,48].

Treatment of denture stomatitis consists mainly in adopting strict methods for oral and denture hygiene, with removal of the denture overnight and soaking it in an antiseptic solution, such as chlorhexidine mouthwash. Considering the frequent Candida colonization, antifungal agents, usually as topical application, are recommended either when the yeasts have been isolated or in the absence of a favorable response to the previous interventions [14,44]. Additionally, denture deficiencies and other risk factors should be identified and addressed.

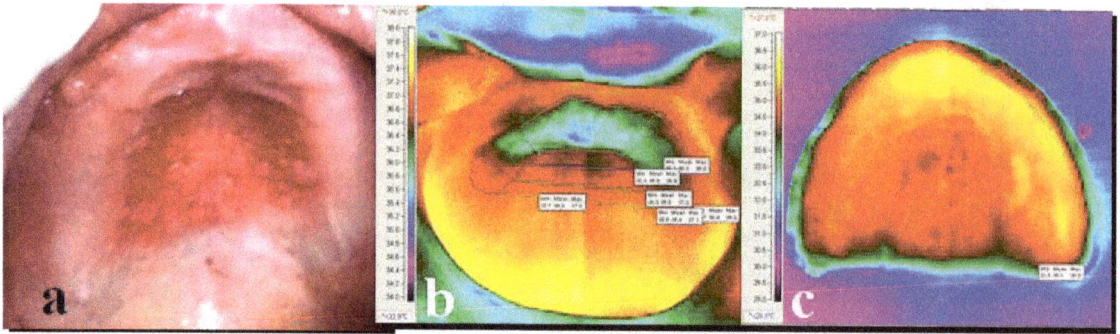

Figure 6. Denture stomatitis – clinical aspect (a); thermography of the oral mucosa (b); thermography of the maxillary denture (c)

4.5. Muscles changes

Edentulousness and dentures can lead to muscle changes, which are mainly an adaptation to the anatomical and functional changes. These can be encountered to the muscle that define the extension of the denture base and the neutral zone and play a role in the denture stability and retention (lips, cheeks and tongue), to masticatory muscles and to the muscles of facial expression.

Etiology. The muscle changes are linked to multiple interrelated factors. Aging associates loss of muscle tone and skin elasticity, decrease of the muscular mass and the force of contraction. The edentulism and the alveolar bone resorption induce major anatomical changes, with muscular consequences. Changing the support for the soft tissues causes the retraction of the lips and cheeks, and the muscular attachment changes in relation to the bone resorption. In severe forms of bone resorption, the muscles are inserted up to the ridge crest and the tongue, due to loss of the guiding offered by the teeth, changes gradually its shape, position and tonicity [49]. The patient's skeletal pattern associates muscular particularities also in the edentulous patient. In skeletal class II patients the tongue is hyperkinetic and has an elevated position that negatively influences the denture stability. In skeletal class III patients the tongue is less active and has a low position. An excessively large tongue, with a retracted position can be observed in edentulous patients that had not been treated for a long period of time. Patients with combination syndrome and skeletal class II with a retrognathic mandible show a tendency towards a protruded mandibular position. Certain systemic alterations, as degenerative and autoimmune conditions, vascular accidents, paresis, burns, traumatisms, nutritional status alterations as protein deficiencies, associate muscular changes.

Prosthetic treatment deficiencies favor abnormal muscular changes. Increased vertical dimension of occlusion and ill-fitting dentures cause muscle spasms, habitual and involuntary movements. Oversized anterior buccal flange of the maxillary denture associates the overextension of the upper lip, with possible anatomical and functional consequences. Association of posterior artificial tooth wear with over jet or lack of coincidence of maximal intercuspal position and centric relation leads to an abnormal protruded mandibular position, which makes difficult the registration of maxillomandibular relationship (centric relation).

Clinical features. Generally, the clinical aspects are the result of complex muscular changes, such as regarding the tone, volume and attachment of the muscle, combined with neuromuscular coordination and control deficiencies.

The changes in muscle tonus can be seen as hypertonia or hypotonia. Muscle hypertonia (Figure 7) is more obvious in lower lip orbicularis oris muscle and in tongue muscles, and causes instability of the mandibular denture. It occurs in the edentulous patients in relation to prosthetic factors as ill-fitting dentures, to patient's individual characteristics as hypodivergent skeletal class II pattern, to parafunctions as bruxism or some systemic conditions. Muscle hypotonia is more frequent for upper lip orbicularis oris muscle and the buccinator muscle, and it occurs related to ageing, to deficient nutritional status and various systemic conditions. Less favorable condition for denture retention and stability, decrease of the efficiency of self-cleaning and reduced visibility of the anterior maxillary teeth in phonation or smiling are some of the effects of muscle hypotonia.

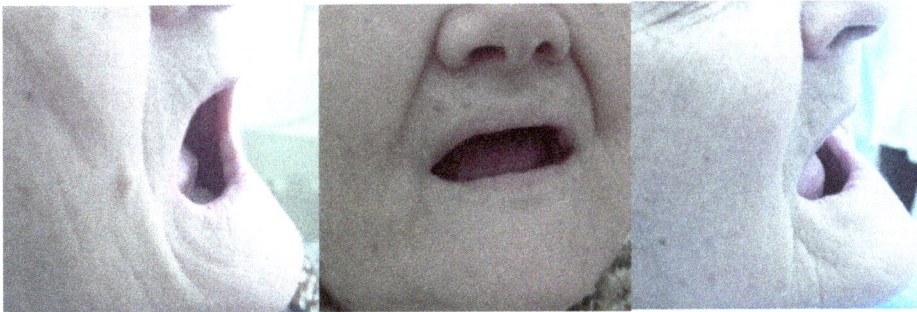

Figure 7. Lower lip orbicularis oris muscle hypertonia, that affects mandibular denture stability\

The changes in volume of the muscles is usually represented by muscular atrophy, which combined with muscular hypotonia, lead to the characteristic facial aspect of old people, with masseter muscle thickness and loose or sagging skin.

Buccinators, orbicularis oris and tongue muscles define the neutral zone, whose accurate limitation is difficult to identify in severe ridge resorption. Changes in the position of the muscle insertions occur, such as high muscle insertions, even on the ridge top (genioglossus and mentalis muscle), with detached oral mucosa. Considering that position of muscle attachments has a major impact to denture base stability and retention, through changes of the denture bearing area, severe ridge resorption with consecutive muscles changes increase the treatment difficulty degree, especially in the mandible.

Muscle force decreasing leads to decrease in the capacity of performing a voluntary act (such as mastication). This occurs in relation to ageing, paresis, depression, denture instability or pain caused by the dentures. Alterations in jaw movements can occur in relation to deficiencies of the prosthetic restorations, as unstable occlusion, denture instability, increased vertical dimension of occlusion or in bruxism. Muscular spasms are encountered in particular situations as in the jaw-closing muscles, related to an increased vertical dimension of occlusion or for jaw-opening muscles related to a decreased vertical dimension of occlusion.

Neuromuscular coordination and control deficiencies, which occur in relation to age and systemic alterations, can increase treatment difficulty and negatively influence the accommodation with the prosthesis. For example, in Parkinson disease a lack of neuromuscular coordination occurs, which leads to difficulties in registration of maxillomandibular relationship and in the insertion and removal of the denture or the overdenture. Abnormal, involuntary, patterned or stereotyped and purposeless orofacial movements (oral dyskinesia) can occur linked to ill-fitting unstable dentures, oral discomfort, and lack of sensory contacts [2]. Facial nerve paresis includes affected unilateral facial musculature movement with asymmetry of facial expression and functional disorders, taste alterations and salivary changes, all having impact on the prosthetic treatment – difficulties in impression taking and in registration of maxillomandibular relationship, reduced masticatory efficiency with unilateral mastication, increased risk of unstable dentures, aesthetic alterations and denture intolerance.

Management. Considering the importance of the muscle factor for the oral functioning, an accurate evaluation should be performed. In some cases, besides the clinical evaluation, additional tests are recommended, such as electromyography or kinesiography, and sometimes special treatment conduct is required [50].

If muscle changes have been identified, these should be taken into account in planning and performing the prosthodontic treatment. In muscle hypertonia, aspects like positioning the artificial teeth in the neutral zone, correct placement of the occlusal plane and correct occlusal relations are essential. In muscle hypotonia, it is recommended to design the buccal flange of the denture with a convex shape and usage of medium viscosity impression materials, in order to have a correct registration of the extension of the denture base and to use the muscle contractions for denture stabilization. Impression taking technique varies according to case's particularities – in patients with protruded tongue at rest, wider movement are required during impression taking, comparing to a retracted tongue, in order to adequately register functional movements (Figure 8).

Extension of denture or overdenture base is limited by the muscle insertions, their encroachment causing, during muscle contraction, movement of the prosthesis. In severe ridge

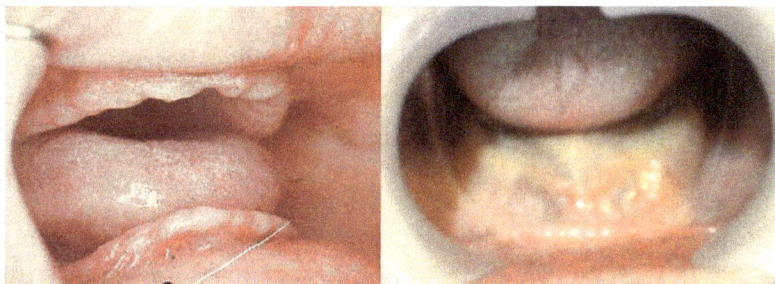

Figure 8. Tongue position at rest – anterior vs. posterior

resorption cases, as for those with muscle insertions on the ridge top, preprosthetic surgery for repositioning of muscle and mucosal attachments is indicated [51].

In neuromuscular coordination and control deficiencies, considering the severe functional alterations, conventional dentures usually don't respond to patient's need and implant overdenture should be chosen instead. Compared to conventional dentures, implant over-dentures provides better functional parameters – exertion of higher masticatory forces promotes better nutrition through the ability to chew harder foods.

Last but not least, manufacturing of a new prosthesis requires an adjustment period for the establishment of the new memory patterns for the masticatory muscles, of about 6 to 8 weeks, aspect that should be mentioned to the patient [52].

4.6. Facial alterations, including esthetic complications

The complete edentulism contributes greatly to the facial aspect known as the aged appearance. Prosthetic treatment needs to adequately address this consequence of edentulism, considering the fact that patients' complaints are frequently related to aesthetic reasons.

Etiology. The facial appearance of the edentulous patient is the result of factors related to complete edentulism and prosthetic treatment, combined with others such as ageing, local and general particularities and medical conditions.

Edentulism associates significant anatomical and functional changes that impact the facial appearance. Lip and cheek support is severely altered by tooth loss and bone resorption. A tendency of increasing the facial concavity occurs in relation to the different pattern of bone resorption of the jaws (centripetal in the maxilla and centrifugal in the mandible). In association with the loss of the occlusal contacts, a counter-clockwise rotation of the mandible, with a decreasing height of the lower third of the face, and sometimes a tendency to a more advanced protruded mandibular position occurs. Facial alterations that are directly linked to edentulism can be considered worsening factors of the esthetic appearance, since there are also preexistent changes in relation to other factors.

As a consequence of aging, there are changes related to the evolution of bones and soft tissues (muscles, fat and skin), in addition to noticeable effects of gravity, with effect on facial esthetics [53]. Systemic health, medication use and behavior (e.g., alcohol and tobacco use) can influence the facial appearance. For example, smoking causes changes particularly in the lower and middle third of the face, like hyperpigmentation and accentuated wrinkles-deeper nasolabial folds, upper lip wrinkles, lower lip vermillion wrinkles, lower lid hyperpigmentation [54]. Premature aged appearance occurs in some diseases like Cutis laxa or glomerulonephritis [55,56].

The prosthetic treatment of the edentulous patient addresses positively some of the previous mentioned facial alteration, but can also contribute to an aged appearance through its deficiencies, as in cases with a decreased vertical dimension of occlusion, a reverse smile line or darker, yellow artificial teeth.

Clinical features. Facial appearance of the edentulous patient registers changes compared to the dentate period, which are mostly found in the lower third of the face (Figure 9).

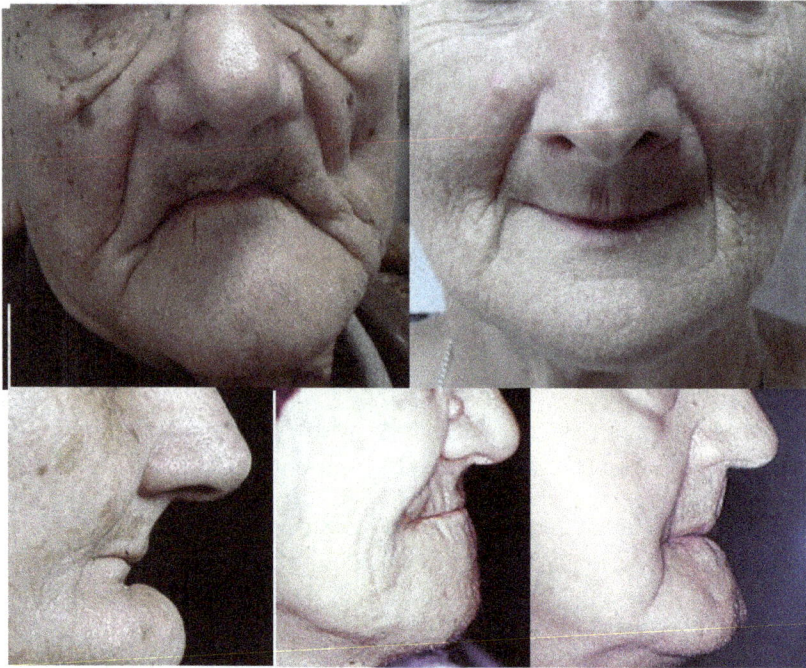

Figure 9. Facial appearance of edentulous patient, with severe bone resorption, without dentures

In edentulous patient, shape and vertical proportions of the face are modified compared to the dentate period. Frequently, edentulous patients have a short face morphotype, appeared in relation to the decrease in the facial lower and total height and the counter-clockwise rotation of the mandible.

Profile changes occur as decreasing its convexity compared to the dentate period. This aspect is due to the different pattern of bone resorption of the jaws and sometimes an advanced protruded mandibular position in the absence of stable occlusion. These changes are more obvious in the skeletal class III patients and are termed as pseudo-class III relation or the old man's prognathism. Profile changes include also modification of nasolabial angle related to nose tip lowering and loss of upper lip support.

Lips register great changes, as reduction of vermilion height and their volume, color modifications, retraction due to support loss, elongation (upper lip) and shortening (lower lip), straight or reversed lip line and low smile line, and reduced lips dynamics that contribute to a decreased teeth exposure during speaking and smiling, which associated a reduction of emotional display, as happiness or sadness [57].

Facial changes related to ageing mark the facial appearance. Lips and cheeks become less prominent and there can be noticed marked folds and wrinkles, loose or sagging skin, changes in the skin texture and hyperpigmentation. These are mainly connected to muscle changes, as hypotonia, and skin changes, as loss of skin elastic recoil.

The prosthetic treatment has a positive impact on the facial esthetics (Figure 10). Generally, it provides a support for the soft tissue, tries to compensate the tooth loss and bone resorption (through the artificial teeth and anterior buccal maxillary flange), ensures a functional vertical dimension of occlusion and give a natural look through exposure of the teeth during smiling or speaking. Some faulty prosthesis or some changes that occurs in time can have a negative impact on facial esthetic. Unpleasant facial appearance can be linked to errors in anterior artificial tooth mounting (too forward, too backward), shade selection (chosen incorrectly, too light, not matching the patient's age), to changes of the artificial teeth over time (through teeth wear the smile line can become reversed, or through aging of the material discolorations can appear). A decreased vertical dimension of occlusion leads to an aged appearance, with deeper perioral folds, and an increased vertical dimension of occlusion associate an unnatural, tensioned look. An overextended buccal flange, encountered more often in the maxillary dentures, leads to an over-supported lip with a tensioned unnatural look. Unstable dentures negatively influence facial appearance through movement while speaking and the facial changes related to protruded mandibular position that many times is associated.

Management. Facial esthetic evaluation must consider changes' severity and causes, in order to properly address them and respond to patients' need and expectations. In order to make an accurate analysis, regular clinical examination (from frontal and lateral view, with and without dentures, in rest and in maximal intercuspal position, during speech and smiling) can be supplemented by radiological examination (cephalometric radiographs) and records from the dentate period, as photos, dental casts, radiographs. The prosthetic rehabilitation of the completely edentulous patient must consider, from an aesthetic point of view, beside the general esthetic principles, also patient's features that are relatively obvious in the dentate period and rather difficult to assess in the edentulous one. The previous should be related to other patient's characteristics (e.g., age, sex, functional particularities, health status) and to prosthodontic biomechanical requirements in order to obtain a good treatment outcome.

4.7. Denture and overdenture biomechanical and technical complications

Removable dental prosthesis are described as having a series of complications in relation to the correctness and accuracy of their planning and execution (extension of the denture base,

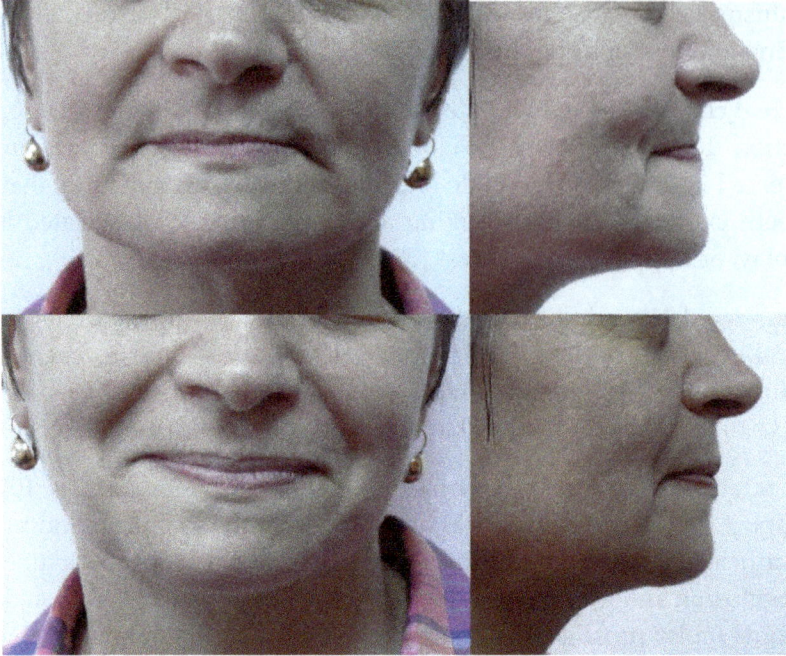

Figure 10. Facial appearance of a recently edentulous patient with and without the dentures

registration of maxillomandibular relationship, mounting of the artificial teeth, occlusal scheme), the technical and biomechanical features of the devices, the properties of the materials used, in conjunction with their evolution in time.

Considering the aims of medical treatments, not properly achieving the prosthodontic treatment goals (denture retention and stability, patient's satisfaction that is liked to aspects like the degree of esthetic and functional rehabilitations and absence of pain) may be considered treatment complications. Removable prosthesis instability can be caused by incorrect denture execution (e.g., overextended flanges, incorrect mounting of the artificial teeth, unstable occlusion), or can occur in time, as a consequence of bone resorption. This issue must be promptly addressed since it can lead to serious complications, such as the fracture of the prosthesis, abutment loss (teeth, implants) and intolerance of the prosthesis. In order to ensure good removable prosthesis stability, the primary aspect that should be consider is its correct execution, mainly regarding the extension of the denture base and artificial teeth mounting. Secondary, usage of denture adhesives, relinings and placement of dental implants should be considered.

The fracture of the removable prosthesis (Figure 11) is a relatively common complication, having numerous risk factors, such as poor denture design, denture instability, teeth or fixed restorations in the opposite jaw, increased mucosal resiliency, previous fractures, accidents (dropping the denture, associated to reduced dexterity), material properties and changes in time, flexural fatigue or other impact factors. Its management includes identifying the cause and the treatment can range from conventionally repairing procedures to reinforcement of the denture base with metal or non-metal products (as glass and polyethylene fibers or net), to changing the previous denture or even the treatment option [58].

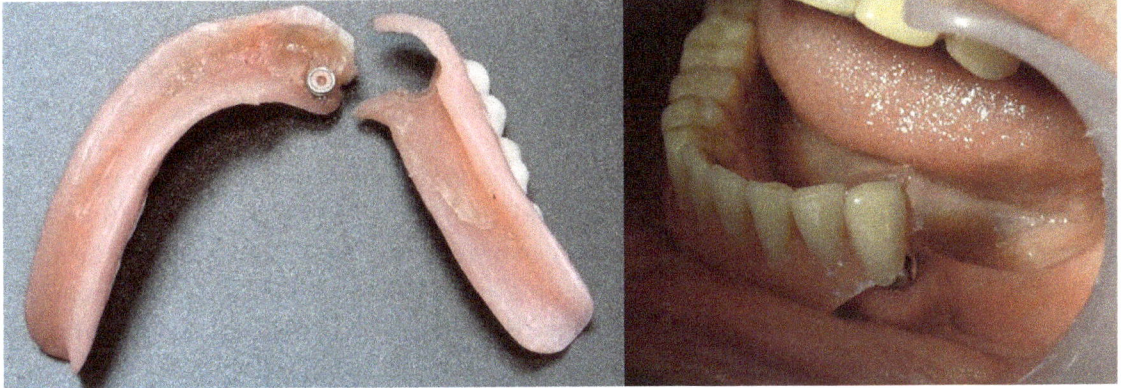

Figure 11. Overdenture fracture at the attachment site

The complications associated to the properties of the material used, mainly polymethylmethacrylate (PMMA), are linked to changes that appears during their evolution in time, as discolorations, artificial teeth wear, increased porosity and decrease flexural strength. Considering their functional and aesthetic impact, denture and overdenture treatment should be renewed at approximately every 5 years.

Additionally, signs of combination syndrome can appear when mandibular overdentures (supported or retained by roots or dental implants) are opposed by an edentulous maxilla. In this situation the masticatory field moves anteriorly, favoring the instability of the maxillary denture and the increased bone resorption rate in the anterior maxilla. This iatrogenic effect can be managed by using implants also in the maxilla, aiming to address or prevent this functional consequence and the destructive process of the oral structures [59].

4.8. Teeth complications, with root overdentures

The root overdentures can have teeth related complications, mainly due to primary or recurrent caries, periradicular lesions developed by vital teeth, endodontically lesions developed by endodontically treated teeth due to loss of the restoration sealing the root canal, periodontitis or root fracture [60]. Their management is dependent of the problem type, in most severe forms tooth loss and recurrent failure of prosthodontic treatment occurring. It is important to preserve the roots as a prevention factor for bone resorption and due their positive impact on the oral functioning [61]. Patients' awareness, instruction and motivation regarding maintaining a proper oral hygiene are essential considering that is the main factor for periodontal disease and caries control. When caries occur, it is important to identify them quickly in order to have high a high success rate for the treatment. Topical fluoridation or coverage with metallic caps can be performed preventively for patients with a high caries risk. For the periodontal disease it is recommended to use Chlorhexidine 0.12% mouthwash twice daily. Also, the removal of the denture overnight and maintenance of proper denture hygiene are recommended. If tooth mobility appears, it can be addressed by reducing the tooth height, which leads to an increase in the crown to root ratio. The risk of root fracture is higher in endodontically treated teeth and when the magnitude of occlusal forces is higher, as in denture instability, bruxism, increased vertical dimension of occlusion, when teeth or fixed prosthesis in the opposite jaw. Preventively, thimble crowns can be used.

4.9. Implants complications, with implant overdentures

For the implant overdenture, the implants complications can be related to the treatment planning (insufficient implant number), implant positioning (surgical complications can appear, such as nerve or blood vessel injuries, penetration of the maxillary sinus or the nasal cavity, hemorrhages or pain) and their evolution (post-insertion infections, compromised survival or implant loss associated deficient osseointegration, peri-implantitis, implant fracture) [62].

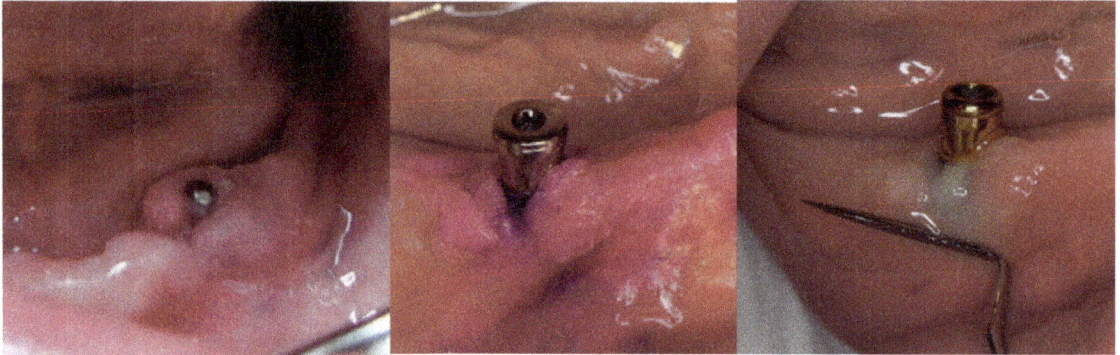

Figure 12. Peri-implant soft tissue lesions-clinical aspect

Therefore, treatment planning considering the fundamental principles of removable implant prosthodontics, overdenture design and execution, maintenance procedures, regular check-ups are all essential for prevention or adequate management of treatment complications. Implant problems are differently addressed according to their type and severity, ranging from simple denture adjustments and enhancing the oral hygiene, to denture relinings or replacement of the denture, to inserting new implants. An important aspect to consider is that implant failure is more common in the maxilla than the mandible, consequently being favorable to place more implants in the upper jaw.

Mandibular implant overdenture is generally considered as being a good predictable treatment, its major implant complication, namely implant loss usually occurring in the first year of function [63,64]. Therefore, regular check-ups are absolutely necessary in this period, for an early intervention that ensures the best prognosis. It is recommended that the dentists performs periodically an accurate evaluation of the implants and surrounding soft tissue regarding the peri-implant marginal bone loss, implant mobility, peri-implant soft tissue, peri-implant bleeding, implant sensitivity during function, result of implant percussion test, plaque accumulation. The overdentures must be verified regarding the overdenture base that is in direct contact with the implant, as risk factor for peri-implant soft tissue complications, regarding the occlusion and maxillomandibular relationship whose faults may be related to exerting increased pressure on implants, as risk factor for implant failure, as its stability and hygiene. Other aspects, like the prosthetic treatment on the opposite jaw (an unstable denture as antagonist can produce excessive forces on the implants) and parafunctions should be checked.

4.10. Attachment system complication, with overdentures

Attachment system complications can occur as a consequence of an incorrect treatment planning, improper treatment conduct (e.g., errors during placement of the retentive housing in the overdenture base) or related to their changes that occur in time, during functioning (e.g., loosening or damage). These vary according to the type of attachment system, e.g., bar, ball, Locator. Most frequent attachment system complications, with overdentures, are: decreased prosthesis retention due to deactivation, detachment, damage or loss of the retentive housing; abutment screw loosening or fracture; fracture of the attachment system components (e.g., bar or clip fracture); soft tissue lesions as hyperplasia under the bar or peri-implant mucositis.

The management of attachment system complications varies according to the attachment system used and the complication type. Technical complications are more common for bar than ball attachments, and both of them are more common compared to locator system [65,66]. Usually low severity complications occurs, such as loss of rubber ring and matrix deactivation, which need to be promptly addressed since they cause overdenture instability with possible negative impact on the dental implants. A more severe complication is bar fracture, that requires increased clinical time and expenses to be resolved, considering that usually the overdenture must be replaced. In elderly edentulous patients simpler prosthetic reconstructions, with complications that require decreased time and money are preferred. Thus, if the option of implant overdenture has been selected, the ball attachment system can be more appropriate than the bar attachment system, due to the more simple maintenance procedures and easier replacement of the implant if necessary.

4.11. Patient satisfaction and quality of life

The conventional dentures are the most common treatment option for the edentulous patients, and usually register good results in terms of patient's satisfaction. Dissatisfaction reasons most claimed by patients are related to denture instability, improper mastication, esthetic deficiency and phonation problems [67]. Denture intolerance is usually connected to subjective factors (the patient's needs and expectations, psychological type, misconceptions) or objective factors (denture instability, pain, functional deficiencies).

The root or implant overdenture have improved retention that contributes to physical and psychological comfort. According to the current evidence, mandibular implant overdentures provide a higher satisfaction and oral health related quality of life compared to conventional denture, but there is uncertainty about the true magnitude of difference between the two [68].

5. Conclusions

Dentures and overdentures, the most frequently used treatment options for the complete edentulism, have complications that are related to patient and prostheses features. Patient's general and local conditions and behavior must be acknowledged as their manifestations, interactions and impact on the prosthetic treatment. Removable implant prosthodontics principles should be well-known and respected during prosthesis execution. The previous, additional to regular check-ups, represent the basis of the prevention removable prosthesis complications.

Denture and overdenture complications are partially similar, differences being related to design particularities, biomechanical aspects and execution procedures. Addressing them depends on their nature and severity, requiring a specific medical conduct. Often simple clinical interventions are needed, but sometimes complex procedures with increased clinical, biological and financial costs must be considered in order to achieve a medical result that corresponds to the current medical standards and patient needs and expectations.

Author details

Elena Preoteasa[1*], Cristina Teodora Preoteasa[2], Laura Iosif[1], Catalina Murariu Magureanu[1] and Marina Imre[1]

*Address all correspondence to: dr_elena_preoteasa@yahoo.com

1 Department of Prosthodontics, Faculty of Dental Medicine, Carol Davila University of Medicine and Pharmacy, Bucharest, Romania

2 Department of Oral Diagnosis, Ergonomics, Scientific Research Methodology, Faculty of Dental Medicine, Carol Davila University of Medicine and Pharmacy, Bucharest, Romania

References

[1] Carlsson GE, Omar R. The Future of Complete Dentures in Oral Rehabilitation. A Critical Review. Journal of Oral Rehabilitation 2010;37(2): 143-156.

[2] Emami E, de Souza RF, Kabawat M, Feine JS. The Impact of Edentulism on Oral and General Health. International Journal of Dentistry 2013; 2013. DOI: 10.1155/2013/498305 (accesed 1 September 2014).

[3] Cunha-Cruz J, Hujoel PP, Nadanovsky P. Secular Trends in Socio-Economic Disparities in Edentulism: USA, 1972–2001. Journal of Dental Research 2007;86(2): 131–13.

[4] Beltrán-Aguilar ED, Barker LK, Canto MT, Dye BA, Gooch BF, Griffin SO, Hyman J, Jaramillo F, Kingman A, Nowjack-Raymer R, Selwitz RH, Wu T. Surveillance for Dental Caries, Dental Sealants, Tooth Retention, Edentulism, and Enamel Fluorosis--United States, 1988-1994 and 1999-2002. Morbidity and Mortality Weekly Report. Surveillance Summaries 2005;54(3): 1-43.

[5] Vos T, Flaxman AD, Naghavi M, Lozano R, Michaud C, Ezzati M, Shibuya K, et al. Years Lived with Disability (YLDs) for 1160 Sequelae of 289 Diseases and Injuries 1990-2010: A Systematic Analysis for the Global Burden of Disease Study 2010. Lancet 2012; 380(9859): 2163-96. DOI: 10.1016/S0140-6736(12)61729-2 (accesed 1 September 2014).

[6] Felton DA. Edentulism and Comorbid Factors. Journal of Prosthodontics 2009;18(2): 88–96.

[7] World Health Organization. International Classification of Functioning, Disability and Health. Geneva, Switzerland. World Health Organization; 2001.

[8] O' Reilly E. Treatment Options for Our Edentulous Patients. http://www.burlington-dentalclinic.ie/wp-content/uploads/2012/10/Dr-Eddie-OReilly-Edentulous-Patients.pdf (accesed 1 September 2014).

[9] Suarez-Sanchez OR. Evaluating Epidemiological Properties of the American College of Prosthodontists (ACP) Prosthodontic Diagnostic Index for Complete Edentulism (PDI-CE)(PDI-Study). Harvard School of Dental Medicine; 2007.

[10] Papadaki E, Anastassiadou V. Elderly Complete Denture Wearers: A Social Approach to Tooth Loss. Gerodontology 2012; 29(2):e721-7. DOI: 10.1111/j. 1741-2358.2011.00550.x. (accesed 14 September 2014).

[11] Dye BA, Tan S, Smith V, Lewis BG, Barker LK, Thornton-Evans G, Eke PI, Beltrán-Aguilar ED, Horowitz AM, Li CH. Trends in Oral Health Status: United States, 1988-1994 and 1999-2004. Vital Health Stat 11. 2007;Apr. (248): 1-92.

[12] Douglass CW, Shih A, Ostry L. Will There Be a Need for Complete Dentures in the United States in 2020? Journal of Prosthetic Dentistry 2002;87(1): 5–8.

[13] Osterberg T, Carlsson GE. Dental State, Prosthodontic Treatment and Chewing Ability-a Study of Five cohorts of 70-Year-Old Subjects. Journal of Oral Rehabilitation 2007;34(8): 553-9.

[14] Felton D, Cooper L, Duqum I, Minsley G, Guckes A, Haug S, Meredith P et al. Evidence-Based Guidelines for the Care and Maintenance of Complete Dentures: a Publication of the American College of Prosthodontists. Journal of the American Dental Association 2011;142(Suppl 1): 1S-20S.

[15] Thompson GW, Kreisel PS. The Impact of the Demographics of Aging and the Edentulous Condition on Dental Care Services. Journal of Prosthetic Dentistry 1998;79(1): 56-9.

[16] American College of Prosthodontists (ACP). The Prosthodontic Diagnostic Index for Complete Edentulism (PDI-CE). http://ww-w.gotoapro.org/assets/1/7/Complete_Edentulism_Checklist.pdf (accesed 1 September 2014).

[17] Al-Zubeidi MI, Payne AG. Mandibular Overdentures: A Review of Treatment Philosophy and Prosthodontic Maintenance. New Zealand Dental Journal 2007;103(4): 88-97.

[18] Kiyak HA, Reichmuth M. Barriers to and Enablers of Older Adults' Use of Dental Services. Journal of Dental Education 2005; 69(9): 975-6.

[19] [19]. Montini T, Tseng TY, Patel H, Shelley D. Barriers to Dental Services for Older Adults. American Journal of Health Behaviour 2014;38(5): 781-8.

[20] Wismeijer D, Ten BC, Schulten EA. Notes Concerning an Overdenture on 2 Implants as the Standard for Treating an Edentulous Mandible. Nederlands Tijdschrift Voor Tandheelkunde 2011;118(12): 633-9.

[21] Sutton AF, Glenny AM, McCord JF. Interventions for Replacing Missing Teeth: Denture Chewing Surface Designs in Edentulous People. The Cochrane Database of Sysematic Reviews 2005;25(1). DOI: 10.1002/14651858.CD004941.pub2 (accesed 1 September 2014).

[22] Preoteasa CT, Nabil Sultan A, Popa L, Ionescu E, Iosif, L, Ghica, MV, Preoteasa E. Wettability of Some Dental Materials. Optoelectronics and Advanced Materials – Rapid Communications 2011; 5(8): 874-8.

[23] Preoteasa E, Imre M, Preoteasa CT. A 3-Year Follow-up Study of Overdentures Retained by Mini–Dental Implants. The International Journal of Oral & Maxillofacial Implants 2014; 29(5). 1034-41.

[24] Carlsson GE. Clinical Morbidity and Sequelae of Treatment with Complete Dentures. Journal of Prosthetic Dentistry 1998;79(1): 17-23.

[25] Petersen PE, Kandelman D, Arpin S, Ogawa H. Global Oral Health of Older People-Call for Public Health Action. Community Dental Health 2010;27(4 Suppl 2): 257-67.

[26] Hummel SK, Wilson MA, Marker VA, Nunn ME. Quality of Removable Partial Dentures Worn by the Adult U.S. Population. Journal of Prosthetic Dentistry 2002;88(1): 37-43.

[27] Pietrokovski J, Harfin J, Levy F. The Influence of Age and Denture Wear on the Size of Edentulous Structures. Gerodontology 2003;20(2): 100-5.

[28] Fitzpatrick AL, Powe NR, Cooper LS, Ives DG, Robbins JA. Barriers to Health Care Access Among the Elderly and Who Perceives Them. American Journal of Public Health 2004; 94(10):1788-94.

[29] Dolan TA, Atchison KA. Implications of Access, Utilization and Need for Oral Health Care by the Non-Institutionalized and Institutionalized Elderly on the Dental Delivery System. Journal of Dental Education 1993;57(12): 876-87.

[30] Dolan TA, Atchison K, Huynh TN. Access to Dental Care Among Older Adults in the United States. Journal of dental Education 2005; 69(9): 961-74.

[31] Health and Behavior. The Interplay of Biological, Behavioral, and Societal Influences. Institute of Medicine (US) Committee on Health and Behavior: Research, Practice, and Policy. Washington DC. National Academies Press (US); 2001. http://www.ncbi.nlm.nih.gov/books/NBK43743/ (accesed 1 September 2014).

[32] Barratt A. Evidence Based Medicine and Shared Decision Making: The Challenge of Getting Both Evidence and Preferences Into Health Care. Patient Education and Counseling 2008;73(3): 407-12.

[33] Graber T, Eliades T, Athanasiou AE. Risk Management in Orthodontics: Expers' Guide to Malpractice. Chicago: Quintessence Publishing Co; 2004.

[34] Berglundh T, Persson L, Klinge B. A Systematic Review of the Incidence of Biological and Technical Complications in Implant Dentistry Reported in Prospective Longitudinal Studies of at least 5 Years. Journal of Clinical Periodontology 2002;29 (Suppl 3): 197-212.

[35] Misch K, Wang H. Implant Surgery Complications: Etiology and Treatment. Implant Dentistry 2008; 17(2): 159-68.

[36] Atwood DA. Reduction of Residual Ridges: A Major Disease Entity. Journal of Prosthetic Dentistry 1971;26(3): 266-79.

[37] Thomason JM, Kelly SA, Bendkowski A, Ellis JS.Two implant retained overdentures--a review of the literature supporting the McGill and York consensus statements. Journal of Dentistry 2012;40(1):22-34.

[38] Budtz-Jörgensen E. Oral Mucosal Lesions Associated with the Wearing of Removable Dentures. Journal of Oral Pathology 1981; 10(2): 65-80.

[39] Dunlap CL, Barker CF. A Guide to Common Oral Lesions. http://dentistry.umkc.edu/Practicing_Communities/asset/OralLesions (accessed 23 July 2014).

[40] Coelho CM, Sousa YT, Daré AM. Denture-Related Oral Mucosal Lesions in a Brazilian School of Dentistry. Journal of Oral Rehabilitation 2004;31(2): 135-9.

[41] Sudarshan R, Sree Vijayabala G, Prem Kumar KS. Inflammatory Hyperplasia of the Oral Cavity. Archives Medical Review Journal. 2012; 21(4): 299-307.

[42] Canger EM, Celenk P, Kayipmaz S. Denture-Related Hyperplasia: A Clinical Study of a Turkish Population Group. Brazilian Dental Journal 2009; 20(3): 243-8.

[43] European Association of Oral Medicine (EAOM). Denture Related Stomatitis. http://www.eaom.eu/empty_24.html (accesed 1 September 2014).

[44] Gendreau L, Loewy ZG. Epidemiology and Etiology of Denture Stomatitis. Journal of Prosthodontics 2011; 20(4): 251-60.

[45] Petersen PE, Yamamoto T. Improving the Oral Health of Older People: The Approach of the WHO Global Oral Health Programme. Community Dentistry and Oral Epidemiology 2005;33(2): 81-92.

[46] Shulman JD, Rivera-Hidalgo F, Beach MM. Risk Factors Associated with Denture Stomatitis in the United States. Journal of Oral Pathology and Medicine 2005 34(6): 340-6.

[47] Lylajam S, Prasanath V. Denture Stomatitis-Etiological Factors and Management. Journal of Clinical Dentistry 2011;2(1): 9-11.

[48] Preoteasa E, Iosif L, Amza O, Preoteasa CT, Dumitrascu C. Thermography, an Imagistic Method in Investigation of the Oral Mucosa Status in Complete Denture Wearers. Journal of Optoelectronics and Advanced Materials 2010;12(11): 2333–4.

[49] Pietrokovski J, Kaffe I, Arensburg B. Retromolar Ridge in Edentulous Patients: Clinical Considerations. Journal of Prosthodontics 2007;16(6): 502-6.

[50] Melescanu Imre M, Preoteasa E, Tancu A, Preoteasa CT. Imaging Technique for the Complete Edentulous Patient Treated Conventionally or With Mini Implant Overdenture. Jornal of Medicine and Life 2013;6(1): 86-92.

[51] Cawood JI, Stoelinga PJ. International Research Group on Reconstructive Preprosthetic Surgery. Consensus Report. International Journal of Oral Maxillofacial Surgery 2000;29(3): 159-62.

[52] Goiato MC, Filho HG, Dos Santos DM, Barão VA, Júnior AC. Insertion and Follow-Up of Complete Dentures: A Literature Review. Gerodontology 2011;28(3): 197-204.

[53] Nkengne A, Bertin C. Aging and Facial Changes--Documenting Clinical Signs, Part 1: Clinical Changes of the Aging Face. Skinmed 2012;10(5): 284-289.

[54] Okada HC, Alleyne B, Varghai K, Kinder K, Guyuron B. Facial Changes Caused by Smoking: A Comparison Between Smoking and Nonsmoking Identical Twins. Plastic and Reconstructive Surgery 2013;132(5): 1085-92.

[55] Mataix J, Bañuls J, Lucas A, Pastor N, Betlloch I. Prematurely Aged Appearance. Clinical and Experimental Dermatology 2006;31(6): 833-4.

[56] Joss N, Boulton-Jones JM, More I. Premature Ageing and Glomerulonephritis. Nephrology Dialisis Transplantation 2001;16(3): 615-8.

[57] Tupac R, et al. Parameters of Care for the Speciality of Prosthodontics. Jornal of pros-thodontics. Implant, Esthetic, and Reconstructive Dentistry. Official Journal of The American College of Prosthodontists 2005;14(4)Suppl: 1-103.

[58] Preoteasa E, Murariu CM, Ionescu E, Preoteasa CT. Acrylic Resin Reinforcement With Metallic and Nonmetallic Inserts. Revista Medico-Chirurgicala a Societatii de Medici si Naturalisti din Iasi 2007; 111(2): 487-93.

[59] Kreisler M, Behneke N, Behneke A, d'Hoedt B. Residual Ridge Resorption in the Edentulous Maxila in Patients With Implant-Supported Mandibular Overdentures: An 8-Years Retrospective Study. International Journal of Prosthodontics 2003;16(3): 265-300.

[60] Ettinger RL, Qian F. Postprocedural Problems in An Overdenture Population: A Lon-gitudinal Study. Journal of Endodontics 2004; 30(5): 310-4.

[61] Crum RJ, Rooney GE Jr. Alveolar Boneloss in Overdentures: A 5-Years Study. Jour-nal of Prosthetic Dentistry 1978; 40(6): 610-3.

[62] Preoteasa E, Meleşcanu-Imre M, Preoteasa CT, Marin M, Lerner H. Aspects of Oral Morphology as decision factors in mini-implant supported overdenture. Romanian Journal of Morphoogy and Embryology 2010;51(2): 309-14.

[63] Burns DR. Mandibular Implant Overdenture Treatment: Consensus and Controver-sy. Journal of Prosthodontics 2000;9(1): 37-46.

[64] Eckert SE, Choi YG, Sánchez AR, Koka S. Comparison of Dental Implant Systems: Quality of Clinical Evidence and Prediction of 5-Year Survival. The International Journal of Oral & Maxillofacial Implants 2005; 20(3):406-15.

[65] Gotfredsen K1, Holm B. Implant-Supported Mandibular Overdentures Retained With Ball Or Bar Attachments: A Randomized Prospective 5-Year Study. Internation-al Journal of Prosthodontics 2000;13(2): 125-30.

[66] Cakarer S, Can T, Yaltirik M, Keskin C. Complications Associated with the Ball, Bar And Locator Attachments for Implant-Supported Overdentures. Medicina Oral, Pa-toogial Oral Y Cirurgia Bucal 2011;16(7): e953-9.

[67] Preoteasa E, Marin M, Imre M, Lerner H, Preoteasa CT. Patients' Satisfaction With Conventional Dentures and Mini Implant Anchored Overdentures. Revista Medico-Chirurgicala a Societatii de Medici si Naturisti din Iasi 2012;116(1): 310-16.

[68] Emami E, Heydecke G, Rompré PH, de Grandmont P, Feine JS. Impact of Implant Support for Mandibular Dentures on Satisfaction, Oral and General Health-Related Quality of Life: A Meta-Analysis of Randomized-Controlled Trials. Clinical Oral Im-plants Research 2009; 20(6): 533-44.

Ultrasonic Instrumentation

Ana Isabel García-Kass,
Juan Antonio García-Núñez and
Victoriano Serrano-Cuenca

1. Introduction

Although ultrasounds (US) were discovered in the 18th Century due to their use in animal kingdom, they were not manufactured until the 19th Century, when certain devices facilitating the reproduction of these non audible for human sounds were developed. They constitute rare frequencies with several properties. First of all they were developed for their use in navy and in medicine. In the 20th Century it was noticed that they could have uses in dentistry, so the first applications for calculus removal were initiated, taking advantage of their mechanical energy and cavitation effect. The different possibilities achieved by conventional US together with those of sonicators, of lower frequency but with similar effects, resulted in a fast development of these technologies.

Since Michigan longitudinal studies demonstrated that the open flap radicular instrumentation techniques were in a long term as effective as the closed ones, the latter were developed, so treatment of periodontitis suffered a change of paradigm. From that moment on, periodontal treatment involved less open flaps and more mechanical treatments, limiting surgeries to very concrete cases, in order to enable access to the deepest pockets and furcations. The result was a reduction in discomfort for patients and a better long term prognosis. Prevention gained more importance and supportive periodontal therapies were regularly done adjusting them to the individual necessities of each patient, depending on the type of periodontitis and the severity of the case. To reduce the number of surgeries, it was crucial to develop instruments able to reach deep pockets. Small curettes and microcurettes were developed, and later on special ultrasonic tips which allowed the instrumentation of pockets of difficult access for Gracey and Universal curettes. Even when effectuating periodontal surgery, clinicians preferred US rather than curettes for the narrow furcations´ instrumentation. The fewer fatigue of the professional and the efficacy of the results have favoured the great development of these instruments during the last years.

A new progress occurred in dentistry with the introduction of piezoelectric US. These US produced less discomfort in patients, and with the development of special tips imitating microcurettes, deep and narrow pockets instrumentation was possible without doing surgery. With the important development of implant rehabilitations during the last twenty years and the subsequent peri-implantitis, the necessity of new instruments has arisen, as traditional and teflon curettes are not suitable for this purpose. To solve this problem, tips of teflon and other materials have emerged to facilitate the elimination of deposits settled over the irregular implants´ surface, with controversial results.

The use of US in endodontics was introduced later to clean and disinfect root canals. It is quite useful basically to make easier the access to the root canals in certain conditions, in endodontic retreatments and to clean before the sealing of the root canal. One of the latest US applications in dentistry is in surgery, as they avoid discomfort of rotary instruments while preserving the soft tissues. The cut precision allows their use in implants´ surgery, ostectomies and especially in those techniques where tearing of soft tissues could be produced due to their proximity, i.e., sinus lift procedures. These techniques are in continuous progress; they are linked to piezo-electric US and to those new materials allowing their use in favourable conditions.

The aim of this chapter is to revise the physical principles of US, the materials used and the historical evolution, their basic uses in perio and endodontics, as well as their efficacy when comparing with other techniques and finally the possibilities in maxilar surgery. Other less frequent applications are also mentioned.

2. History and physics of ultrasounds

Before 1700 man was unaware of ultrasounds because their frequency is below human´s audible frequency. In 1700, Spallanzani described their use by bats when flying and capturing their preys. Later on, it was demonstrated that other animal species had the same faculties, and in the 19th Century, with the discovery of Doppler effect about deformation of light waves in movement, it was observed that this property could also be applied to ultrasounds. In fact, they are sound waves that are not audible for men due to their high frequency (Figure 1).

At the end of the 19th Century, the Curie brothers [1] described the piezoelectric effect (from greek *piezein*, mechanic pressure) of several crystals, property used later for the fabrication of ultrasonic devices with new characteristics. At this time, in 1883, Galton develops a high frequency whistle to find out the human hearing limit, and from that moment on ultrasounds (US) for different applications are developed. Although the first ultrasonic apparatus date from 1950, the first commercial application for dentistry was in periodontics in 1957 with Cavitron®, developed by Dentsply for doing prophylaxis and calculus removal. Its name comes from the cavitation effect produced by ultrasounds when working with water. When a liquid flows through a region where pressure is lower than its steam pressure, the liquid boils and produces

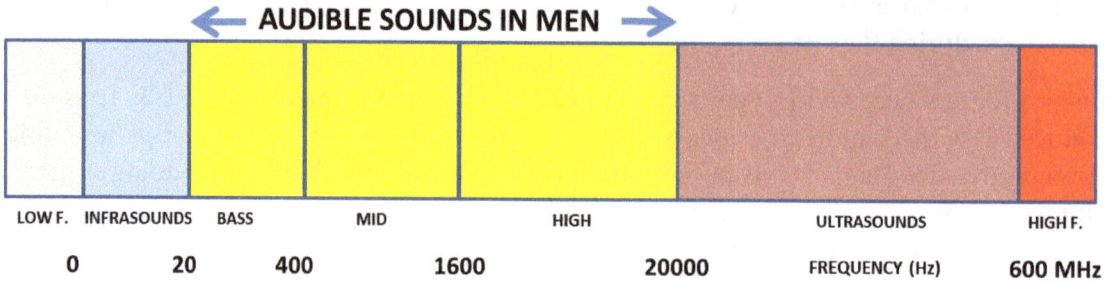

Figure 1. Human audition and ultrasound frequencies in Hz

vapour bubbles. The bubbles will be carried to a higher pressure area, where the steam returns immediately to the liquid phase, imploding the bubbles suddenly. Thus, a change from liquid to gaseous phase takes place, and again to liquid phase with water dissociation and formation of H^+ and OH^- (Figure 2).

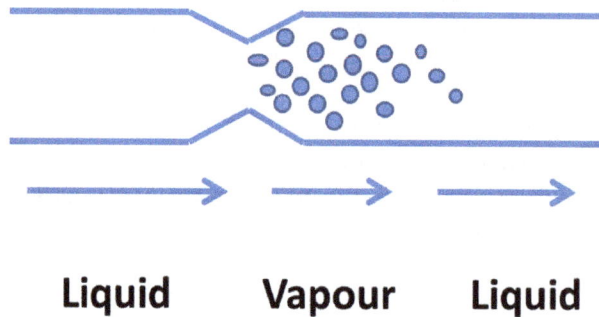

Liquid   Vapour   Liquid

Figure 2. Representation of cavitation effect

Cavitation is defined as the formation of submicroscopic cavities or vacuums as a result of the vibration of a fluid due to the high frequency alternating movement of the tip of an instrument. When these vacuums implode, shock waves which spread through the medium are generated and produce energy (heat) release [2].

The basis of the ultrasonic action consists of an electric generator transmitting vibrations to the tip of the device with frequencies of 25,000 to 30,000 Hz, whose shock waves generate pressures and depressions which detach the calculus and break water molecules by the cavitation phenomenon. To the effect of cavitation it adds an acoustic streaming, with a great cleaning and bactericidal action, which potentiates the bactericidal effect of cavitation, effect that can increase adding an antiseptic product to the irrigation fluid.

There are two types of ultrasonic devices: the classical ones, laminated or magnetostrictive, with elliptical oscillation of the tip, and the piezoelectric ones, of quartz with lineal oscillation. Laminated US are based on the Joule magnetostriction phenomenon. According to this phenomenon, several ferromagnetic materials get deformed when they go through a magnetic field. The deformation degree depends on the material employed, the magnetization strength, the previous treatment of the material and the temperature. The metallic sheets are situated in the handle, i.e. in the handpiece where the insert is placed (Figure 3).

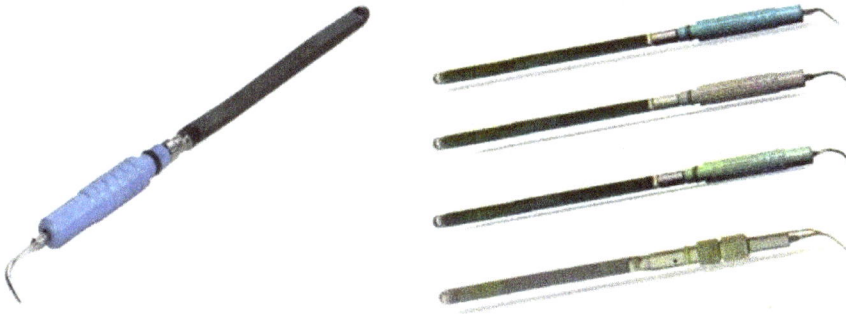

Figure 3. Laminated US device and several ultrasonic inserts for Cavitron

Piezoelectric US (Figure 4) are based on quartz clock principles. When applying an alternating current to the ceramic/quartz discs, changes in polarity produce expansion and contraction trasmitting the oscillation to the tip, applicator or insert. The sound thus generated, presents the same intensity, frequency and wavelength than the material employed in its fabrication (quartz, zinc blende, sodium borate...). Nowadays, the most used crystals are ceramic zirconate discs, which are less sensitive to temperature and blows.

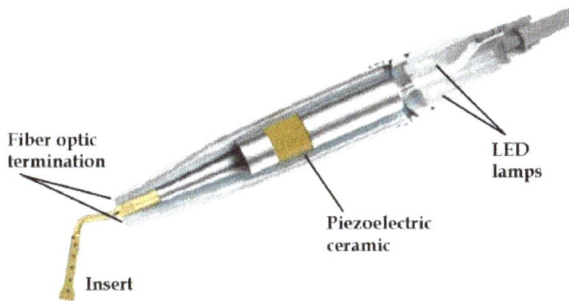

Figure 4. Piezoelectric US for surgery. Modified from Variosurg (NSK) catalogue

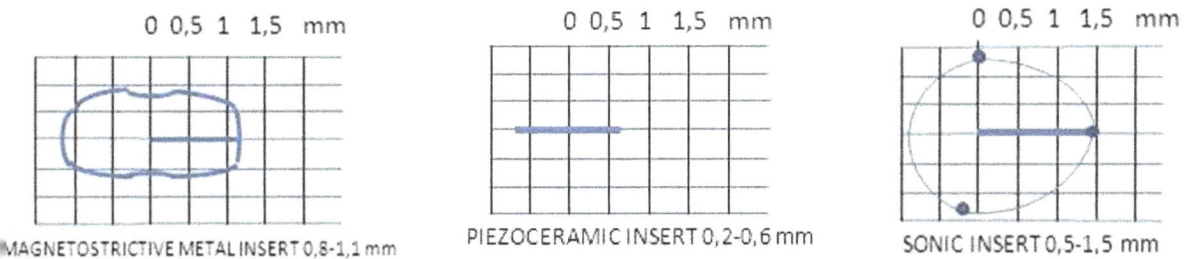

Figure 5. Oscillation of magnetostrictive US, piezoceramic US and sonicators

3. Biologic actions

US present several effects over the tissues which vary depending on the time, type of US and way of application. These effects are mechanical, thermal, biological, chemical, massage and placebo.

1. Mechanical effects. The most important, as vibration favours the removal of calculus, biofilm and of the cementum surface, damaged by bacterial toxins and sometimes contaminated by bacteria (Figure 6). Inside the root canals, US clean the pulpal detritus.

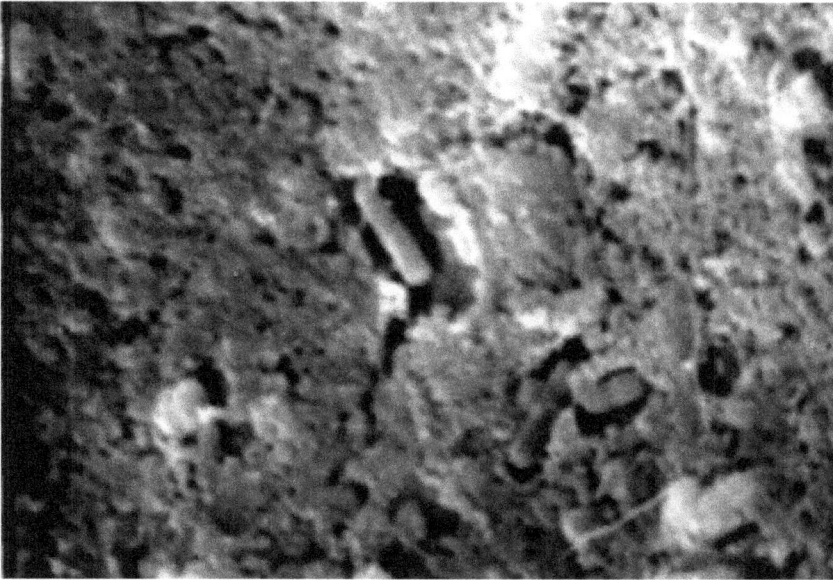

Figure 6. Bacterial presence inside cementum in periodontitis. Original magnification SEM x3000. Bacteria can be iden-tified supragingivally, in the epithelial junction and in apical areas of cementum

2. Thermal effects. US are a way of energy and thus, during their application, heat is generated. This heat can be useful, as it favours the cleaning of the treated area and the elimination of detritus, blood debris, biofilm and calculus; but if it is excessive it could burn the tissues, especially gingiva and periostium. This is the reason why it is crucial to control the irrigation system, checking for possible obstructions of applicator/insert.

3. Biological effects. US produce an increase in permeability of the cellular membrane, known as phonophoresis, which facilitates the cellular function, and thus the recuperation of the inflamed soft tissues.

4. Chemical effects. Ultrasonic vibration favours the chemical processes in the area in which they are applied. Biological exchanges among the treated tissues improve; in addition, an increase of the blood supply takes place, helping to reduce inflammation and to facilitate the arrival of blood cells and anti-inflammatory mediators, favouring tissue normality. It

also produces oxidation and macromolecule depolymerization phenomena, due to the ions release.

5. The massage and placebo effects, also associated to US, are of less interest in our field, but they should not be forgotten.

Due to the cavitation effect and the acoustic micro-streaming produced by oscillatory movements of ultrasonic inserts, US are used in humans in different ways for diagnosis and treatment. In the oral cavity they are mainly used for root instrumentation in periodontics, and less in endodontics, ostectomy, and sinus lift procedures. There are also other less frequent applications that we shall describe.

4. US in periodontics and implants

It is well known that periodontal disease is based on the presence of a mature biofilm with more than 700 bacterial species, being only a fraction of them related to periodontitis. The progression of the disease depends on the periodontopathogens, but also on the patient's immune system and its response to bacterial aggression. The elimination of bacteria, their toxins and calculus produced by saliva, is essential to keep under control the disease. Once local factors are removed, a strict hygiene is required, as well as a supportive periodontal treatment program, in order to eliminate calculus and subgingival biofilm, which is the main responsible of the bone and attachment loss and is formed shortly after its elimination.

Treatment was traditionally based on the mechanical elimination of plaque and calculus, which facilitate biofilm's survival, mainly using hand instruments and US, directly or by an open flap procedure. Longitudinal studies of the decades of 70's and 80's, showed that even most periodontally advanced cases, well treated and maintained, remained stable through the years [3], versus those patients who did not receive any treatment, who suffered a considerable tooth loss and worsening of periodontal parameters [4].

Since Michigan longitudinal studies [5-7] demonstrated that the open flap radicular instrumentation techniques were in a long term as effective as the closed ones [7], the latter were developed, so treatment of periodontitis suffered a change of paradigm. From that moment on, periodontal treatment involved less open flaps and more mechanical treatments, limiting surgeries to very concrete cases, in order to enable access to the most deep pockets and furcations [8]. The result was a reduction in discomfort for patients and a better long term prognosis. Prevention gained more importance and supportive periodontal therapies were regularly done adjusting them to the individual necessities of each patient, depending on the type of periodontitis and the severity of the case.

To reduce the number of surgeries, it was crucial to develop instruments able to reach deep pockets. Small curettes and microcurettes were developed, and later on special ultrasonic tips which allowed the instrumentation of pockets of difficult access for Gracey and Universal curettes.

The first device used in periodontal prophylaxis was Cavitron®, introduced in 1957 by Dentsply (USA). With the important development of implant rehabilitations during the last twenty years and the subsequent peri-implantitis, the necessity of new instruments has arisen, as traditional and teflon curettes are not suitable for this purpose. Ultrasonic instruments are very comfortable to use, they produce less fatigue in the operator than curettes and allow the combination of different tips and products in order to improve the treatment efficacy. Several authors [9] even demonstrate better results when instrumentation is done with US instead of curettes.

During the 80's, we demonstrated in several publications that prophylaxis done *in vitro* with US resulted at least equal or even more effective than with curettes [10, 11] (Figure 7).

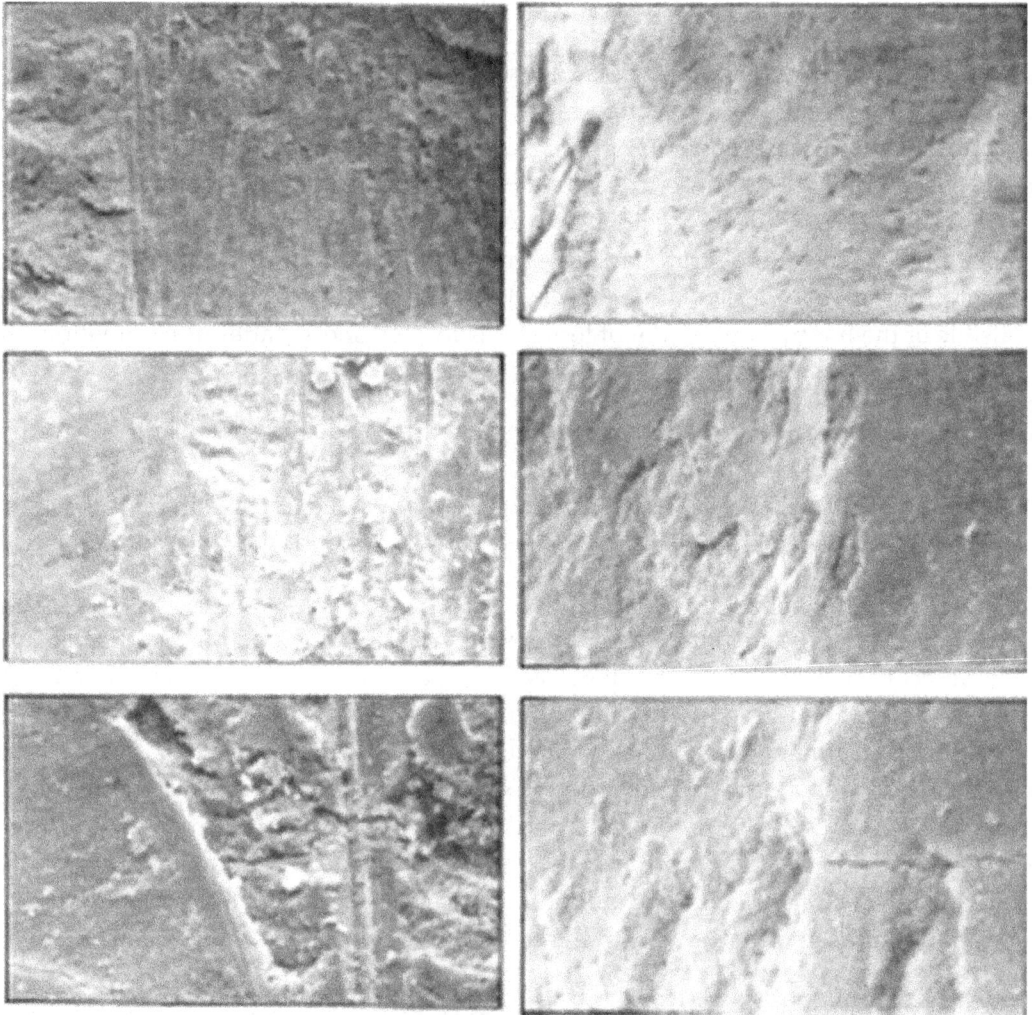

Figure 7. Cementum of the same tooth treated with curettes (left) and US (right). Original magnification SEM x352, x1136 and x3000

In Drisko´s 1993 review, it is suggested that a thorough radicular debridement can be achieved without overinstrumentation, using certain sonic and ultrasonic scalers. The evaluation of residual plaque and calculus after hand and mechanical instrumentation with sonic and ultrasonic scalers, shows that sonic and US instruments obtain similar, and in some cases, better results than those obtained with manual instrumentation. When comparing modified ultrasonic inserts with unmodified ultrasonic inserts and manual scalers, it is observed that the modified ones generate smoother surfaces, better plaque and calculus removal, less damage and better access to the bottom of the pocket, which together with a less operating time lead to a lower fatigue [12].

Several years later, another review of the same author shows that US, through their cavitation effect, are able to eliminate toxins from the cementum surface without damaging it. This, together with the irrigation action, improves healing, as it is not necessary an excessive instrumentation of cementum to achieve satisfactory results. The additional benefits of the chemical irrigation during ultrasonic instrumentation are the weakly attached subgingival plaque removal and a better access to difficult areas such as narrow and deep pockets, root grooves and furcations. Thus, microultrasonic tips, of smaller diameter, allow the penetration 1 mm farther than manual instruments [13].

In a position paper of 2000, US and sonicators were compared, reaching similar results than hand instruments in terms of plaque, calculus and endotoxins removal. Ultrasonic scalers used at medium power produced less damage in root surfaces than manual instruments or sonicators. Furcations seemed to be more accesible when using sonic or ultrasonic scalers than when using manual instruments. It was still not clear if root roughness was more or less pronounced when using US or curettes, and if the roughness produced in radicular cement affected long term wound healing. Although the aim of root instrumentation is the highest as possible elimination of calculus and toxins, it is necessary to preserve cementum. According to the reviewed papers, toxins remain in the root surface, thus being easily removed with US. One of the main problems of the intervention with US and sonicators is the aerosols production, which involves the risk of transmitting infectious diseases, therefore it is essential the use of barriers against aerosols. Concerning the use of chemical agents there is no evidence of their additional clinical benefit [14].

To avoid the potential damage of the cementum surface done by sonic and US instruments and curettes, and looking after an effective treatment of the root surface, a sonic instrument covered by teflon was introduced in order to compare it with the standard instrumentation and with Per-io-Tor in extracted teeth. Per-io-Tor and the mentioned sonic instrument seemed to be adequate for soft deposits' elimination in the root surface, but not for calculus removal [15].

Another study compared *in vivo* the effect of two piezoelectric US, Vector scaler and Enac scaler, with a hand scaler. Instrumentation was completed until the obtaining of a hard surface. Roughness, amount of remaining calculus and loss of dental substance were examined by SEM. Vectorial US provided a smooth root surface with minimal dental substance loss [16].

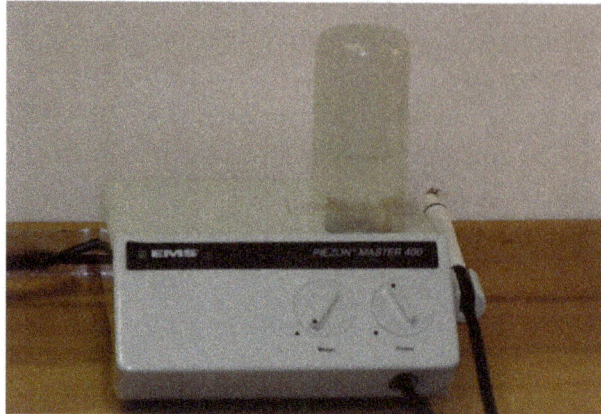

Figure 8. EMS piezoelectric US Piezon Master

The effects of US were described in 1969 by Clark [17]: they depend on the vibratory movement amplitude, the pressure applied, the instrument´s tip sharpness, and the tip´s application angle and time by surface unit. Their effects condition the way of use: they should be used at 40-50% of their power to avoid the metal fatigue and to favour the long-term duration of device and tip, they should be applied tangentially (parallel to the root surface) to avoid damage in the cementum surface (Figure 9), they should never be applied with the tip perpendicular to the cementum and the tip should be in a continuous movement (Figure 10) in order to avoid the production of holes in enamel and cementum. To avoid an excessive increase of temperature, the irrigation should be abundant (Figure 11), and to achieve an optimal efficacy the most suitable tip should be selected for each indication. It should be taken into account that it is different to work over a thick layer of supragingival calculus than over a thin subgingival layer, which is more adhered. This is the reason why large tips are used for superficial calculus, small tips for subgingival calculus, curette-like for scaling and thin and long for narrow and deep pockets (Figure 11).

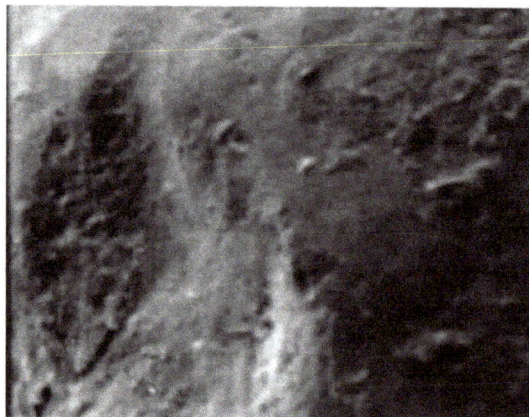

Figure 9. Hole in cementum due to a wrong ultrasonic instrumentation. Original magnification x600

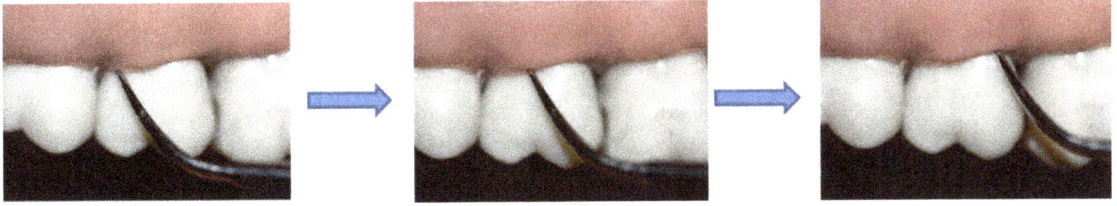

Figure 10. Insert application and displacement for calculus removal

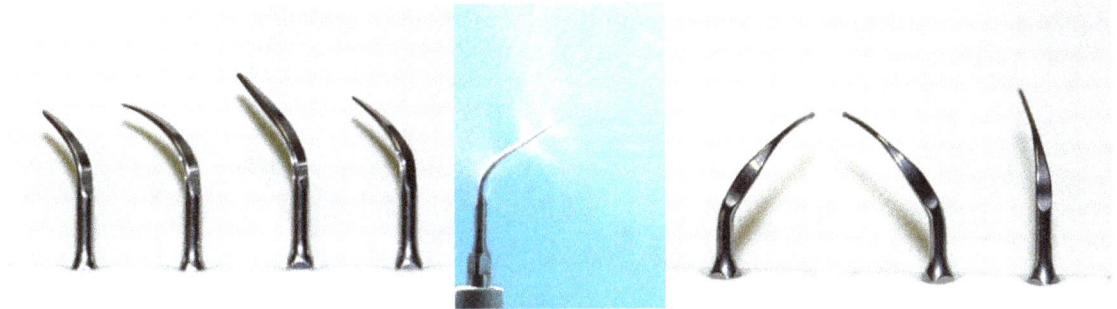

Figure 11. Supra (left) and thin subgingival (right) ultrasonic tips should always work with abundant irrigation

When US are used with complementary water tank and an antiseptic liquid, it is convenient to wash the whole circuit with demineralized water after its use, so the obstruction of tubes with the substances used is avoided. In case of using only water, it is recommended to fill in the deposit with low mineralized water, in order to facilitate the cleaning and prevent obstructions in tubes and inserts.

Due to their lineal oscillation over the dental surface, the actual rounded-tip piezoelectric US, reduce abrasion and obtain a uniform and smooth surface. With 32.000 oscillations per second, they are autoregulated and their cavitation effect and acoustic streaming reduce discomfort and have limited effects over gingival epithelium (Figure 12).

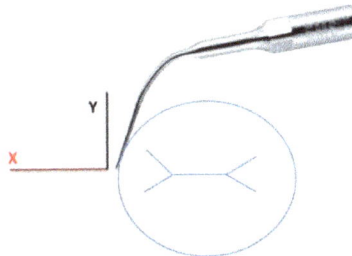

Figure 12. Vector decomposition of ultrasonic oscillation

Some of these US may incorporate two bottles, one for the bactericidal agent and the other for water for clearing or cleaning. They are also equipped with perio and endodontic tips.

Ultrasounds present few contraindications. They are not recommended in children except in very concrete cases. They should be avoided in the proximity of composite resins, as they could produce roughness or even detachment of the filling. They should not be used directly over ceramic partial fixed prosthesis or veneers, as ceramic could detach or break. In patients with certain types of pacemakers, interferences could be produced with inhibition and increase of the stimulation frequency. It is recommended the intermittent use of ultrasounds, avoiding the support of instruments over the generator as well as deprogramming the frequency modulation during the sessions. With a magnet, the pacemaker, which usually works at demand mode, converts into fixed-rate, not being sensitive to electromagnetic fields. In case of non sensible to electromagnetic interferences pacemakers, US could be used in the same way as in patients without pacemakers. Another option in these patients is the use of sonicators (Figure 13) because they use an air flow so they don´t generate electromagnetic fields.

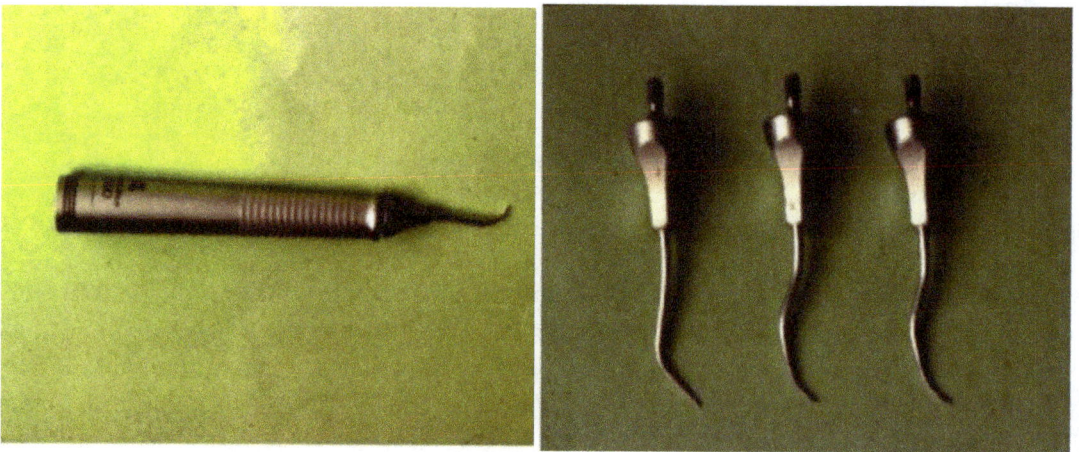

Figure 13. Sonicator and varied tips

These instruments present certain advantages and disadvantages in relation to ultrasounds. Their oscillation frequency is much lower, of 2,000 Hz, because the oscillation is produced by the air that arrives directly from the equipment and generates an orbital oscillation in the application tip. Their efficacy is similar to that of ultrasounds, but they can only use water instead of antiseptic liquids and the set of tips is much more reduced than the ultrasounds.

Ultrasounds are used as preventive and complementary to surgery treatment in implants. In this case the tip should not be metallic but of teflon, in order to avoid the damage of the implants´ surface (Figure 14).

Fox *et al.* compared plastic and metal curettes in titanium implants in an *in vitro* study. Plastic instruments produced an insignificant alteration of the implants´ surface after instrumentation, in contrast with metal instruments, which significantly altered this surface [18].

Something similar occurs when using Piezoelectric Ultrasonic Scalers with carbon, plastic and metallic tips on titanium implants. Remaining plaque and calculus index seemed to be similar with the three treatments. When using a laser profilometer and a laser scanning electron

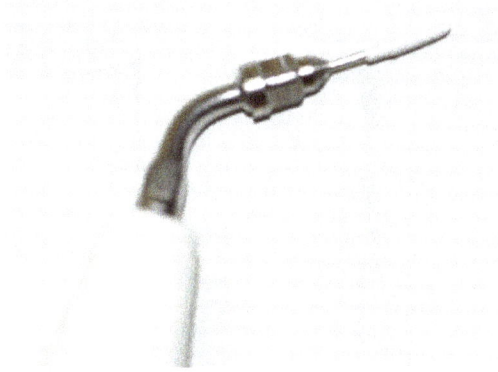

Figure 14. EMS Teflon insert for implants' instrumentation

microscope to evaluate the treated abutment surface characteristics, implants treated with carbon and plastic tips presented smoother surfaces than those treated with metallic tips, which were more damaged [19].

5. US in endodontics

US were incorporated into this field in 1957 when Richman used them for root canal cleaning and instrumentation [20]. In 1976, Martin improved endodontic treatment adding simultaneous irrigation, but its commercialization and use only were extended from 1980 by Martin *et al.* [21]. There are sonic apparatus in which special files are used, and several ultrasonic devices which work with standard files, with the usual colours and diameters (Figure 15).

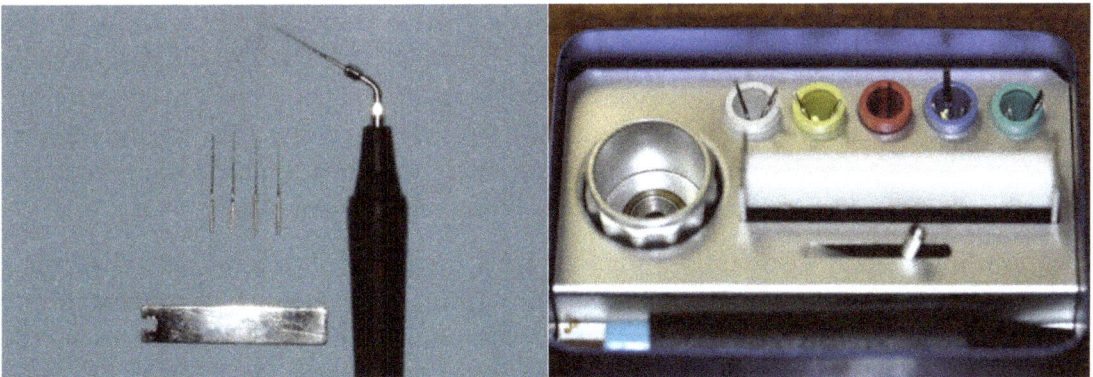

Figure 15. EMS ultrasonic handle and several endodontic K-files.

In endodontics US work by a transversal vibration, with a characteristic pattern of nodes and antinodes along the file's length (Figure 16) [22, 23], and may work in two different ways: with simultaneous ultrasonic instrumentation and irrigation (UI) or with passive ultrasonic irrigation (PUI), which works in an alternating way.

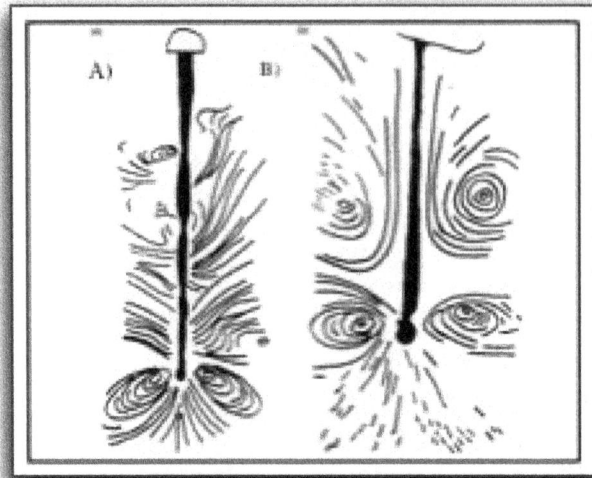

Figure 16. Diagrammatic representation of the current observed in ultrasonic (A) and sonic (B) activated files [24].

As for ultrasonic instrumentation UI, it is discussed if the root canals thus instrumented are significantly cleaner than those prepared with files in the usual way. Some authors support UI cleaning is better [25-29], while other studies affirm the cleaning is similar [30-36]. For Ruddle, these differences could be due to the limited space available in the root canal to let the ultrasonic vibration [37]. Also the lack of space could be responsible of the lesions produced during ultrasonic instrumentation, such as perforations and deficient root canal preparations [38]. This is the reason why this technique is only recommended after the complete root canal preparation [39], by what is known as PUI.

Passive ultrasonic irrigation was described by Weller [40] as a technique in which the effect of the ultrasonic tip reduces the risk of contact with the root canal surface, thus reducing the risk of perforation, while the cavitation and cleaning effects are preserved. As the root canal has already been prepared, the file moves freely and the irrigant penetrates easily in the apical area of the root canal system [41]. In this technique two ways of irrigation may be used: continuous or discontinuous, in which irrigation works intermittently after each ultrasonic cycle. Both of them allow control of irrigation, so they seem to be equally efficient [42].

Sonic instruments may also be used for root canal therapy with similar results. Jensen *et al.* compare the sonic and ultrasonic cleaning efficacy after manual instrumentation in molars with curved roots. Results are analysed with photomicrographs with a grid in order to quantify the debris and evaluate the root canal cleaning level in the three groups. Sonic and ultrasonic treated molars after manual instrumentation seemed to be cleaner than those only manually treated, while the level of cleaning among sonic and ultrasonically treated molars was similar [43].

Another recent *in vitro* study compares the ability of different ultrasound irrigation procedures to eliminate debris and to open the dentine tubules. Previously instrumented with mechanical rotatory technique single-rooted extracted teeth are treated with US. The amount of debris and the number of open dentinal tubules were established by SEM. In the apical third, ultrasonic activation of the irrigation with Irrisafe tips seemed to be the most effective method to eliminate debris and open dentinal tubules [44].

According to Martí-Bowen *et al.*, the use of US in periapical surgery with retrograde filling, it is feasible to reach difficult access root canals with sacrifice of few root tissue. Nowadays, good results are obtained in teeth with periapical pathology which previously were condemned to failure [45].

Van der Sluis *et al.* summarize the potential uses of US in endodontics with the following options: to improve the endodontic access (for example elimination of calcifications), irrigation of root canals, to remove broken posts and other obstructions inside the root canals, humectation with sealer of the root canal walls, guttapercha condensation of the obturations of root canals, mineral trioxide aggregate (MTA) application, endodontic surgery, and increase of the dentinal permeability in dental bleaching [46]; also to break fillings due to their shock effect, to remove old fillings and make easier the access to root canals, and in endodontic retreatments. There are available different applicators with the most adequate form for each use (Figures 17, 18).

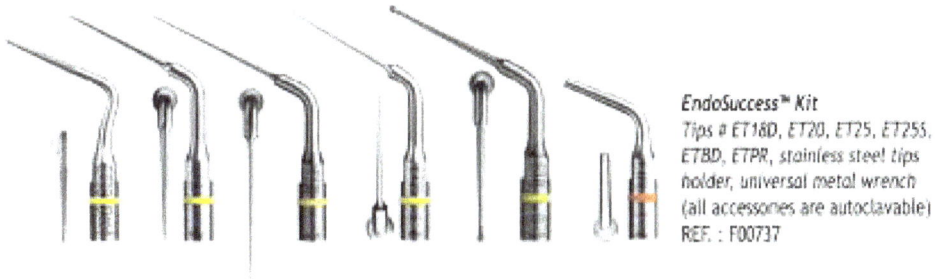

EndoSuccess™ Kit
Tips # ET18D, ET20, ET25, ET25S,
ETBD, ETPR, stainless steel tips
holder, universal metal wrench
(all accessories are autoclavable)
REF. : F00737

Figure 17. Satelec EndoSuccess Retreatment Kit. From left to right, tips for dentinal overhangs, calcificatons or filling materials elimination; for treatments in the coronal third; for treatments in the medium and apical thirds; for retreatment in coronal third and isthmus; for canal probing; and for loosening of posts and crowns. (Courtesy of Satelec, Merignac Cedex, France)

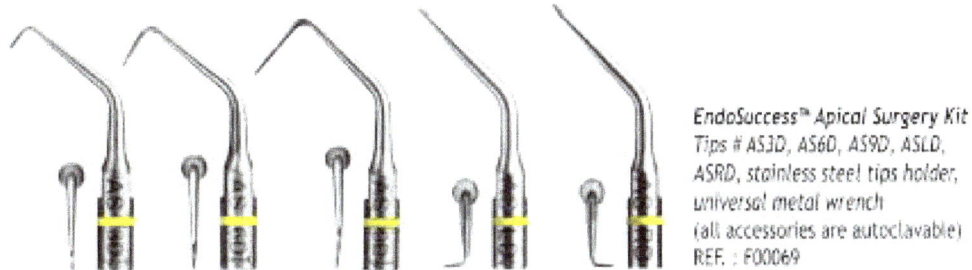

EndoSuccess™ Apical Surgery Kit
Tips # AS3D, AS6D, AS9D, ASLD,
ASRD, stainless steel tips holder,
universal metal wrench
(all accessories are autoclavable)
REF. : F00069

Figure 18. Satelec EndoSuccess Apical Surgery Kit. From left to right, universal apical surgery tip; second instrument; complicated cases (up to the coronal third), premolar left-orientated tip; premolar right orientated tip. (Courtesy of Satelec, Merignac Cedex, France)

6. US in surgery

Another application of US in dentistry is in oral and maxillofacial surgery to cut hard tissues. Experimental studies show that their application present better histological results than the rotary techniques. The precision of the cut with the different available inserts allows their use in our specialization in different fields such as general oral surgery, osseous grafts and implantology.

Although initially their use was reduced to sinus lift procedures, because they preserve the sinus membrane, their use has been extended to obtain bone grafts, osseous distraction and cortical split procedures, inferior dental nerve surgery, implant surgeries, extractions, etc. These biophotonic equipments allow changes in vibration's frequency from standard mode, with constant vibrations and frequency (used over soft tissues), to surgery mode (for hard tissues), where the modulation of amplitude and continuous vibration improves the efficacy over bone. Several applicators are designed for each osseous intervention (Figure 19).

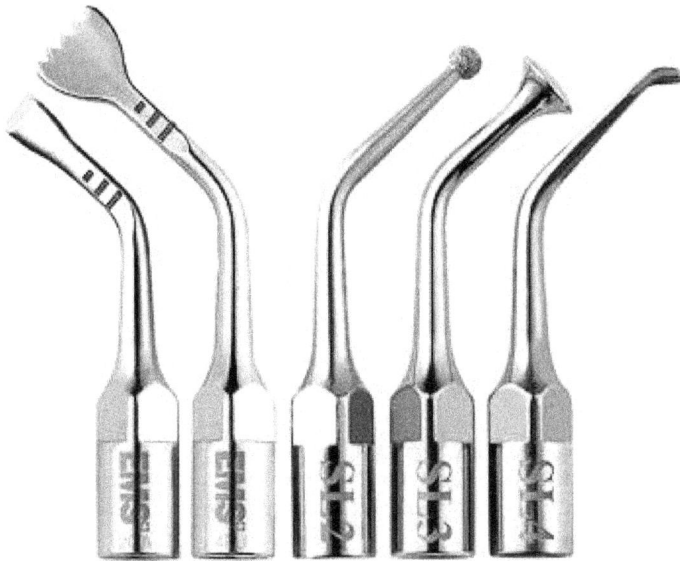

Figure 19. EMS Piezon Master Surgery US presents tips (from left to right) for vertical non-traumatic osseous incision, horizontal non-traumatic osseous incision, non-traumatic osteotomy, detachment of Schneider's membrane during sinus lift procedures and obtaining of bone fragments for bone augmentation.

The tips are different depending on the application: they present multiple lateral impact for surgery; curved, thin and scalpel-like for osteotomy; thin for non-traumatic extractions; cone-shaped diamond covered and calibrated for guiding during preparation; rounded or flat, diamond covered or scaler-shaped for sinus lift procedures. There are multiple surgical possibilities, as it is possible to do thin incisions for grafts, cysts elimination, sinus lift procedures with alveolar or lateral access, extractions, osteoplasties, osteotomies and other.

The advantages justifying their use are less bleeding and thus better visibility during the intervention, higher cut precision than with traditional instruments and less increase of temperature, less discomfort for patients as ultrasonic vibration is less noisy than drilling, and especially that the action over the soft tissues is minimal when they are accidentally applied over them, without tearing them up.

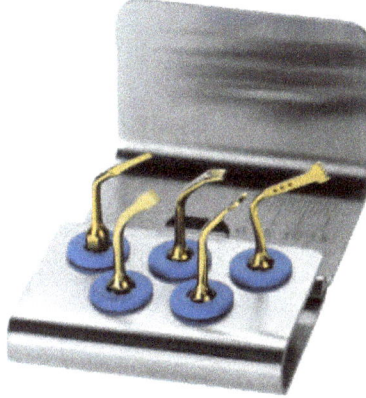

Basic Kit Piezosurgery

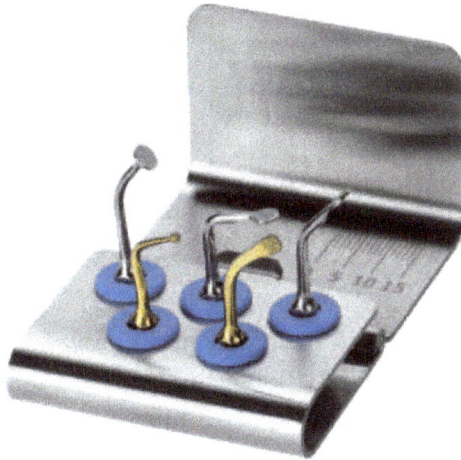

Figure 20. Mectron Piezosurgery´s basic surgery and sinus lift procedure kits.

The action of the tip is effectuated by two mechanical effects: direct and indirect. In the direct mechanical effect, the tissues in contact with the tip are under a very high frequency. It is the effect of a hammer working only over the hard tissues. In the indirect one, positive and negative pressures are generated over the fluids; they are known as cavitation, and they displace the osseous tissue and potentiate the mechanical effects. This produces localized osseous destruction in a continuous or discontinuous way, being the surgeon who decides one or another possibility depending on the osseous density and the required refrigeration. This makes the cut selective without neither microscopic osseous nor soft tissue alterations. Refrigeration should be abundant with saline solution, in order to avoid heating and wash up the field to obtain a better vision.

Kits are usually available for each type of indication. The insert size and angulation allow the use depending on the necessities of the case. There are basic kits, kits for surgery, osseous distraction, implants, endodontic surgery, alveolar and lateral sinus lift procedures, osteoplasy and ostectomy, etc (Figure 20).

7. US trays

US trays deserve to be mentioned. Their utilization is essential in the dental office as intermediate step between the washing with soap and the sterilization of instrumental. They allow the elimination of organic debris that remain adhered in the instrument gaps facilitating the sterilization (Figure 21).

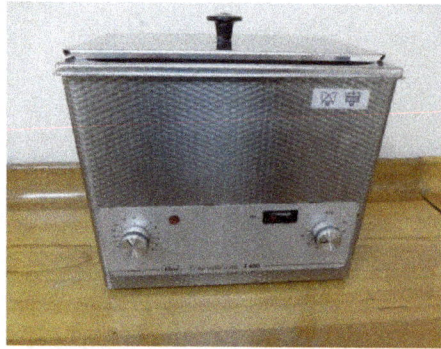

Figure 21. US tray.

Other applications of ultrasounds in Dentistry are removal of broken screws in implants, posts and crowns removal, etc. (Figure 22), but these applications are less frequent, they are not standardized and each professional acts according to his guidelines.

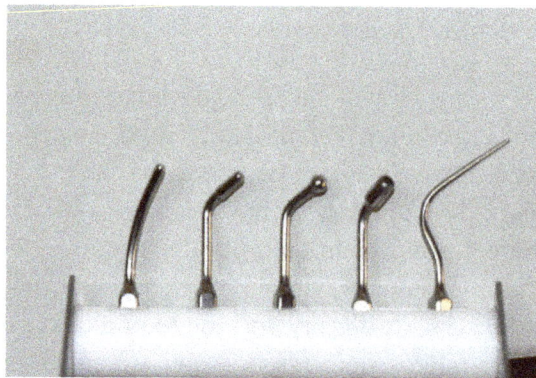

Figure 22. Set of diverse US tips

8. Conclusion

The evolution of US in dentistry during the last 65 years has been revised. The first laminated devices, only used for supragingival and slightly subgingival tartrectomies, have lead to sonicators and newer piezoelectric US with multiple inserts which allow the performance of tartrectomies reducing patient's discomfort and subgingival instrumentation. The variety of available tips lets us choose those which better adapt to our necessities and to the clinical situation, even in cases of periimplantitis. In endodontics, tips to facilitate the access, to clean the root canal and to carry out retreatments are available.

The industry offers the clinician optimal possibilities to achieve retrograde fillings more difficult or even impossible to carry out with other techniques. Among the latest applications, new possibilities emerge to effectuate certain surgical treatments, sinus lift procedures, implants placement, removal of fillings and crowns and other clinical situations.

Taking into account the great advance in US technology during the last years, it is reasonable to anticipate a great future for these devices. We are commited to regularly revisit the literature in order to know new opportunities provided by technology so the most suitable device is used in each clinical situation.

Author details

Ana Isabel García-Kass, Juan Antonio García-Núñez[*] and Victoriano Serrano-Cuenca

*Address all correspondence to: garcinu@odon.ucm.es

Department of Stomatology III, School of Dentistry, Complutense University of Madrid, Madrid, Spain

References

[1] Curie J, Curie P. Dévélopements par presión de l'électricité polaire dans les cristaux hémièdres à faces inclinées. In: Editeurs G-V, ed. Compte rendu hebdomadaire des séances de l'Académie des Sciences. Paris, 1880.

[2] American Association of endodontist Glossary, 6° Ed Chicago, 1998.

[3] Lindhe J, Nyman S. Long-term maintenance of patients treated for advanced perio-dontal disease. J Clin Periodontol 1984: 11: 504-514.

[4] Becker W, Berg L, Becker B. Untreated periodontal disease: a longitudinal study. J Periodontol 1979: 50: 234-244.

[5]   Ramfjord S, Knowles J, Nissle R, Shick R, Burgett F. Longitudinal study of periodontal therapy. J Periodontol 1973: 44: 66-77.

[6]   Knowles J, Burgett F, Nissle R, Shick R, Morrison E, Ramfjord S. Results of periodontal treatment related to pocket depth and attachment level. Eight years. J Periodontol 1979: 50:225-33.

[7]   Ramfjord S, Caffesse R, Morrison E, et al. 4 modalities of periodontal treatment compared over 5 years. J Clin Periodontol 1987: 14: 445-452.

[8]   Rateitschak-Pluss E, Schwarz J, Guggenheim R, Duggelin M, Rateitschak K. Non-surgical periodontal treatment: where are the limits? An SEM study. J Clin Periodontol 1992: 19: 240-244.

[9]   Matia J, Bissada N, Maybury J, Ricchetti P. Efficiency of scaling of the molar furcation area with and without surgical access. Int J Periodontics Restorative Dent 1986: 6: 24-35.

[10] Bascones-Martínez A, García-Núñez J, Herrera I, et al. MEB en superficies dentarias tratadas con diferentes aparatos de limpieza. Prof Dental 1983: 11: 5-12.

[11] García-Núñez J, Ramos-Navarro J, Cerero-Lapiedra R, Esparza-Gómez G. Resultado de las técnicas de profilaxis a la luz de la MEB. Av Odontoestomatol 1986: 7: 83-86.

[12] Drisko C. Scaling and root planing without overinstrumentation: hand versus power-driven scalers. Curr Opin Periodontol 1993: 78-88.

[13] Drisko C. Root instrumentation. Power-driven versus manual scalers, which one? Dent Clin North Am 1998: 42: 229-244.

[14] Drisko C, Cochran D, Blieden T, et al. Position paper: sonic and ultrasonic scalers in periodontics. Research, Science and Therapy Committee of the American Academy of Periodontology. J Periodontol 2000: 71: 1792-1801.

[15] Kocher T, Langenbeck M, Rühling A, Plagmann H. Subgingival polishing with a teflon-coated sonic scaler insert in comparison to conventional instruments as assessed on extracted teeth. (I) Residual deposits. J Clin Periodontol 2000: 27: 243-249.

[16] Kawashima H, Sato S, Kishida M, Ito K. A comparison of root surface instrumentation using two piezoelectric ultrasonic scalers and a hand scaler in vivo. J Periodontal Res 2007: 42: 90-95.

[17] Clark S. The ultrasonic dental unit: a guide for the clinical application of ultrasonics in dentistry and in dental hygiene. J Periodontol 1969: 40: 621-629.

[18] Fox S, Moriarty J, Kusy R. The effects of scaling a titanium implant surface with metal and plastic instruments: an in vitro study. J Periodontol 1990: 61: 485-490.

[19] Kawashima H, Sato S, Kishida M, Yagi H, Matsumoto K, Ito K. Treatment of titanium dental implants with three piezoelectric ultrasonic scalers: an in vivo study. J Periodontol 2007: 78: 1689-1694.

[20] Richman R. The use of ultrasonics in root canal therapy and root resection. Med Dent J 1957: 12: 12-18.

[21] Martin H, Cunningham W, Norris J, Cotton W. Ultrasonic versus hand filing of dentin: a quantitative study. Oral Surg Oral Med Oral Pathol 1980: 49: 79-81.

[22] Walmsley A. Ultrasound and root canal treatment: the need for scientific evaluation. Int Endod J 1987: 20: 105-111.

[23] Walmsley A, Williams A. Effects of constraint on the oscillatory pattern of endosonic files. J Endod 1989: 15: 189-194.

[24] Lumley P, Walmsley A, Laird W. Streaming patterns produced around endosonic files. Int Endod J 1991: 24: 290-297.

[25] Cunningham W, Martin H. A scanning electron microscope evaluation of root canal debridement with the endosonic ultrasonic synergistic system. Oral Surg 1982: 53: 527-531.

[26] Cunningham W, Martin H. Endosonics-the ultrasonic synergistic system of endodontics. Endod Dent Traumatol 1985: 1: 201-206.

[27] Stamos D, Sadeghi E, Haasch G, Gerstein H. An in vitro comparison study to quantitate the debridement ability of hand, sonic, and ultrasonic instrumentation. J Endod 1987: 13: 434-440.

[28] Lev R, Reader A, Beck M, Meyers W. An in vitro comparison of the step-back technique versus a step-back/ultrasonic technique for 1 and 3 minutes. J Endod 1987: 13: 523-530.

[29] Archer R, Reader A, Nist R, Beck M, Meyers W. An in vivo evaluation of the efficacy of ultrasound after step-back preparation in mandibular molars. J Endod 1992: 18: 549-552.

[30] Reynolds W, Madison S, Walton R, Krell K, Rittman B. An in vitro histological comparison of the step-back, sonic, and ultrasonic instrumentation techniques in small, curved root canals. J Endod 1987: 13: 307-314.

[31] Goldman M, White R, Moser C, Tanca J. A comparison of three methods of cleaning and shaping the root canal in vitro. J Endod 1988: 14: 7-12.

[32] Baker M, Ashrafi S, Van Cura J, Remeikis N. Ultrasonic compared with hand instrumentation: a scanning electron microscope study. J Endod 1988: 14: 435-440.

[33] Pugh R, Goerig A, Glaser C, Luciano W. A comparison of four endodontic vibratory systems. Gen Dent 1989: 37: 296-301.

[34] Walker T, del Río C. Histological evaluation of ultrasonic and sonic instrumentation of curved root canals. J Endod 1989: 15: 49-59.

[35] Ahmad M, Pitt Ford T, Crum L. Ultrasonic debridement of root canals: acoustic streaming and its possible role. J Endod 1987: 13: 490-499.

[36] Goodman A, Reader A, Beck M, Melfi R, Meyers W. An in vitro comparison of the efficacy of the step-back technique versus a step-back/ultrasonic technique in human mandibular molars. J Endod 1985: 11: 249-256.

[37] Ruddle C. Endodontic disinfection: tsunami irrigation. Endo Prac 2008: 2008: 7-16.

[38] Lumley P, Walmsley A, Walton R, Rippin J. Effect of precurving endosonic files on the amount of debris and smear layer remaining in curved root canals. J Endod 1992: 18: 616-619.

[39] Zehnder M. Root canal irrigants. J Endod 2006: 32: 389-398.

[40] Weller R, Brady J, Bernier W. Efficacy of ultrasonic cleaning. J Endod 1980: 6: 740-743.

[41] Krell K, Johnson R, Madison S. Irrigation patterns during ultrasonic canal instrumentation. Part I. K-type files. J Endod 1988: 14: 65-68.

[42] van der Sluis L, Gambarini G, Wu M, Wesselink P. The influence of volume, type of irrigant and flushing method on removing artificially placed dentine debris from the apical root canal during passive ultrasonic irrigation. Int Endod J 2006: 39: 472-476.

[43] Jensen S, Walker T, Hutter J, Nicoll B. Comparison of the cleaning efficacy of passive sonic activation and passive ultrasonic activation after hand instrumentation in molar root canals J Endod 1999: 25: 735-738.

[44] Mozo S, Llena C, Chieffi N, Forner L, Ferrari M. Effectiveness of passive ultrasonic irrigation in improving elimination of smear layer and opening dentinal tubules. J Clin Exp Dent 2014: 6: 47-52.

[45] Martí-Bowen E, Peñarrocha-Diago M, García-Mira B. Periapical surgery using the ultrasound technique and silver amalgam retrograde filling. A study of 71 teeth with 100 canals. Med Oral Patol Oral Cir Bucal 2005: 10: 67-73.

[46] van der Sluis L, Cristescu R. Ultraschall in der Endodontie. Die Quintessenz 2009: 60: 1281-1292.

Panoramic Radiography — Diagnosis of Relevant Structures That Might Compromise Oral and General Health of the Patient

Ticiana Sidorenko de Oliveira Capote,
Marcela de Almeida Gonçalves,
Andrea Gonçalves and Marcelo Gonçalves

1. Introduction

The chapter provides information about panoramic radiography, showing the principal indications, advantages and disadvantages of this examination. Moreover, focus is given to some anatomical variations that can be detected on panoramic radiographs such as bifid mandibular canal, retromolar canal, and alterations such as calcified stylohyoid complex, arterial calcifications, phleboliths, sialolithiasis and tonsilloliths. Such structures/alterations are not reasons for indication of panoramic radiography, but they are radiographic findings, being important their identification, indication of more accurate examinations, and even referring to other professionals. Therefore, a literature review was conducted, citing relevant anatomy textbooks and scientific papers, and it was illustrated with panoramic radiographs showing these described structures/alterations.

2. Indications and contraindications of panoramic radiographs

Panoramic radiography is a radiologic technique that provides an overview of the jaws and surrounding structures. It is frequently indicated when professionals want to evaluate some structures such as unerupted third molars, orthodontic treatment, tooth development, developmental abnormalities, trauma, large lesions, and others [1, 2]. The panoramic radiograph allows the dental professional to view a large area of the maxilla and mandible on a single film [2].

The panoramic radiography is frequently used as initial diagnostic image of some alterations and based on it, the professional will verify the need of other more detailed and more accurate examinations [1].

If you have a full-mouth series, the panoramic radiography shows no more or little useful information for a patient receiving general dental care [1].

Some contraindications of panoramic radiographs are clinical situations that require detail and definition, such as carious lesions, visualization of alveolar crests, level of root canal filling [3], periodontal disease or periapical lesions [2].

In dental clinical practice, panoramic radiography is one of the most indicated radiographic examinations by dentists because it provides a general overview of dentomaxilomandibular structures and it is not so costly for patients.

3. Advantages and disadvantages of panoramic radiography

Panoramic radiography has many advantages including short time for the procedure, greater patient acceptance and cooperation, overall coverage of the dental arches and associated structures (more anatomic structures can be viewed on a panoramic film than on a complete intraoral radiograph series), simplicity, low patient radiation dose [2, 4]. The dose to the patient is approximately ten times less than full-mouth survey using the long cone and E+ film and it is four times less than four bitewings using the long round cone and E+ film [4].

The panoramic radiograph is less confusing to the patient than a series of small separate intraoral radiographs, making it easier for the dentist to explain the diagnosis and treatment plan to the patient [5].

The panoramic radiograph is an excellent imaging modality in patients with trismus or trauma, because such patients cannot open their mouths and this is not needed to take a panoramic film [4]. It is an excellent projection of diverse structures on a single film, which no other imaging system can achieve. Individual structures may be imaged by other methods, once pathologic conditions have been detected using the panoramic radiography [3, 4].

Nevertheless, this radiographic examination presents a lack of details and resolution of some structures due to overlapping of anatomical structures in the image, mild distortion and magnification [1, 3]. Objects of interest that are located outside the focal trough (it is the area of the dental anatomy that is reproduced distinctly on the panoramic radiograph) [5] are not seen [2], and artifacts are commom and may easily be misterpreted [5].

These features limit the indications of panoramic radiographs in cases where details and accurate measurements are needed [1, 3].

4. Anatomical variations observed on panoramic radiographs

The term "normal" in Anatomy refers to the shape and position most frequently found in individuals, that is, the typical shape. Anatomical variation is the deviation from the normal that does not bring any noticeable functional disorder [6].

Not very unusual, the bifid mandibular canals are observed on panoramic radiographs (Figure 1).

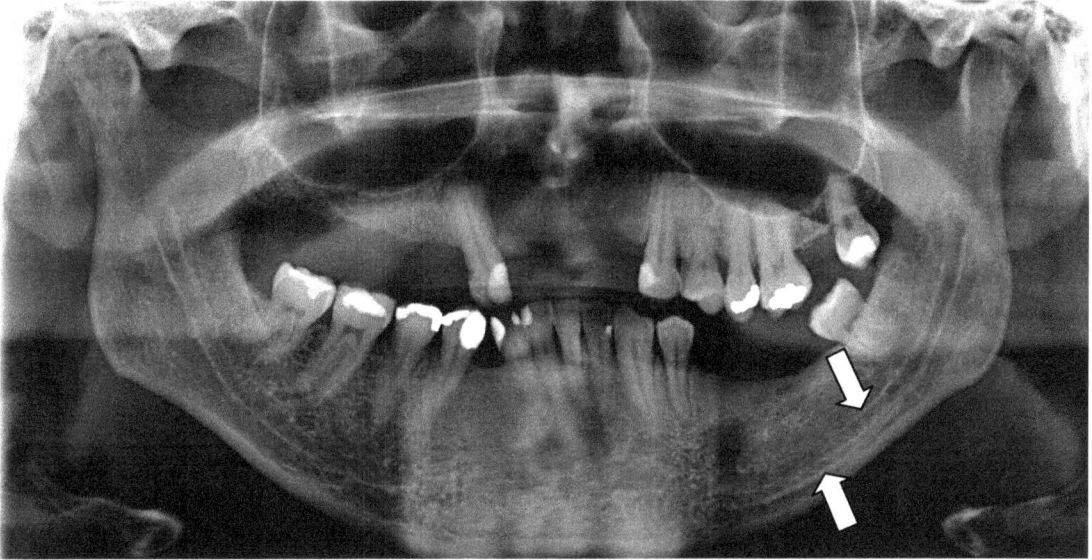

Figure 1. Digital panoramic radiography with a bifid mandibular canal image on the left side.

There are different frequencies and shapes in the literature.

Only 4 panoramic radiographs (0.08%) from 5,000 were highly suggestive of bifurcation [7]. Seven cases (0.35%) from 2,012 radiographs presented a suggestive image of a double mandibular canal [8]. From 700 panoramic radiographs evaluation, 3 cases (0.43%) showed bifid mandibular canal [9]. Duplication or division of the mandibular canal was found in 33 individuals (0.9%) from the 3,612 evaluated panoramic radiographs [10]. It is important to observe the presence of bifid mandibular canals to prevent potential complications during surgical dental procedures. A total of 6,000 panoramic radiographs were studied, and there were 57 bifid mandibular canals (0.95%) [11].

Three main patterns of duplication were found radiographically [10]. The first variety (Type 1) consisted of two canals originating from one foramen. The second variety of duplication or division (Type 2) was produced by a short upper canal extending to the second molar or third molar teeth. Type 3 was seen as two mandibular canals of equal dimensions apparently arising from separate foramina in the mandibular ramus and joining together to form one canal in the molar region of the body of the mandible. Other variations (Type 4) included duplication or division of the canal, apparent partial or complete absence of the canal or lack of symmetry.

The most common supplemental mandibular canals are duplicate canals commencing from a single mandibular foramen and the least common arising from two distinctly separate foramina [10]. A different classification was used by reference [9], which verified that type III (the canal is located close to the lower border of the mandible) is the most common, followed by the type II (the canal is noted between the apices of the first and second molars and the lower border of the mandible) and the type I (the canal is in close contact with the apices of the first and the second molars).

No great difference in frequency between males and females was found by reference [10] and there was no statistical significance between sex and types of the mandibular canal in the study of reference [9]. Women presented more bifid mandibular canals than men (63.5% vs. 36.5%) [8].

When bifid mandibular canals were evaluated by cone beam computed tomography (CBCT), a higher frequency was found. An incidence of 15.6% from 301 mandible sides was observed by [12] and, in a recent study an incidence of 10.2% was found in CBCT of 1933 patients [13]. However, different results were found by reference [8]. In their study, computed axial tomography was used in 3 of the 7 cases with apparent double inferior alveolar nerve images on panoramic radiographs. The existence of a bifid canal could only be confirmed in 2 of these patients. The authors suggested that the true incidence of bifid mandibular canals might be lower than reported by other studies. The possible causes underlying a false double-canal radiograph may include the imprint of the mylohyoid nerve on the internal mandibular surface where it separates from the inferior alveolar nerve and travels to the floor of the mouth [8, 14, 15]. Another explanation could be the radiologic osteocondensation image produced by the insertion of the mylohyoid muscle into the internal mandibular surface, with a distribution parallel to the dental canal [8, 16].

Bifurcation of the mandibular nerve may be a cause of inadequate anesthesia in a small percentage of cases [7, 8]. One of the seven patients who presented bifid mandibular canals on panoramic radiographs commented that her dentist had experienced problems in performing inferior alveolar nerve block in the past. Another patient had no such problems, and the remaining five patients had either never undergone anesthesia or remembered no associated problems [8]. This problem is usually resolved by performing inferior alveolar nerve anesthesia at a somewhat higher level (the so-called "Gow-Gates" technique) [8, 17]. Other possible complications can occur during surgery of the lower third molar, in orthognathic or reconstructive mandibular surgery, and in the placement of dental implants [8, 18], because of possible damage to an unidentified second mandibular canal [8].

Another anatomical variation that can be observed on panoramic radiographs is the retromolar canal, and it can be considered a type of mandibular canal division.

Retromolar canal has been observed in dry mandibles, cadaveric dissections, panoramic radiographs and cone beam computed tomography. Variability in the prevalence of the retromolar canal is also verified in different studies, 1.7% [19], 12.19% [20], 12.9% [21], 14.08% [22], 17% [23], 18% [24], 21.9% [25], 25% [26], 26.58% [27] (studies with dry mandibles); 5.8% [28], 16.8% [29] (studies with panoramic radiography); 16% [30], 75.4% in individuals assessed by tomography exams, 72% in cadavers [31], 52.5% [13], 75.4% [32] (studies with computed tomography).

In the retromolar canals there were found striated muscle fibers, myelinated nerve fibers and blood vessels [26]. In the retromolar canal an artery was found, being the branch of the inferior alveolar artery, and the existing nerve derived from the inferior alveolar nerve and went to the third-molar region, the retromolar triangle mucosa, the buccal mucosa, the vestibular gingiva of the premolar region and inferior molars [33]. Accessory canals in the retromolar region are functionally important in providing the neural and/or vascular components of the mandible [34]. Figure 2 shows one retromolar canal bilaterally.

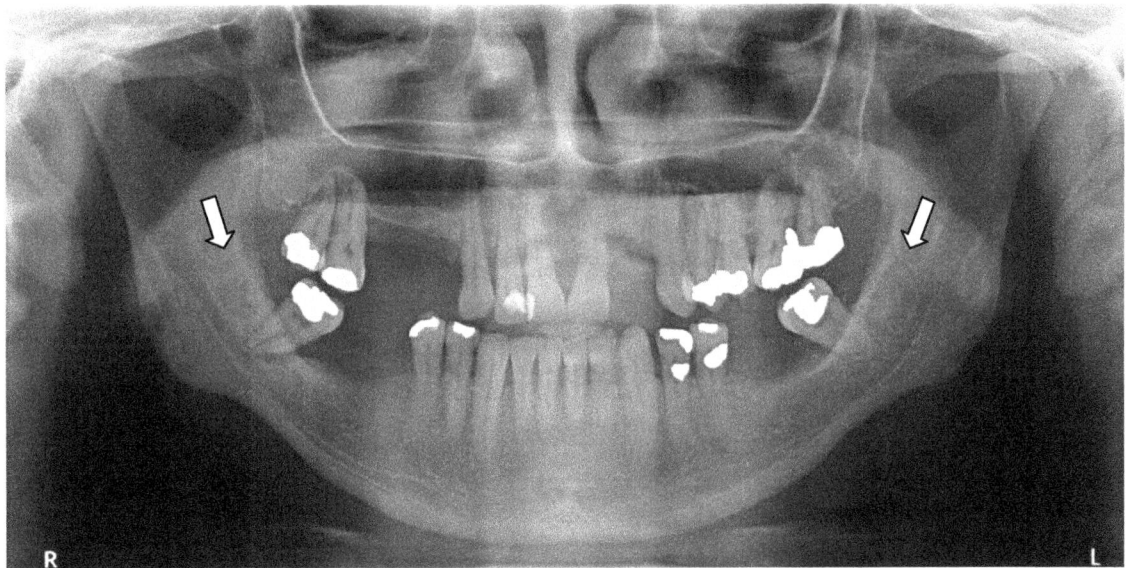

Figure 2. Digital panoramic radiography presenting a retromolar canal image on both sides.

Therefore, the content of the mandibular retromolar canal, usually of nerve fibers and/or blood vessels, is very important for surgical and anesthetic procedures involving the retromolar area. The confirmation of retromolar foramen and canal locations prior to surgical procedures, such as extraction of an impacted molar and bone harvesting as a donor site for bone graft surgery [35]. Complications such as traumatic neuroma, paraesthesia, and bleeding could arise because of failure to recognize the presence of mandibular canal variation [36, 37].

Studies have demonstrated the advantage of computed tomography over panoramic radiography in identification of anatomical variations [30, 36, 38].

It is clinically significant to accurately localize a bifid mandibular canal before dentoalveolar surgery especially when their presence is suspected by panoramic radiography [39]. Therefore, when professionals have suspicious of accessory mandibular canals on panoramic radiography, computed tomography should be done to confirm them and avoid complications.

5. Alterations observed on panoramic radiographs that might compromise oral and general health

Due to the broad coverage of panoramic radiographs, sometimes we can visualize some structures that affect more than the patient's oral health, but also general health. Many changes are asymptomatic and can be identified casually, as when the panoramic radiography is required for dental evaluation.

Among them, there are the calcified stylohyoid complex, arterial calcifications and other soft tissue calcifications.

5.1. Calcified stylohyoid complex

The styloid process is a cylindrical bone originated on the temporal bone [40-44] in front of the stylomastoid foramen [41-43], being located between the internal and external carotid arteries and laterally to the tonsillar fossa [43, 45, 46].

According to reference [47], elongated styloid process defines a styloid process that is longer than normal and thus associated with calcification of the process and its ligament, but some authors preferred the term calcified stylohyoid complex to describe the elongated process with advanced calcification [47].

The stylohyoid ligament is attached to the lesser horn of the hyoid bone [43, 48] and the calcification of the stylohyoid complex includes the stylohyoid ligament which connects the styloid process to the lesser horn of the hyoid bone [43].

The etiology of elongated styloid process is unknown [40, 43-45, 49, 50]. It was suggested that calcified styloihyoid complex could be resulted from local chronic irritations, history of trauma, endocrine disorders in female at menopause, persistence of mesenchymal elements, bone tissue growth and mechanical stress or trauma during stylohyoid ligament development [40, 43, 45, 46, 49], although no significant difference between females at menopause or not were showed [43]. A case report of twins suggested a possibility that calcified stylohyoid complex might be originated from genetic factors [44].

Only one report commented about the positive correlation that was found between the length of the styloid process and serum calcium concentration, heel bone density and body height and weight [47]. Previous studies reported difference in age for calcified stylohyoid ligament [51], i.e., the length increased with the age [41-43, 52], and its occurrence is rare in children [46]. Thus, dentists should pay attention not only for pathosis of the teeth and jaws, but also for information on general health conditions [47].

The measurements of the calcified stylohyoid complex on the panoramic radiography consist on the distance from the point where the styloid process left the tympanic plate to the tip of the process, involving mineralized parts of the ligament [42, 47, 50].

The literature reports that calcified styloid process is considered normal when it does not extend below the mandibular foramen. It is considered elongated when it extends below the mandibular foramen [51]. Finally, calcification of the stylohyoid ligament occurs when the calcification extends below the mandibular foramen and does not appear to be continuous with the base of the skull [51]. Figure 3 presents a panoramic radiography showing a calcified stylohyoid complex on both sides.

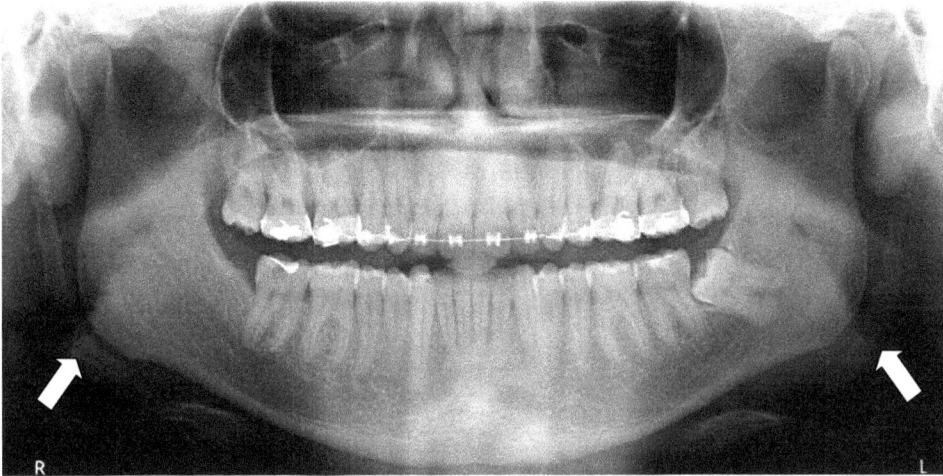

Figure 3. Digital panoramic radiography with a calcified stylohyoid complex on both sides. On the right side we can observe the stylohyoid ligament calcification near the hyoid bone. On the left side a fragmented stylohyoid ligament calcification can be seen.

Cervicalpharyngeal pain is classified into 3 entities: Eagle syndrome, stylohyoid syndrome and pseudostylohyoid syndrome [46]. Eagle's syndrome comprises elongated styloid process when it causes clinical symptoms, including dysphagia, foreign body sensation [45, 46, 48, 50, 53, 54], odynophagia, hypersalivation, and more rarely, temporary voice changes [53]. Eagle syndrome needs a history of trauma or neck surgery and painful symptoms on clinical palpation of the elongation or ossification of the stylohyoid process complex [46]. It may also cause stroke when compresses carotid arteries [40].

Stylohyoid syndrome does not comprise a history of trauma or surgery [46], and it occurs due to the compression of the internal and external carotid arteries and vascular structures [43, 53], resulting in a persistent pain to the carotid region, as headache, chronic neck pain, pain upon head movement and pain radiating to the eye [53]. It also shows radiographic elongation or ossification of the stylohyoid process complex [46] and it affects patients older than 40 years [46, 48]. This condition is more prevalent than Eagle syndrome [48].

In pseudostylohyoid syndrome there is no evidence of any elongation or ossification, but the patient describes the symptoms [46].

In Eagle syndrome, the styloid process is longer than 25mm [46]; from 25mm to 30mm it is considered elongated [42], although it varies in length in different people and even on the two sides of the same person [41, 42]. There is a significant prevalence for men concerning the styloid process length [42, 47]. However, there was no difference between sexes on the pattern distribution of calcified stylohyoid complex [43, 47, 51, 52]. The calcified stylohyoid complex bilaterally is prevalent [1, 41-43, 49, 52].

Radiographic imaging may include panoramic radiography, lateral cephalometry, Towne projection film, or computed tomogragphy (CT) scan [42, 43, 45, 46, 48, 53].

Calcified stylohyoid complex is usually visualized on panoramic radiography [1, 40, 51] as an incidental finding [49], as a long, thin, radiopaque process that is thicker at its base, posteriorly to the external acoustic meatus, with a trajectory downward and forward [1, 46]. A thicker calcified stylohyoid complex is uncommon. Figure 4 presents a very thick calcified stylohyoid complex.

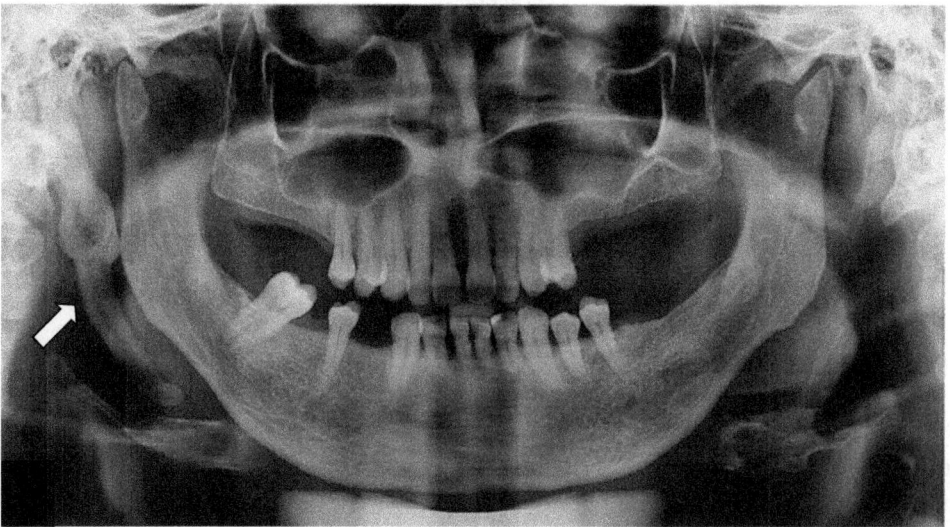

Figure 4. Digital panoramic radiography shows a thick calcified stylohyoid complex on the right side.

Panoramic radiography is the best imaging modality to visualize the styloid process bilaterally [42, 45] in patients with or without symptoms, and helps avoid misinterpretation of symptoms as tonsillar pain or dental pain, pharyngeal or muscular origin [42]. Panoramic radiography may be the first choice as imaging modality, because of its availability, low cost, diagnostic performance, and less patient dose compared to other imaging methods [43]. Nevertheless, panoramic radiography is not appropriate for measuring the length, and to show direction and anatomical variation of calcified stylohyoid complex compared to the multislice computed tomography [40, 46, 48, 54] and cone beam computed tomography do [43].

Data from clinical history, physical and radiographic examination must be considered when diagnosing Eagle's syndrome [46, 47, 54]. In the physical examination the calcified stylohyoid complex can be palpated on the tonsillar fossa as a hard and pointed structure [45, 49, 54].

The differentiation diagnosis of styloid ligament calcification may include calcified carotid artery atheromas, pheboliths and lymph node calcification [47] and for symptomatic elongated styloid process may comprise temporomandibular joint disorder, glossopharyngeal and trigeminal neuralgias, temporal arteritis, migraine, myofacial pain, atypical odontalgia, sialadenitis, sialolithiasis, cervical arthritis and tumors [46, 49], pain secondary to unerupted or impacted third molars, histaminic headache [46].

Most patients with calcified stylohyoid complex are asymptomatic [1, 44, 52] and no treatment is required [1]. The first choice of treatment is the use of analgesics and anti-inflammatory medications [46, 49]. However, for severe symptomatic patients with Eagle's syndrome the surgical excision of the stylohyoid complex is recommended [1, 44, 46, 54]. Regardless the cervicalpharyngeal pain it is important for the dentist who is involved in the diagnosis and treatment of these syndromes to identify on the panoramic radiography the calcified stylo-hyoid complex and to refer the patient to a specialized team.

5.2. Arterial calcifications

The common carotid artery originates from the aorta artery and in the height of the upper edge of the thyroid cartilage branches into two terminal branches: internal and external carotid artery. The identification of the point of bifurcation is often located 3 cm below the lower edge of the mandible [55].

It is considered a dystrophic calcification where there are deposited calcium salts in chronically inflamed or necrotic tissues. The presence of an atheromatous plaque in the extracranial carotid vascular path is the main cause for vasculocerebral embolism and obstructive diseases [1].

Carotid artery atherosclerotic plaques develop when fatty substances, cholesterol, platelets, cellular waste products, and calcium are deposited in the lining of the artery [56]. Some risk factors for atherosclerosis are: diabetes mellitus, obesity, hypertension, smoking, inadequate diet, chronic kidney disease and menopause among others [57].

Panoramic radiographs, obtained during professional dental examinations, are a potential method for early detection of Calcified Carotid Artery Atheroma (CCAA) [58]. Patients found to have carotid calcification on panoramic radiographs should be referred for cerebrovascular and cardiovascular evaluation and aggressive management of vascular risk factors [59]. Patients who have risk factors and CCAA on panoramic radiographs have a higher chance of suffering a vascular event compared with patients without image CCAA on panoramic radiographs, indicating that the incidental finding of calcifications on a panoramic dental radiograph is a powerful marker for future adverse, nonfatal, vascular events, with cardio-vascular events being more common than cerebrovascular events [56].

The prevalence of CCAA in HIV+patients was assessed by reference [60] through review of medical records and on panoramic radiography and the authors concluded that infection and the treatment used to treat HIV infection can influence the identification of CCAA. Thus, a careful examination of panoramic radiographs in these patients is recommended and the need for further studies related to the subject is reinforced.

Authors [61] observed hypertension as the major risk factor associated with carotid artery calcification followed by diabetes mellitus and hyperlipidemia in the Thai population. A standard panoramic dental radiography detected the presence of calcified cervical carotid artery disease in approximately 31% of postmenopausal women with no history of transient ischemic attack or stroke. It was demonstrated that hypertension was a significant risk factor for the development of atheromas [62]. Other authors [63] observed that patients who had evidence of calcified carotid plaque on panoramic radiographs had lower incidence of diabetes mellitus and hyperlipidemia but were more likely to have stroke, compared with patients with negative panoramic radiography for calcification.

The utility of observing calcification will obviously depend on the prevalence and amount of calcium within these lesions, which varies according to each patient [64].

A high interobserver agreement (92.4%) on the detection of carotid artery calcification (CAC) on panoramic radiographs of male patients above 50 years old was observed by reference [65]. No significant difference in the prevalence CCA in HIV+patients using conventional and digital panoramic radiograph was found [60]. Authors [66] emphasized that digital panoramic radiograph allow low intensity calcifications to be visualized due to the possibility of changing the contrast, density and expansion.

Radiographically, calcified carotid atheroma is initially developed at the bifurcation of arteries, soft tissues of the neck, and adjacent to the greater horn of the hyoid bone and the cervical vertebrae C3 and C4 or the intervertebral space between them. They are radiopaque, usually multiple and irregularly shaped, with a vertical distribution and they have an internally heterogeneous radiopacity [1]. The shape varies from circular to mostly linear with irregular margins and appears punctate containing areas of radiolucencies [67]. Figures 5 and 6 present panoramic radiographs with images suggesting the presence of atheromas.

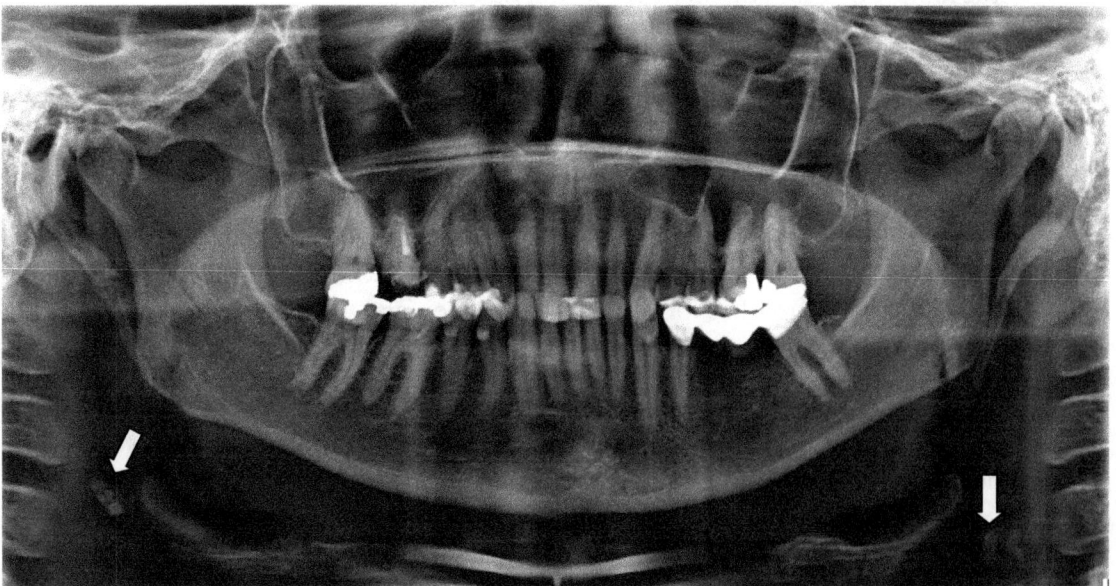

Figure 5. Digital panoramic radiography with images suggesting the presence of atheroma on both sides.

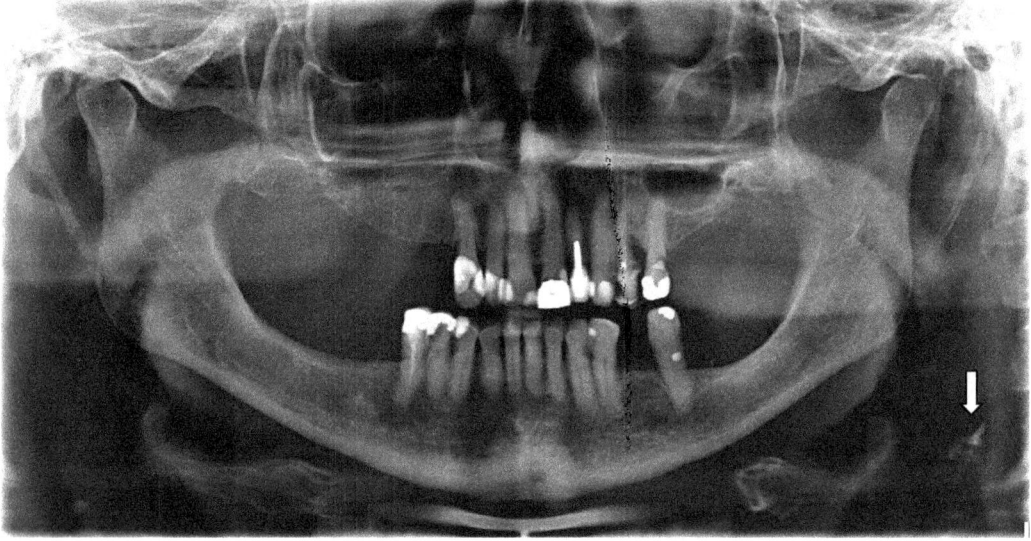

Figure 6. Digital panoramic radiography with image suggesting the presence of atheroma on left side.

Panoramic radiographs of a 67-year-old white woman were evaluated, and observed the presence of multiple, irregular, nonhomogenous radiopacities lying overboth the right and the left carotid bifurcations [64]. The calcifications were located inferior to the angle of the mandible and the tip of the hyoid bone, and to the top tip of the thyroid cartilage and the C3, C4 and C5 vertebrae [64]. Other authors [61] evaluated panoramic radiographs in 1370 patients and reported the presence of calcified carotid artery as irregular, heterogenous, vertcolinear or circular radiopaque lower to the neck at the level of the C3 and C4 intervertebral junction in the Thai population. The carotid artery calcifications were located within the soft tissues of the neck, approximately 2 centimeters inferior and posterior to the angle of the mandible, at about the level of the lower margin of the third cervical vertebra [62].

The differential diagnosis of CCAA image can be performed with several nearby anatomical structures such as the hyoid bone, styloid process, especially the thyroid cartilage and triticeous cartilage.

The triticeous cartilage often occurs in each lateral thyrohyoid ligament forming the edges of the thyrohyoid membrane [68].

The calcified triticeous cartilage can be confused with an atheromatous plaque but the shape, outline and location help in discriminating the triticeous cartilage from calcification in the carotid arteries [1, 67].

Triticeous cartilages and calcified carotid atheromas are located in a similar region on panoramic radiographs; the shape and outline help in differentiating these 2 calcifications in the neck. Triticeous cartilage is specifically located between the greater horn of the hyoid and superior horn of the thyroid cartilage, and the shape is mostly well-defined oval, with a smooth, well-defined corticated border [67]. Figure 7 shows a panoramic radiography with triticeous cartilages on both sides.

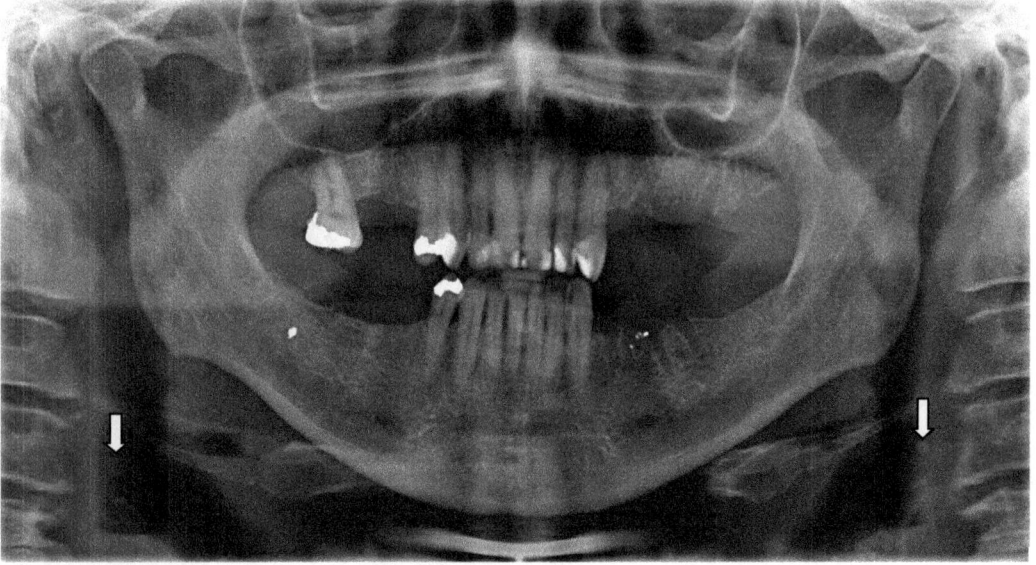

Figure 7. Digital panoramic radiography with image suggesting triticeous cartilage on both sides (between the greater horn of the hyoid and superior horn of the thyroid cartilage).

Authors [57] emphasized that although the panoramic radiography is not the test of choice, it is possible to identify atheroma in the carotid artery and therefore the dentist may instruct the patient to seek medical advice as soon as possible.

In order to confirm the presence of CACs, advanced imaging techniques such as duplex ultrasound, magnetic resonance imaging, and angiography should be performed [61].

The reliability of digital panoramic radiographs in detecting atheroma in the carotid artery was assessed [69] and the authors compared with ultrasound examinations. The results showed that digital panoramic radiography has a high level of agreement with ultrasonography with 76% of sensitivity and 98.66% of specificity. The authors concluded that the panoramic radiograph should not be routinely used in the detection of calcified carotid atheromatous plaques although when detected on a routine dental examination it is very useful.

The image of CCAA on panoramic radiograph was confirmed utilizing duplex ultra-sonography, which revealed carotid artery stenosis (CAS) [64]. The authors suggested that calcifications seen lying over the carotid bifurcation on panoramic radiographs should prompt further evaluation for CAS.

The dystrophic calcification of the tunica intima resulting in CCAA can be distinguished radiographically from another calcified form of arteriosclerosis, medial artery arteriosclerosis (MAA) or Mönckeberg's medial calcific sclerosis. The calcification in MAA is generalized because it affects the tunica media of medium and smaller muscular arteries. Calcifications are typically diffuse, multiple, and circumferential along the wall of the arterial vessel. MAA may be an indicator of peripheral artery disease, including diabetes mellitus or chronic kidney disease. MAA is generally observed in the limbs and rarely reported in the head and neck [70]. MAA can be identified on the panoramic radiography when the facial artery is affected.

According to reference [71], the panoramic radiography can be the first auxiliary in diagnosis for detecting facial artery calcification in patients in hemodialysis. The authors suggested that more studies should be performed, in order to determine the incidence of that alteration in those patients.

Radiographically, the calcium deposited in the arterial wall outlines the artery contour, being identified as a pair of parallel, thin radiopaque lines, or with circular aspect, depending on the evaluated view [1].

5.3. Sialolithiasis

Sialolithiasis is the most common disease of the salivary glands [72-74] characterized by obstruction of salivary secretion by a calculus, associated with swelling, pain [72, 75, 76] and infection of the affected gland [75]. More than 80% of the salivary gland calculi occurs in the submandibular gland [1, 72, 74-78] and 5%-20% in the parotid gland [72, 75-78] and rarely in the sublingual gland and the minor salivary glands (1% to 2%) [72, 75-77]. It is common in adults (1.2% of the population), with a male predominance [1, 72, 74, 76, 77], although previous investigators cited that sialolithisis occurs more frequently in white woman [73]. Children are rarely involved and sialolithiasis is more frequently in the third to the sixth decades of life [72, 74-77].

Patients with sialolithiasis may complain of moderate to intense pain when it involves the duct of a major salivary gland, particularly at mealtimes, when salivary flow is stimulated [1, 73], associated with enlargement of the gland [73].

Sialoliths are stones found within the ducts of salivary glands [1] and may be single or multiple [72, 76]. Single sialolith is more common seen [1, 79]. Figure 8 shows a panoramic radiography with a single sialolith on the right side in the submandibular gland. They measure from 1 mm to less than 1 cm [72, 74, 75]. Giant sialoliths are rare, bigger than 3.5 cm and also occur in male patients and are commonly located in the submandibular gland [74].

According to reference [74], several factors seem to be involved in the development of salivary calculi in the submandibular gland tissues such as: the submandibular excretory duct is wider in diameter and longer than the Stensen's duct; the secretion against gravity [74, 77]; the secretion is more alkaline compared with pH of the parotid saliva; the submandibular saliva contains a higher quantity of mucin proteins, while parotid saliva is entirely serous; then its saliva presents high calcium and phosphate content [73, 74, 77].

Initial events that contribute for the formation of a nidus that later will be the site for the precipitation of mineral salts contained in the salivary secretion include infection, inflammation, physical trauma, salivary stagnation, introduction of foreign bodies and the presence of desquamated ephitelial cells [73, 74].

The likely mechanism of sialolith formation in the sublingual gland is mechanical trauma with mucus extravasation, which serves as a nidus for stone formation [77]. In summary, the formation of a sialolith requires salivary stagnation, a nidus and a precipitation of salivary salts [75].

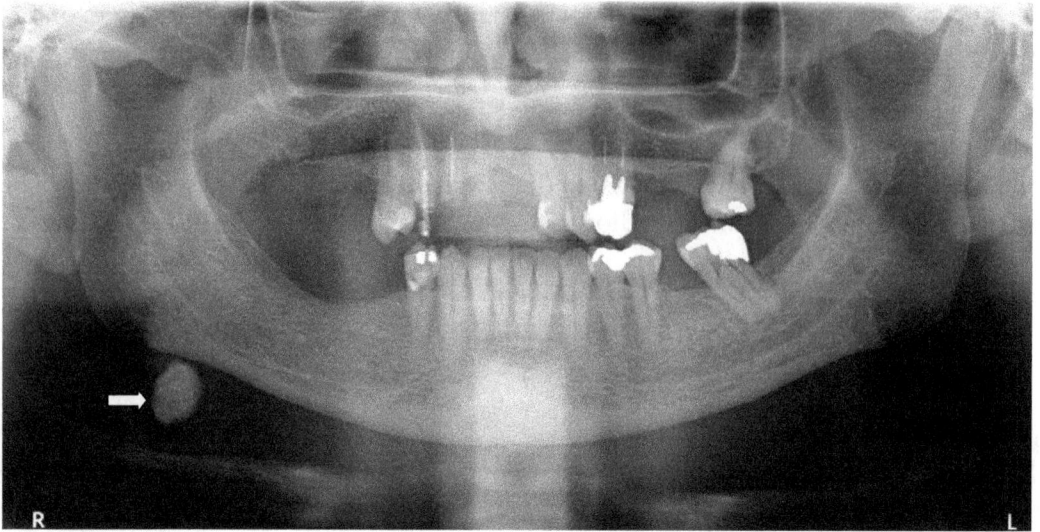

Figure 8. Digital panoramic radiography with image suggesting a single sialolith in the right submandibular gland.

Depending on the sialolith size and calcification degree, it can be visible in conventional radiographs. In panoramic radiography, the calcification image may appear superimposed on the mandible; therefore, it may be mistaken by an intrabone lesion [73]. Plain film radiography demonstrates dystrophic calcifications and the possible involvement of adjcent osseous structures [1].

Panoramic radiography usually shows sialoliths in the submandibular gland if they are located in the posterior duct [1]. If calculi can not be visualized in conventional radiographs, other imaging examinations may be necessary [73]. Sialography is used to evaluate obstructive and inflammatory conditions of the ductal system. If the patient is allergic to the iodine contrast agent used in sialography, the alternative imaging examination is ultrasonography or scintilography [1].

Computed tomography or magnetic resonance imaging are appropriate if the sialography suggests the presence of a space-occupying mass [1]. According to previous investigation, panoramic radiography and CT scan estimation appeared to be somewhat closer to the surgical specimen size [75].

Sialoliths in the sublingual gland are usually round or oval shaped. However, stones in Wharton's duct may be elongated. Parotid stones are usually smaller and more often multiple [77]. A single mass of calcification of the parotid gland with a calcification of part of its duct can be seen in the Figure 9.

Giant sublingual sialolith was previous described as a large single calcified mass in sublingual area on panoramic radiography. Giant sublingual sialolith has already been associated with dysphagia as well as eating and speaking difficulty [76]

Sialolith is usually homogeneously radiopaque, although it can show evidence of multiple layers of calcification if large [1, 79]. Salivary stones are usually shaped by the duct and then

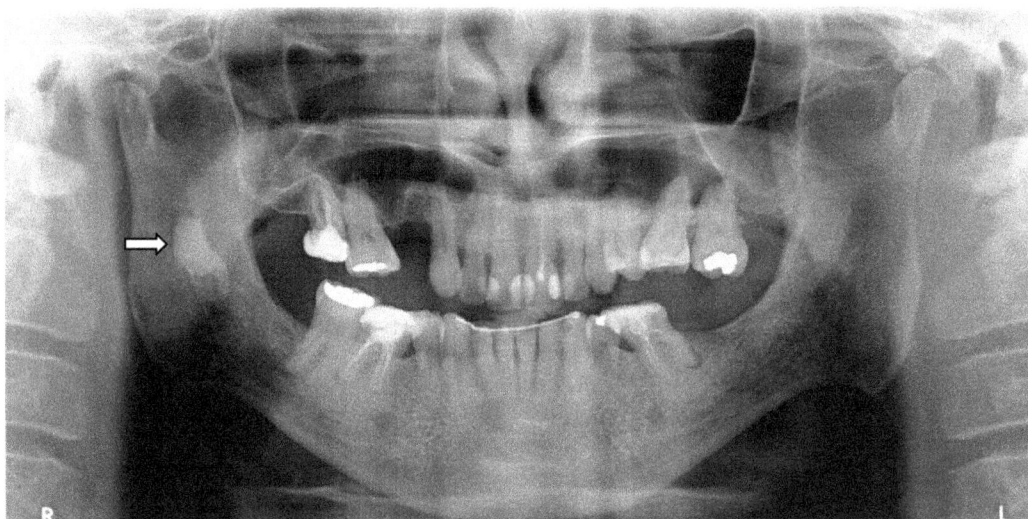

Figure 9. Digital panoramic radiography showing a image suggesting a calcification in the right parotid gland and in its duct.

they are elongated [77, 79]. Sialoliths are more likely localized in the Wharton's duct (submandibular gland) than in the Stensen's duct (parotid gland) [79]. Figure 10 shows calcifications in the submandibular and parotid glands.

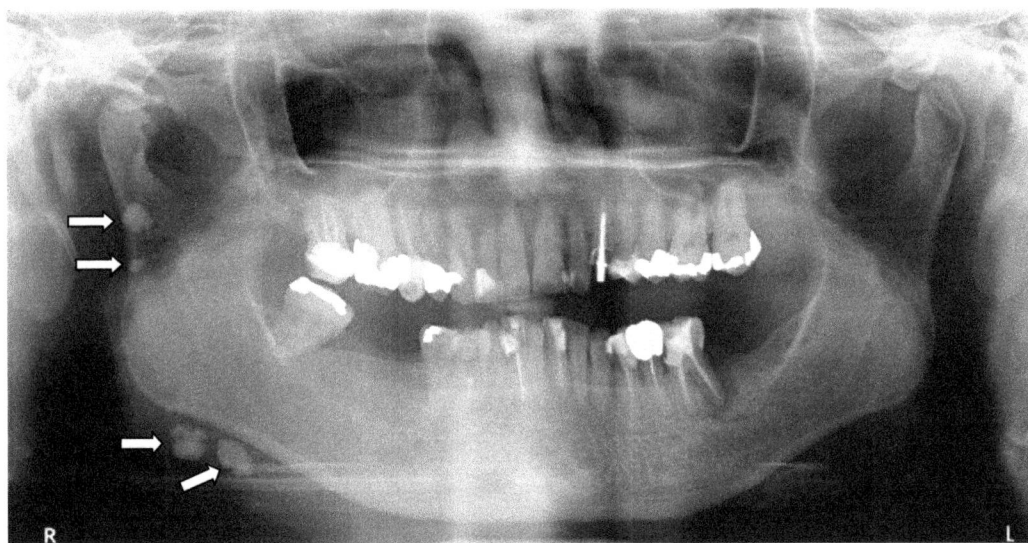

Figure 10. Digital panoramic radiography with image suggesting calcifications in the right submandibular and parotid glands.

A previous report described 3 cases with multiple microliths in their parotid parenchyma in Sjögren's syndrome showing panoramic radiography with many spots-like calcifications observed around the gonial angle and in the posterior part of the ramus [78]. According to previous publication, parotid calculi are frequently seen about halfway up on the ramus and may be multiple [80] as cited above. We can observe a panoramic radiography with multiple microliths in the parotid gland on both sides in the Figure 11.

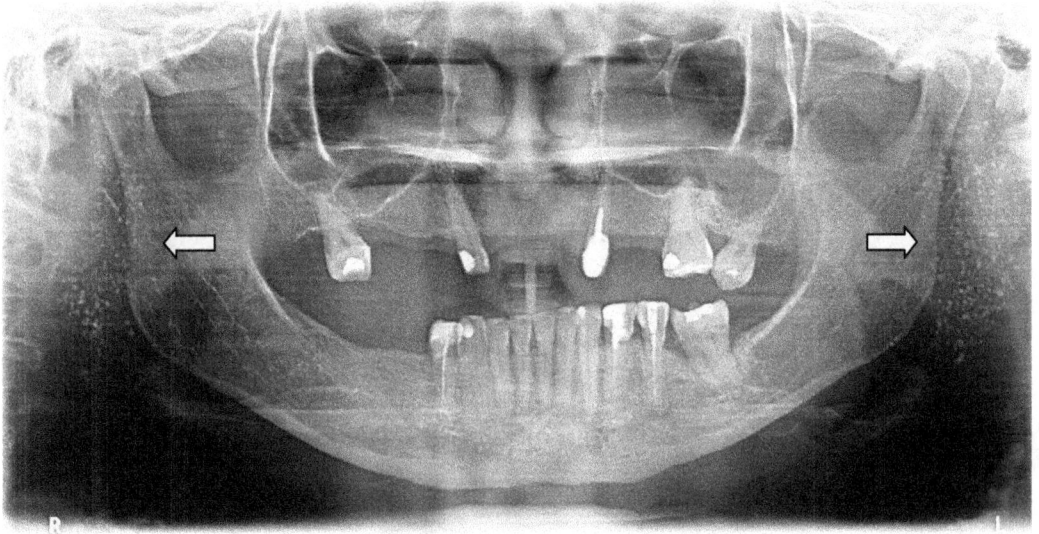

Figure 11. Digital panoramic radiography with image suggesting multiple microliths in the parotid gland on both sides.

Although this report is about panoramic radiography, previous investigations comment about cone beam computed tomography (CBCT) and reported that for visualization of the delicate structures of the parotid and submandibular salivary glands and for identification of sialoliths and single ductal strictures, CBCT sialography may be better than plain film sialography [81]. CBCT is the preferable imaging modality for salivary calculus diagnosis considering its high diagnostic-information-to-radiation-dose ratio [82] and to show the shapes of stones more clearly [75].

Vascular malformation with phleboliths must be included in the differential diagnosis of salivary gland obstruction and magnetic resonance imaging may be able to distinguish between them, but sialography is the most effective diagnostic modality to this differentiation [79].

According to [72], sialolithiasis treatment depends on the localization of the salivary calculus [72, 73]. The sialolith should be removed via a transoral sialolithotomy avoing sialadenectomy. Intraglandular sialoliths necessitate sialadenectomy [73, 75]. Solitary sialoliths usually do not recur [72].

5.4. Phleboliths

Phleboliths are idiopathic calcification (or calcinosis) that results from deposition of calcium in the normal tissue. This calcification results from deposition of calcium in the normal tissue, despite normal serum levels of calcium and phosphate [1]. Phleboliths are calcified thrombi

found within vascular channels, often in the presence of hemangiomas or vascular malformations. They may originate from injury to a vessel wall or result from stagnation of the flow of
blood [83, 84]. A case of intramuscular hemangioma was related by reference [85], where it
was observed the large number of phleboliths of the tongue due to the long-term presence of
hemangioma and stagnant blood flow. The authors [86], when reporting an intramuscular
hemangioma also suggested that the cause of the large number of phleboliths is the long-term
presence of hemangioma and stagnant blood.

The presence of vascular anomalies in the head and neck has a great importance for the
professionals working in this area, since any procedure performed in this region without the
due caution may trigger the onset of an emergency, as bleeding, which can lead to the patient's
death. Therefore, there is a need to conduct a thorough diagnosis in order to help in the
discovery of the existence of these defects, so that such situations are avoided [87]. Those
authors reviewed the charts of 108 patients with vascular anomalies and observed in 31% of
the cases that the changes were in the region of the mouth and tongue, being the period of
childhood and adolescence the most affected (64%).

Clinically, the vascular changes may have a swollen soft tissue, which is throbbing and with
its modified coloration and some noises when auscultating [1].

A case of a patient with multiple swellings on the surface and in the mouth with a purplish
coloration in intraoral examination was reported by reference [88]. Radiographic examination
showed small phleboliths in the left submandibular region, and ultrasound also showed
calcifications. Histological examination showed that the characteristics are originated from
venous malformation. Three cases of hemangioma of the head and neck varying like the clinical
characteristics presented were presented by reference [89], however some commonalities
between them could be noticed as swelling, absence of pulse or noise, and two cases showed
discoloration.

Phleboliths calcification starts in the center of the thrombus and consists of apatite crystals of
calcium phosphate and carbonate [1]. Initially, calcification of the thrombus occurs, forming
the core of the phlebolith. The fibrinous component then undergoes secondary calcification
and becomes attached. Repetition of this process causes enlargement of the phlebolith [86].

Radiographically, the phlebolith features radiopaque, rounded or oval image measuring more
than 6mm in diameter and uniform periphery. Internally, it can present a homogeneous
radiopacity, but it commonly presents a laminated appearance with a target aspect [1]. A
patient with an oral mixed mucosal and submucosal venous malformation with multiple
phleboliths, which the panoramic radiograph revealed multiple round-to-oval radiopaque
bodies located in the soft tissues of the left retromolar trigone. Those structures had a laminated
pattern and were interpreted as phleboliths [90].

A patient presented a small mass that contained calcification in the anterior part of the masseter
muscle and the plain radiograph showed a round, uniformly radiopaque lesion [91]. The same
was observed by other authors [92], who reported about a patient with a masseteric intramuscular hemangioma, which other than a mild facial asymmetry, was subjectively asymptomatic.
This diagnosis could not be reached without computed tomography (CT) scan that identified

the presence of the calcified body confirmed by the panoramic radiograph. The patient did not exhibit the lamellated feature of a phlebolith. MRI with contrast was ordered for further evaluation and diagnosis that clearly visualized an enhanced vascular lesion within the left masseter muscle, and confirmed the presence and location of the phlebolith. However, phleboliths are not easily recognized in magnetic resonance image (MRI) film because of their very low signal intensity. They are best identified on plain radiograph and CT scan. Authors [93] observed in occlusal radiograph of a patient with vascular malformation, two oval radiopaque images, diagnosed after microscopic examination as being phlebolith.

Studies about hemangiomas and venous malformations associating imaging methods have been reported in literature aiming to improve the diagnosis of these changes and the presence of phleboliths. CT was used in 3 cases that revealed phleboliths so no other imaging was considered to be necessary [89]. Phlebolith was observed on radiography and ultrasonography of paranasal sinus [88]. Plain x-rays may also help with the diagnosis because of the typical appearance of the calcified bodies and computed tomography, magnetic ressonance, and ultrasonography are more useful for making an accurate diagnosis [91]. A case of intramuscular hemangioma and another one of vascular malformation presenting phleboliths by the use of sialography and occlusal radiographs was presented by reference [84]. Occlusal radiography and Doppler ultrasonography also were used in a case of vascular malformation [93].

The radiographic image of phlebolith can be similar to a sialolith [1]. Phleboliths are usually multiple, with oval shape, randomly located and lamellated [92]. Figure 12 shows a panoramic radiography with multiple phleboliths on the right side.

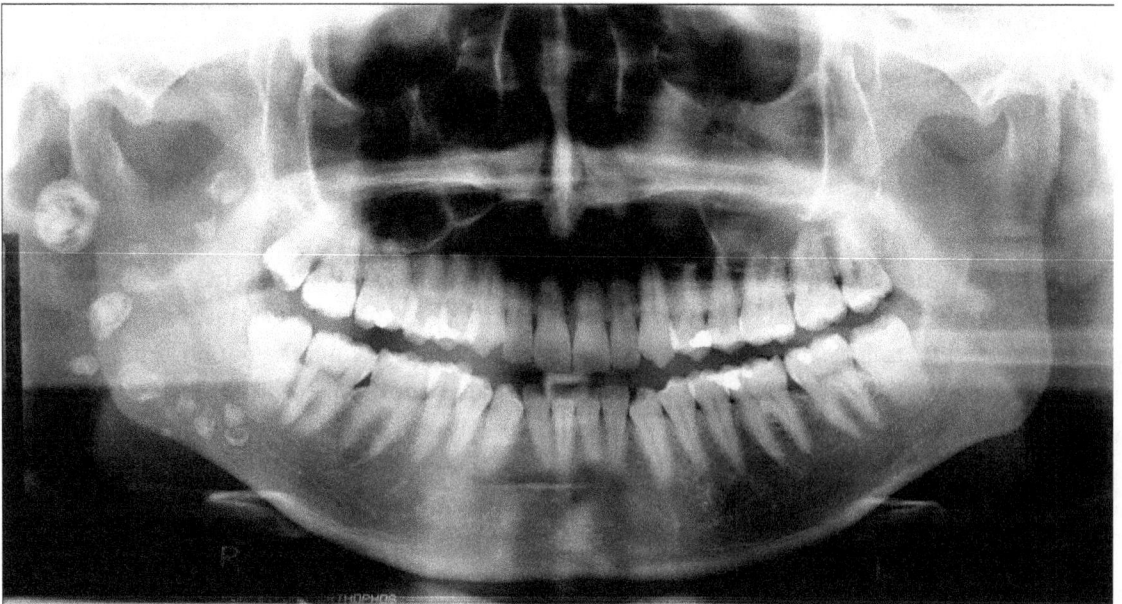

Figure 12. Panoramic radiography with image suggesting multiple phleboliths on the right side.

The sialoliths are frequently elliptically or elongated shaped due to the anatomic contour of the salivary duct [90, 92]. According to reference [90], sialography usually reveals a filling defect at the site of the salivary calculus, whereas phleboliths appear to be external to the duct system [90]. A case of recurrent episodes of pain and swelling in the right submandibular region was reported by reference [79]. Radiopaque images were identified in occlusal and panoramic radiographs, being diagnosed as sialoliths. The sialendoscopy was indicated and no intraductal stones were detected. A vascular network of capillaries was detected in all the ductal lumen altering the sialolithiasis diagnostic to a vascular malformation with phleboliths. The authors concluded that the vascular malformation obstructing the duct of the salivary gland is overlooked by physicians, and that phleboliths may be confounded with sialoliths.

5.5. Tonsilloliths

Tonsilloliths are calcifications within a tonsillar crypt, which involve primarily the palatine tonsil caused by dystrophic calcification as a result of chronic inflammation [94]. Small concretions are not uncommon findings especially in the aged population [95], however large tonsillar concretions occur with a much lower incidence [95-98].

The prevalence of tonsilloliths (measuring above 2 mm) in 1524 patients attending the oral and maxillofacial radiology clinic of The University of Iowa was observed to be 8.14% by reference [99]. The age range of subjects was 9.2–87 years (mean 52.6 years), the average size of tonsillolith was 4mm (range: 3–11 mm), with no sex predilection.

The large tonsilloliths occur in males and females equally [98, 100], and on the fifth decade of life [100]. Tonsilloliths in children are rare and they are more common in young adults with long stories of recurrent tonsillar inflammation [98, 100].

The exact etiology and pathogenesis is unknown. Repeated episodes of inflammation may produce fibrosis at the openings of the tonsillar crypts. Bacterial and epithelial debris then accumulates within these crypts and contributes to the formation of retention cysts. Calcification occurs subsequent to the deposition of inorganic salts and the enlargement of the formed concretion takes place gradually. The tonsilloliths derive their phosphate and carbonate of lime and magnesia from saliva secreted by salivary glands [94-98, 101]. The mineral content of tonsilloliths can be composed by phosphorus, calcium, carbonate or magnesium [95].

On the panoramic radiography, tonsilloliths commonly appear as multiple, small, and ill-defined radiopacities [99]. On the other hand, other authors [94] described tonsilloliths as usually being single and unilateral, but occasionally they may be multiple or bilateral. Tonsilloliths should be the first differential diagnosis when multiple opaque lesions with ill-defined borders, which are superimposed on the palatal uvula and the ramus are detected on the panoramic radiography [94]. The radiographic appearance of tonsilloliths was predominantly multiple and well defined (62.90%) and the single, well-defined tonsillolith in a similar location constituted 28.23% in the study of reference [99]. The authors verified that the majority of the cases were located in the lower one third of the mandibular ramus (93.55%). Figures 13 and 14 shows panoramic radiographs with multiple tonsilloliths in the lower one third of the mandibular ramus on both sides.

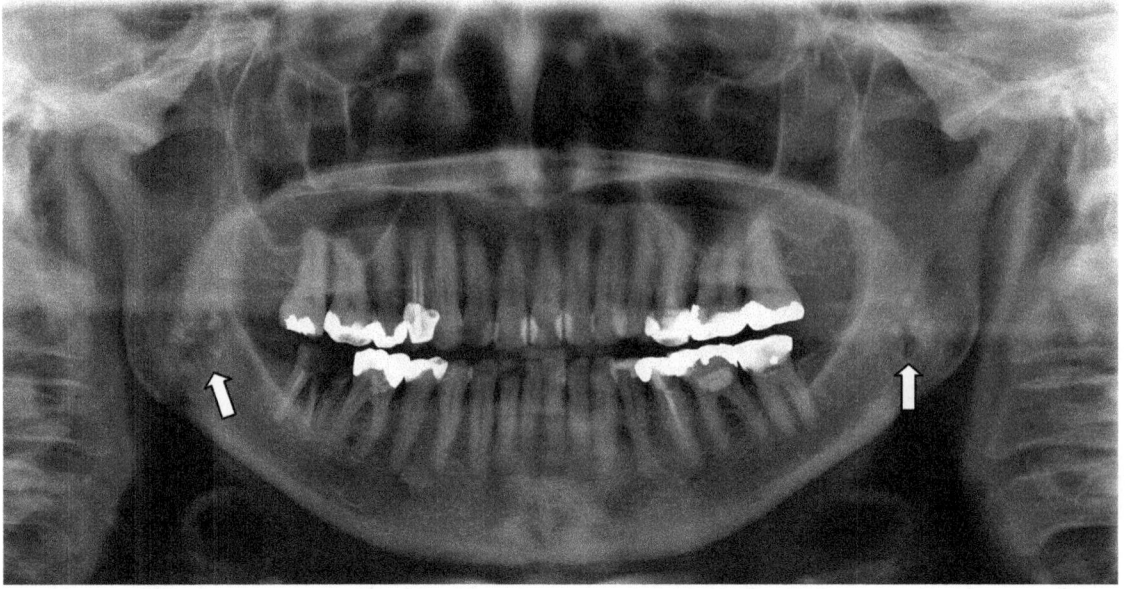

Figure 13. Digital panoramic radiography with image suggesting multiple tonsilloliths in the lower one third of the mandibular ramus on both sides.

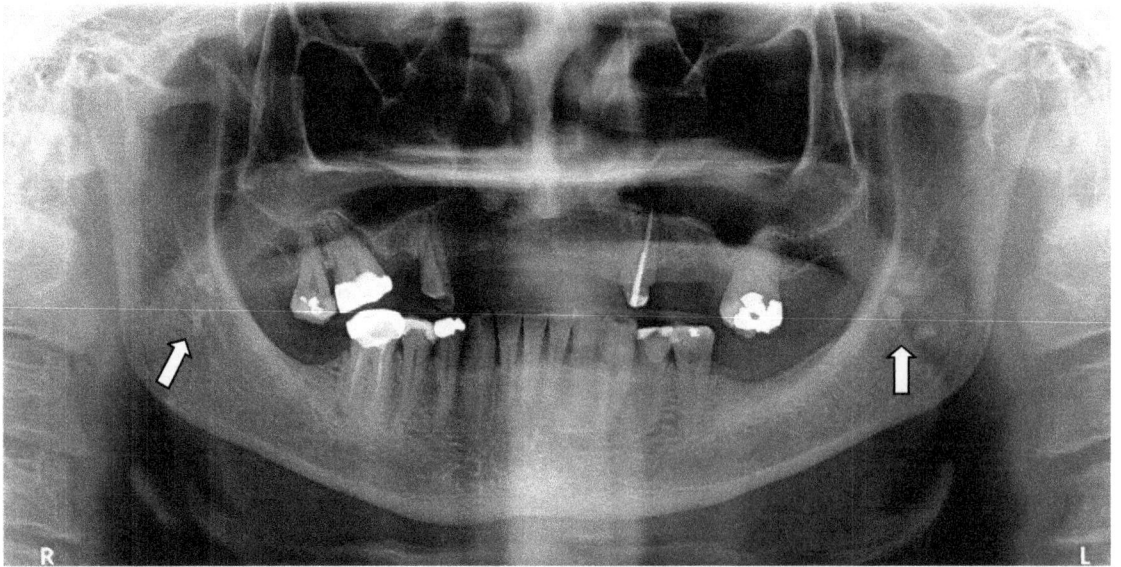

Figure 14. Digital panoramic radiography with image suggesting multiple tonsilloliths in the lower one third of the mandibular ramus on both sides.

Calcifications in the carotid arterial, lymph nodes, salivary gland and stylohyoid ligament are some of the differential diagnosis that might be considered [101].

On the clinical examination, it should be considered malignancy or calcified granulomatous disease such as tertiary syphilis, tuberculosis and deep fungal infection as differential diagnosis [98].

When no predisposing causes can be discovered (like chronic obstructive sialolithiasis of the salivary glands, past medical history of kidney stone), the medical history represents the most important element to recognise the tendency of some patients to develop calcifications, as in the case reported [96]. The observations in the study of [99] do not support any correlations between tonsilloliths and calcifications in other body organs, tissues, or ducts.

Patients with tonsilloliths may be asymptomatic probably when the calcifications have small size [101], and their lesions discovered incidentally on panoramic radiographs or they can present pain or soreness, dysphagia, halitosis, otalgia, infection, a foreign body-like sensation, irritable cough, difficulty in swallowing, bad/altered taste [94-96, 98-100].

Incidental findings of large tonsilloliths are reported using panoramic radiography [96, 98, 100]. The panoramic radiography helps to observe the location of opacities, but considering its two-dimensional limitations, a computed tomography or cone beam computed tomography scan is necessary to accurately position the calcifications [96, 100].

Treatment is usually removal of concretions by curettage and larger lesions may require local excision [96, 98, 99]. If there is evidence of chronic tonsillitis, tonsillectomy offers definitive therapy; however it is advisable to postpone tonsillectomy until all acute symptoms have subsided [98].

The diagnosis of tonsillar calculi, exploring their etiology, evaluating them for removal, and not dismissing them as clinically insignificant it is important because of the significant morbidity via chronic infection, pain, and/or swallowing abnormalities, with the potential of further pulmonary complications [95].

6. Conclusion

Panoramic radiograph is a radiological technique that provides an overview of the jaws and adjacent structures. Asymptomatic patients may show anatomical variations or alterations that may be randomly displayed on panoramic radiographs. These alterations may contribute to clinical complications and damage the patient's oral and general health. Therefore, it is of utmost importance that dentists be able to recognize the evidence of these variations and alterations on panoramic radiographs and request additional examinations that provide a more accurate diagnosis. Thus, we conclude that the panoramic radiograph, within its limitations, contributes effectively to the initial diagnosis of anatomic variations and alterations, and the dental professional can identify the risks and refer their patients to a specialist.

Author details

Ticiana Sidorenko de Oliveira Capote[1*], Marcela de Almeida Gonçalves[1],
Andrea Gonçalves[2] and Marcelo Gonçalves[2]

*Address all correspondence to: ticiana@foar.unesp.br

1 Dental School at Araraquara, Univ. Estadual Paulista, UNESP, Department of Morphology, Araraquara, São Paulo, Brazil

2 Dental School at Araraquara, Univ. Estadual Paulista, UNESP, Department of Diagnostic and Surgery, Araraquara, São Paulo, Brazil

References

[1] White SC, Pharoa MJ. Oral Radiology: Principles and Interpretation. 5th ed. Saint Louis: Mosby; 2007.

[2] Haring JI, Jansen L. Dental radiography: principles and techniques. 2nd ed. Philadelphia: Saunders; 2000. 569 p.

[3] Alvares LC, Tavano O. Curso de radiologia em odontologia. 4th ed. São Paulo, Brazil: Livraria Santos Editora Ltda; 2002. 248 p.

[4] Langland OE, Langlais RP, Preece JW. Principles of dental imaging. 2nd ed. Lippincott Williams & Wilkins; 2002. 459 p.

[5] De Lyre WR, Johnson ON. Essentials of dental radiography for dental assistants and hygienists. 4th ed. Norwalk, Conn.: Appleton & Lange; 1990. xvii, 446 p.

[6] Aumuller G. Anatomia. Rio de Janeiro: Guanabara Koogan; 2009.

[7] Grover PS, Lorton L. Bifid mandibular nerve as a possible cause of inadequate anesthesia in the mandible. Journal of oral and maxillofacial surgery : official journal of the American Association of Oral and Maxillofacial Surgeons 1983;41(3):177-179.

[8] Sanchis JM, Penarrocha M, Soler F. Bifid mandibular canal. Journal of oral and maxillofacial surgery : official journal of the American Association of Oral and Maxillofacial Surgeons 2003;61(4):422-424.

[9] Zografos J, Kolokoudias M, Papadakis E. [The types of the mandibular canal]. To Helleniko periodiko gia stomatike & gnathoprosopike cheirourgike / episemo organo tes Hetaireias Stomatognathoprosopikes Cheirourgikes. The Greek Journal of Oral & Maxillofacial Surgery 1990;5(1):17-20.

[10] Nortje CJ, Farman AG, Grotepass FW. Variations in the normal anatomy of the inferi-
or dental (mandibular) canal: a retrospective study of panoramic radiographs from
3612 routine dental patients. The British Journal of Oral Surgery 1977;15(1):55-63.

[11] Langlais RP, Broadus R, Glass BJ. Bifid mandibular canals in panoramic radiographs.
Journal of the American Dental Association 1985;110(6):923-926.

[12] Kuribayashi A, Watanabe H, Imaizumi A, Tantanapornkul W, Katakami K, Kura-
bayashi T. Bifid mandibular canals: cone beam computed tomography evaluation.
Dentomaxillofacial Radiology 2010;39(4):235-239.

[13] Kang JH, Lee KS, Oh MG, Choi HY, Lee SR, Oh SH, et al. The incidence and configu-
ration of the bifid mandibular canal in Koreans by using cone-beam computed tomography. Imaging Science in Dentistry 2014;44(1):53-60.

[14] Wilson S, Johns P, Fuller PM. The inferior alveolar and mylohyoid nerves: an anatomic study and relationship to local anesthesia of the anterior mandibular teeth.
Journal of the American Dental Association 1984;108(3):350-352.

[15] Sillanpaa M, Vuori V, Lehtinen R. The mylohyoid nerve and mandibular anesthesia.
International Journal of Oral and Maxillofacial Surgery 1988;17(3):206-207.

[16] Kiersch TA, Jordan JE. Duplication of the mandibular canal. Oral Surgery, Oral Medicine, and Oral Pathology 1973;35(1):133-134.

[17] Meechan JG. How to overcome failed local anaesthesia. British Dental Journal
1999;186(1):15-20.

[18] Quattrone G, Furlini E, Bianciotto M. [Bilateral bifid mandibular canal. Presentation
of a case]. Minerva Stomatologica 1989;38(11):1183-1185.

[19] Ossenberg NS. Temporal crest canal: case report and statistics on a rare mandibular
variant. Oral Surgery, Oral Medicine, and Oral Pathology 1986;62(1):10-12.

[20] Bilodi AKS, Singh S, Ebenezer DA, Suman P, Kumar K. A study on retromolar foramen and other accessory foramina in human mandibles of Tamil Nadu region. International Journal of Health Sciences and Research 2013;3(10):61-65.

[21] Galdámes IS, Matamala DZ, López MC. Retromolar Canal and Forame prevalence in
dried mandibles and clinical implications. International Journal of Odontostomatolo-
gy 2008;2(2):183-187.

[22] Athavale SA, Vijaywargia M, Deopujari R, Kobayashi K. Bony and cadaveric study
of retromolar region. People's Journal of Scientific Research 2013;6(2):14-18.

[23] Motta-Junior J, Ferreira ML, Matheus RA, Stabile GAV. Forame retromolar: sua re-
percussão clínica e avaliação de 35 mandíbulas secas. Revista de Odontologia da UN-
ESP 2012;41(3):164-168.

[24] Gupta S, Soni A, Singh P. Morphological study of accessory foramina in mandible and its clinical implication. Indian Journal of Oral Sciences 2013;4(1):12-16.

[25] Narayana K, Nayak UA, Ahmed WN, Bhat JB, Devaiah BA. The retromolar foramen and canal in south Indian dry mandibles. European Journal of Anatomy 2002;6(3): 141-146.

[26] Bilecenoglu B, Tuncer N. Clinical and anatomical study of retromolar foramen and canal. Journal of oral and maxillofacial surgery : official journal of the American Association of Oral and Maxillofacial Surgeons 2006;64(10):1493-1497.

[27] Rossi AC, Freire AR, Prado BG, Prado FB, Botacin PR, Caria PHF. Incidence of retromolar foramen in human mandibles: ethinic and clinical aspects. International Journal of Morphology 2012;30(3):1074-1078.

[28] von Arx T, Hanni A, Sendi P, Buser D, Bornstein MM. Radiographic study of the mandibular retromolar canal: an anatomic structure with clinical importance. Journal of Endodontics 2011;37(12):1630-1635.

[29] Muinelo-Lorenzo J, Suarez-Quintanilla JA, Fernandez-Alonso A, Marsillas-Rascado S, Suarez-Cunqueiro MM. Descriptive study of the bifid mandibular canals and retromolar foramina: cone beam CT vs panoramic radiography. Dentomaxillofacial Radiology 2014;43(5):20140090.

[30] Lizio G, Pelliccioni GA, Ghigi G, Fanelli A, Marchetti C. Radiographic assessment of the mandibular retromolar canal using cone-beam computed tomography. Acta Odontologica Scandinavica 2013;71(3-4):650-655.

[31] Schejtman R, Devoto FC, Arias NH. The origin and distribution of the elements of the human mandibular retromolar canal. Archives of Oral Biology 1967;12(11): 1261-1268.

[32] Patil S, Matsuda Y, Nakajima K, Araki K, Okano T. Retromolar canals as observed on cone-beam computed tomography: their incidence, course, and characteristics. Oral Surgery, Oral Medicine, Oral Pathology, and Oral Radiology 2013;115(5):692-699.

[33] Kodera H, Hashimoto I. [A case of mandibular retromolar canal: elements of nerves and arteries in this canal]. Kaibogaku Zasshi Journal of Anatomy 1995;70(1):23-30.

[34] Haveman CW, Tebo HG. Posterior accessory foramina of the human mandible. The Journal of Prosthetic Dentistry 1976;35(4):UNKNOWN.

[35] Kawai T, Asaumi R, Sato I, Kumazawa Y, Yosue T. Observation of the retromolar foramen and canal of the mandible: a CBCT and macroscopic study. Oral Radiology 2012;28(1):10-14.

[36] Kaufman E, Serman NJ, Wang PD. Bilateral mandibular accessory foramina and canals: a case report and review of the literature. Dentomaxillofacial Radiology 2000;29(3):170-175.

[37] Anderson LC, Kosinski TF, Mentag PJ. A review of the intraosseous course of the nerves of the mandible. The Journal of Oral Implantology 1991;17(4):394-403.

[38] Lee J, Yoon S, Kang B. Mandibular canal branches supplying the mandibular third molar observed on cone beam computed tomographic images: reports of four cases. Korean Journal of Oral and Maxillofacial Radiology 2009;39:209-212.

[39] Fukami K, Shiozaki K, Mishima A, Kuribayashi A, Hamada Y, Kobayashi K. Bifid mandibular canal: confirmation of limited cone beam CT findings by gross anatomical and histological investigations. Dentomaxillofacial Radiology 2012;41(6):460-465.

[40] Gokce C, Sisman Y, Sipahioglu M. Styloid Process Elongation or Eagle's Syndrome: Is There Any Role for Ectopic Calcification? European Journal of Dentistry 2008;2(3): 224-228.

[41] MK OC. Calcification in the stylohyoid ligament. Oral Surgery, Oral Medicine, and Oral Pathology 1984;58(5):617-621.

[42] More CB, Asrani MK. Evaluation of the styloid process on digital panoramic radiographs. The Indian Journal of Radiology & Imaging 2010;20(4):261-265.

[43] Alpoz E, Akar GC, Celik S, Govsa F, Lomcali G. Prevalence and pattern of stylohyoid chain complex patterns detected by panoramic radiographs among Turkish population. Surgical and Radiologic Anatomy : SRA 2014;36(1):39-46.

[44] Kim JE, Min JH, Park HR, Choi BR, Choi JW, Huh KH. Severe calcified stylohyoid complex in twins: a case report. Imaging Science in Dentistry 2012;42(2):95-97.

[45] Rizzatti-Barbosa CM, Ribeiro MC, Silva-Concilio LR, Di Hipolito O, Ambrosano GM. Is an elongated stylohyoid process prevalent in the elderly? A radiographic study in a Brazilian population. Gerodontology 2005;22(2):112-115.

[46] Valerio CS, Peyneau PD, de Sousa AC, Cardoso FO, de Oliveira DR, Taitson PF, et al. Stylohyoid syndrome: surgical approach. The Journal of Craniofacial Surgery 2012;23(2):e138-140.

[47] Okabe S, Morimoto Y, Ansai T, Yamada K, Tanaka T, Awano S, et al. Clinical significance and variation of the advanced calcified stylohyoid complex detected by panoramic radiographs among 80-year-old subjects. Dentomaxillofacial Radiology 2006;35(3):191-199.

[48] Kaushik A, Kaushik M, Panwar R, Tanwar R, Garg P, Garg S. Calcified stylohyoid ligaments: A diagnostic dilemma. SRM Journal of Research in Dental Sciences 2012;3(4):275.

[49] Koivumaki A, Marinescu-Gava M, Jarnstedt J, Sandor GK, Wolff J. Trauma induced eagle syndrome. International Journal of Oral and Maxillofacial Surgery 2012;41(3): 350-353.

[50] Sudhakara Reddy R, Sai Kiran C, Sai Madhavi N, Raghavendra MN, Satish A. Prevalence of elongation and calcification patterns of elongated styloid process in south India. Journal of Clinical and Experimental Dentistry 2013;5(1):e30-35.

[51] MacDonald-Jankowski DS. Calcification of the stylohyoid complex in Londoners and Hong Kong Chinese. Dentomaxillofacial Radiology 2001;30(1):35-39.

[52] Ferrario VF, Sigurta D, Daddona A, Dalloca L, Miani A, Tafuro F, et al. Calcification of the stylohyoid ligament: incidence and morphoquantitative evaluations. Oral Surgery, Oral Medicine, and Oral Pathology 1990;69(4):524-529.

[53] Jain S, Bansal A, Paul S, Prashar DV. Styloid-stylohyoid syndrome. Annals of Maxillofacial Surgery 2012;2(1):66-69.

[54] Moon CS, Lee BS, Kwon YD, Choi BJ, Lee JW, Lee HW, et al. Eagle's syndrome: a case report. Journal of the Korean Association of Oral and Maxillofacial Surgeons 2014;40(1):43-47.

[55] Figún ME, Garino RR. Anatomia odontológica funcional e aplicada. São Paulo: Panamericada; 1989. 658 p.

[56] Friedlander AH, Cohen SN. Panoramic radiographic atheromas portend adverse vascular events. Oral Surgery, Oral Medicine, Oral Pathology, Oral Radiology, and Endodontics 2007;103(6):830-835.

[57] Guimaraes Henriques JC, Kreich EM, Helena Baldani M, Luciano M, Cezar de Melo Castilho J, Cesar de Moraes L. Panoramic radiography in the diagnosis of carotid artery atheromas and the associated risk factors. The Open Dentistry Journal 2011;5:79-83.

[58] Bayram B, Uckan S, Acikgoz A, Muderrisoglu H, Aydinalp A. Digital panoramic radiography: a reliable method to diagnose carotid artery atheromas? Dentomaxillofacial Radiology 2006;35(4):266-270.

[59] Cohen SN, Friedlander AH, Jolly DA, Date L. Carotid calcification on panoramic radiographs: an important marker for vascular risk. Oral Surgery, Oral Medicine, Oral Pathology, Oral Radiology, and Endodontics 2002;94(4):510-514.

[60] da Silva NG, Pedreira EN, Tuji FM, Warmling LV, Ortega KL. Prevalence of calcified carotid artery atheromas in panoramic radiographs of HIV-positive patients undergoing antiretroviral treatment: a retrospective study. Oral Surgery, Oral Medicine, and Oral Pathology 2014;117(1):67-74.

[61] Pornprasertsuk-Damrongsri S, Thanakun S. Carotid artery calcification detected on panoramic radiographs in a group of Thai population. Oral Surgery, Oral Medicine, Oral Pathology, Oral Radiology, and Endodontics 2006;101(1):110-115.

[62] Friedlander AH, Altman L. Carotid artery atheromas in postmenopausal women. Their prevalence on panoramic radiographs and their relationship to atherogenic risk factors. Journal of the American Dental Association 2001;132(8):1130-1136.

[63] Griniatsos J, Damaskos S, Tsekouras N, Klonaris C, Georgopoulos S. Correlation of calcified carotid plaques detected by panoramic radiograph with risk factors for stroke development. Oral Surgery, Oral Medicine, Oral Pathology, Oral Radiology, and Endodontics 2009;108(4):600-603.

[64] Almog DM, Illig KA, Khin M, Green RM. Unrecognized carotid artery stenosis discovered by calcifications on a panoramic radiograph. Journal of the American Dental Association 2000;131(11):1593-1597.

[65] Yoon SJ, Shim SK, Lee JS, Kang BC, Lim HJ, Kim MS, et al. Interobserver agreement on the diagnosis of carotid artery calcifications on panoramic radiographs. Imaging Science in Dentistry 2014;44(2):137-141.

[66] Garay I, Netto HD, Olate S. Soft tissue calcified in mandibular angle area observed by means of panoramic radiography. International Journal of Clinical and Experimental Medicine 2014;7(1):51-56.

[67] Ahmad M, Madden R, Perez L. Triticeous cartilage: prevalence on panoramic radiographs and diagnostic criteria. Oral Surgery, Oral Medicine, Oral Pathology, Oral Radiology, and Endodontics 2005;99(2):225-230.

[68] William PL, Warwick R, Dyson M, Bannister LH. Gray Anatomia. 37 ed. Rio de Janeiro: Guanabara Koogan; 1995.

[69] Khambete N, Kumar R, Risbud M, Joshi A. Evaluation of carotid artery atheromatous plaques using digital panoramic radiographs with Doppler sonography as the ground truth. Journal of Oral Biology and Craniofacial Research 2012;2(3):149-153.

[70] MacDonald D, Chan A, Harris A, Vertinsky T, Farman AG, Scarfe WC. Diagnosis and management of calcified carotid artery atheroma: dental perspectives. Oral Surgery, Oral Medicine, Oral Pathology, and Oral Radiology 2012;114(4):533-547.

[71] Miles DA, Craig RM. The calcified facial artery. A report of the panoramic radiographic incidence and appearance. Oral Surgery, Oral Medicine, and Oral Pathology 1983;55(2):214-219.

[72] Eyigor H, Osma U, Yilmaz MD, Selcuk OT. Multiple sialolithiasis in sublingual gland causing dysphagia. The American Journal of Case Reports 2012;13:44-46.

[73] Jardim EC, Ponzoni D, de Carvalho PS, Demetrio MR, Aranega AM. Sialolithiasis of the submandibular gland. The Journal of Craniofacial Surgery 2011;22(3):1128-1131.

[74] Ledesma-Montes C, Garces-Ortiz M, Salcido-Garcia JF, Hernandez-Flores F, Hernandez-Guerrero JC. Giant sialolith: case report and review of the literature. Journal of Oral and Maxillofacial Surgery 2007;65(1):128-130.

[75] Bodner L. Giant salivary gland calculi: diagnostic imaging and surgical management. Oral Surgery, Oral Medicine, Oral Pathology, Oral Radiology, and Endodontics 2002;94(3):320-323.

[76] Gungormus M, Yavuz MS, Yolcu U. Giant sublingual sialolith leading to dysphagia. The Journal of Emergency Medicine 2010;39(3):e129-130.

[77] Hong KH, Yang YS. Sialolithiasis in the sublingual gland. The Journal of Laryngology and Otology 2003;117(11):905-907.

[78] Shimizu M, Yoshiura K, Nakayama E, Kanda S, Nakamura S, Ohyama Y, et al. Multiple sialolithiasis in the parotid gland with Sjogren's syndrome and its sonographic findings--report of 3 cases. Oral Surgery, Oral Medicine, Oral Pathology, Oral Radiology, and Endodontics 2005;99(1):85-92.

[79] Su YX, Liao GQ, Wang L, Liang YJ, Chu M, Zheng GS. Sialoliths or phleboliths? The Laryngoscope 2009;119(7):1344-1347.

[80] Langland OE, Langlais RP, Morris CR. Principles and practice of panoramic radiology : including intraoral radiographic interpretation. Philadelphia: Saunders; 1982. xiv, 458 p.

[81] Jadu FM, Lam EW. A comparative study of the diagnostic capabilities of 2D plain radiograph and 3D cone beam CT sialography. Dentomaxillofacial Radiology 2013;42(1):20110319.

[82] Dreiseidler T, Ritter L, Rothamel D, Neugebauer J, Scheer M, Mischkowski RA. Salivary calculus diagnosis with 3-dimensional cone-beam computed tomography. Oral Surgery, Oral Medicine, Oral Pathology, Oral Radiology, and Endodontics 2010;110(1):94-100.

[83] Shemilt P. The origin of phleboliths. The British Journal of Surgery 1972;59(9): 695-700.

[84] Mandel L, Perrino MA. Phleboliths and the vascular maxillofacial lesion. Journal of Oral and Maxillofacial Surgery 2010;68(8):1973-1976.

[85] Kamatani T, Saito T, Hamada Y, Kondo S, Shirota T, Shintani S. Intramuscular hemangioma with phleboliths of the tongue: A case report. Indian Journal of Dentistry 2014.

[86] Kanaya H, Saito Y, Gama N, Konno W, Hirabayashi H, Haruna S. Intramuscular hemangioma of masseter muscle with prominent formation of phleboliths: a case report. Auris, nasus, larynx 2008;35(4):587-591.

[87] Silva MI, Sassi LM, Rapoport A, Benedito VO, Machado R, Quebur MI. Aspectos clínicos e histológicos das anomalias vasculares da boca. Revista Brasileira de Cirurgia de Cabeça e Pescoço 2004;33(2):63-69.

[88] Chava VR, Shankar AN, Vemanna NS, Cholleti SK. Multiple venous malformations with phleboliths: radiological-pathological correlation. Journal of Clinical Imaging Science 2013;3(Suppl 1):13.

[89] Altug HA, Buyuksoy V, Okcu KM, Dogan N. Hemangiomas of the head and neck with phleboliths: clinical features, diagnostic imaging, and treatment of 3 cases. Oral Surgery, Oral Medicine, Oral Pathology, Oral Radiology, and Endodontics 2007;103(3):e60-64.

[90] Scolozzi P, Laurent F, Lombardi T, Richter M. Intraoral venous malformation presenting with multiple phleboliths. Oral Surgery, Oral Medicine, Oral Pathology, Oral Radiology, and Endodontics 2003;96(2):197-200.

[91] Kato H, Ota Y, Sasaki M, Arai T, Sekido Y, Tsukinoki K. A phlebolith in the anterior portion of the masseter muscle. The Tokai Journal of Experimental and Clinical Medicine 2012;37(1):25-29.

[92] Gordon JS, Mandel L. Masseteric Intramuscular Hemangioma: Case Report. Journal of Oral and Maxillofacial Surgery 2014.

[93] Mohan RP, Dhillon M, Gill N. Intraoral venous malformation with phleboliths. The Saudi Dental Journal 2011;23(3):161-163.

[94] Babu BB, Tejasvi MLA, Avinash CK, B C. Tonsillolith: a panoramic radiograph presentation. Journal of Clinical and Diagnostic Research 2013;7(10):2378-2379.

[95] Cooper MM, Steinberg JJ, Lastra M, Antopol S. Tonsillar calculi. Report of a case and review of the literature. Oral Surgery, Oral Medicine, and Oral Pathology 1983;55(3):239-243.

[96] Giudice M, Cristofaro MG, Fava MG, Giudice A. An unusual tonsillolithiasis in a patient with chronic obstructive sialoadenitis. Dentomaxillofacial Radiology 2005;34(4):247-250.

[97] Mesolella M, Cimmino M, Di Martino M, Criscuoli G, Albanese L, Galli V. Tonsillolith. Case report and review of the literature. Acta Otorhinolaryngologica Italica 2004;24(5):302-307.

[98] Sezer B, Tugsel Z, Bilgen C. An unusual tonsillolith. Oral Surgery, Oral Medicine, Oral Pathology, Oral Radiology, and Endodontics 2003;95(4):471-473.

[99] Bamgbose BO, Ruprecht A, Hellstein J, Timmons S, Qian F. The prevalence of tonsilloliths and other soft tissue calcifications in patients attending oral and maxillofacial radiology clinic of the University of Iowa. International Scholarly Research Notices Dentistry 2014;2014:839635.

[100] Guevara C, Mandel L. Panoramic radiographic demonstration of bilateral tonsilloliths. The New York State Dental Journal 2011;77(3):28-30.

[101]   de Moura MD, Madureira DF, Noman-Ferreira LC, Abdo EN, de Aguiar EG, Freire AR. Tonsillolith: a report of three clinical cases. Medicina Oral, Patologia Oral y Cirugia Bucal 2007;12(2):E130-133.

4

Improving Antimicrobial Activity of Dental Restorative Materials

J.M.F.A. Fernandes, V.A. Menezes,
A.J.R. Albuquerque, M.A.C. Oliveira, K.M.S. Meira,
R.A. Menezes Júnior and F.C. Sampaio

1. Introduction

The oral cavity harbors a great diversity of microbial species that have a strong tendency to colonize dental surfaces, tongue and oral mucosa [1,2]. These accumulations of oral bacteria on dental surfaces are natural forms of biofilm growth in humans. They are also known as dental plaque and in spite of several favorable conditions (e.g. temperature, humidity) these biofilms are constantly challenged by host factors. It is recognized that structural organization of a dental biofilm are influenced by the interplay of many unfavorable and also several favorable ones such as the chemical nature of the substrate and the type of the surface where the biofilm develops [3].

In dentistry, restoration failure is generally attributed to a combination of oral bacteria and inappropriate features of dental materials. Efficient dental restorative materials are important for an adequate recovery of masticatory and esthetic functions. However, these materials are prone to biofilm formation, affecting oral health. It is well accepted that under *in vivo* conditions, rough surfaces attract more biofilm than smooth ones, but the variables that influence bacterial adhesion to dental materials are still a matter of debate.

Dental caries is the most prevalent disease found in the oral cavity of humans. It is regarded as multifactorial chronic and complex disease which is dependent of a cariogenic biofilm [4,5]. Thus, a carious lesion takes some time to develop. However, initial carious lesions are easily and rapidly formed during a three-day of high sucrose regime and poor oral hygiene conditions. So, as long as there is a cariogenic microbial biofilm attached to a dental surface there is a great chance to find a carious lesion on this tooth spot [6]. Growth of oral bacteria on dental surfaces requires adhesion strategies because there is a constant flow of host secretions (e.g. saliva) that can interfere on the ability of planktonic cells (non-attached bacteria). As a result, the formation of the oral biofilm is not homogenous and it contains multiple bacterial species [4,7,8].

Oral bacteria can adhere to hydrophobic as well as to hydrophilic surfaces and many explanatory theories are suggested including the influence of complex electrostatic mechanisms such as van der Waals energy. After biofilm establishment on restorations, surface deterioration of materials (e.g.: resin composites and glass-ionomer cements) will take place facilitating the development of a mature biofilm resulting in dental carious lesions. The microflora from these diseased teeth sites is significantly different from healthy sites on a tooth [10]. The frequent changes in environmental conditions can lead to shifts in biofilm microflora and as a result the microbial homeostasis breaks down in dental plaque (e.g. low pH), and disease occurs.

It must be pointed out that the presence of these oral microbes in the mouth is natural, and is also essential for the normal development of the physiology of the oral cavity [9]. Hence, any antimicrobial strategy has to consider the perspective of restoring some microbial equilibrium and not a complete depletion of oral bacterial from the mouth. Many antimicrobial substances, compounds or mixture of antibacterial agents (e.g. bisbiguanides, metal ions, quaternary ammonium compounds, essential oils) have been successfully formulated into home care products to control oral biofilms. Several investigations have proved their efficacy in controlling the development of oral biofilms despite important drawbacks as tooth staining, bad taste, etc. [3,4]. Moreover, at moderate or high concentrations, these antimicrobial mouthwashes and toothpastes can inhibit bacterial growth in many different modes and truly affect biofilm-forming capacity of some pathogenic traits. Hence, to be considered a successful antimicrobial agent a substance, compound or the mixture of both must be able of maintaining the oral biofilm at "normal" cariogenic bacterial levels which are compatible with the individual oral health. Simultaneously, the material must be effective without any interference on the beneficial properties of the resident oral microflora.

Mouthwashes and toothpastes are accepted methods to deliver antimicrobials into the oral mouth. However, they are completely dependent on the discipline and compliance of the patient to the oral treatment. In addition, many of these antimicrobials are prescribed for short periods to avoid any risk of disturbing the resident oral microflora [3,10]. Hence, one strategy is to incorporate antimicrobials into dental materials. The possibility that dental restorative material may release antimicrobial compounds are regarded as an interesting strategy for overcoming the development of cariogenic dental biofilms and the risk for secondary dental caries. In addition, there is a chance that under less biofilm stress dental materials could increase longevity. This strategy is of great importance since dental restorations properties may be improved if an antibiotic-dental material is used.

The aim of the present review is to shed light on the techniques and effectiveness on improving antibacterial activities of dental restorative materials. The main focus is on incorporation and subsequent slow-release of antimicrobial chemical species, molecules, compounds and low molecular weight antibacterial agents such as metal ions, iodine, antibiotics, chlorhexidine and natural products such as essential oils. The *in vitro* and *in vivo* techniques used in microbiology are also explored taking into account that main bacteria involved are Gram-positive cocci shaped bacteria such as *Streptococcus sobrinus, Streptococcus mutans* and Lactobacillus sp.

2. *In vitro* and *in vivo* techniques for studying biofilms

In 1940´s microbiologists described an interesting phenomenon that occurs when fresh sea water is kept in a glass bottle, the so-called "bottle effect". It was observed that the number of microorganisms attached a glass surface increase while at the same time there is a reduction in free-living microorganisms [11]. This is a relevant historical landmark because it represents the starting point of a paradigm shift that is still valid these days. In fact, only 30 years later, scientific community understood that the biofilm mode of life is the rule rather the exception when bacteria and fungi species are collected, studied and investigated in nature under real life conditions. Biofilms are defined as complex consortia of microorganisms that are attached to a surface that can be of biotic or abiotic nature [12].

The microbial biofilm formation involves a multi-stage process in which bacterial and fungi adhere to the surface. For more details see figure 1 which is based in several reports [13-16].

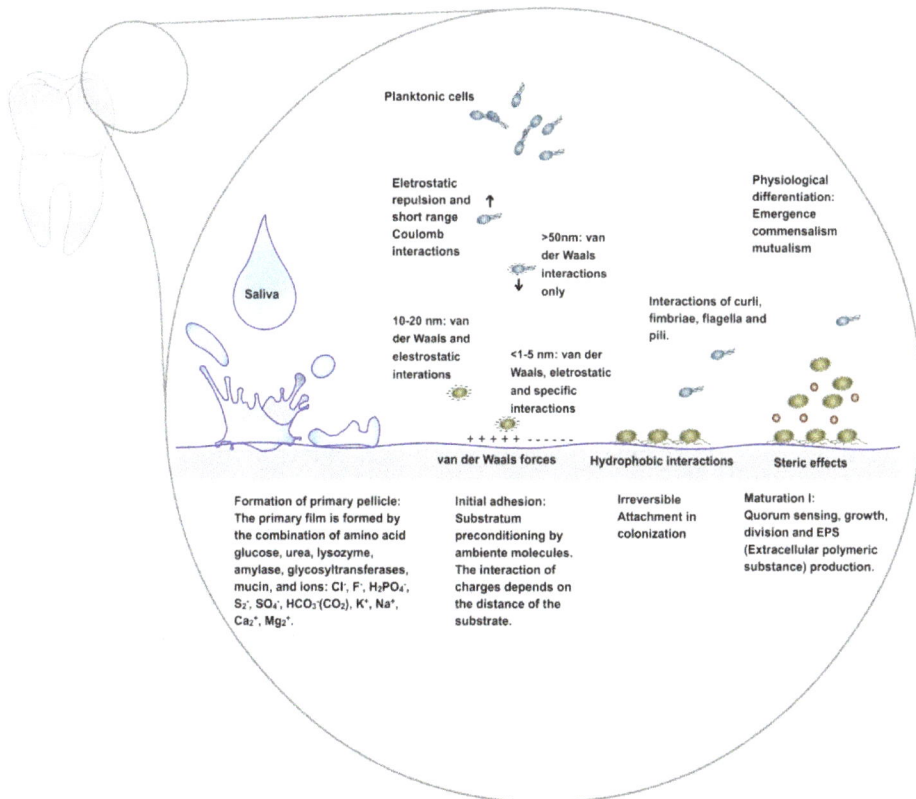

Figure 1. The multi-stage process of biofilm formation by oral microorganisms.

At this stage only weak forces are operating. Therefore it is also known as the initial reversible attachment stage. Subsequently, there is a production of an extracellular matrix (containing polysaccharides, proteins and DNA) that results in a stronger attachment which is also known as the irreversible attachment stage [16]. In general, after attachment, biofilm growth follows two other distinct phases or behavior: spreading and dispersal of microorganisms.

Basically, the attachment process involves equilibrium of electrostatic forces. Microbes and tooth surfaces are negatively charged. As they are immersed in a fluid (saliva) system which is rich in calcium and other counterions, these negative charged surfaces attract and mobilize cations. As a result, a double charged layer is formed (electrical double layer) and this overlap causes a repulsive electrostatic force. Simultaneously, as the bacterium approaches the tooth surface, they also experience a repulsive force (van der Waals force). Finally, the combinations of repulsive and attraction forces known as DLVO theory modulate the microorganism adherence to dental surfaces. This is valid for dental restorative materials as well, and one must consider the fact that it can be more favorable if a porous or irregular surface is facilitating bacterial adherence [3,13-16].

The first bacteria to attach to the acquired pellicle (layer of glycoproteins) on the tooth surface are called the pioneer species (*Streptococcus oralis, Streptococcus mitis, Streptococcus sanguis*). Surprisingly, *S. mutans* is not a first colonizer despite its high cariogenic nature. In fact, *S. mutans* is the most studied bacteria in oral microbiology but under clinical environment one must consider that a multispecies biofilm is operating [3,9].

Historically, in Dentistry, the examination of mature oral biofilms started when electron microscope became available for microbiologists [19]. Later, molecular biological tools became popular and new insights about how microbes attach and develop on tooth surfaces were finally confirmed. One "striking" observation was actually a confirmation of an obvious theory that microbes stick to a surface many benefits are obtained: a) selection of sites where they stay in favorable environments, b) these surfaces may have enough substrate or can contribute to diffuse some nutrient and c) the different species often work together and this consortium provides physical support and protection [20-29].

More recently, zeta potential, confocal laser scanning microscopy (CLSM) together with fluorescence techniques received attention and became useful techniques to study bacteria adhesion to surfaces [29]. In spite of the great evolution in techniques, many limitations have to be considered when comes to the evaluation of an antimicrobial substances against biofilms development. First, there is still the gap of *in vitro* and *in vivo* environments. *In situ* studies can overcome some of these limitations but other drawbacks cannot be ruled out. Most studies on bacteria adhesion to surfaces were carried out under *in vitro* conditions which do not reflect the real life. Secondly, there is the paradox of testing planktonic cells but interpretations are generalized to conditions of biofilm formation. It is well established that biofilms express genes different from those of planktonic cells. Moreover, it has been observed that biofilm cells are generally believed to closely resemble planktonic cells in stationary phase. However, biofilms were found to more closely resemble to planktonic cells at exponentially growing than those of planktonic cells in the stationary phase [19,20]. In addition, it cannot be ruled out the differences between single species biofilm versus multispecies biofilms since under laboratory

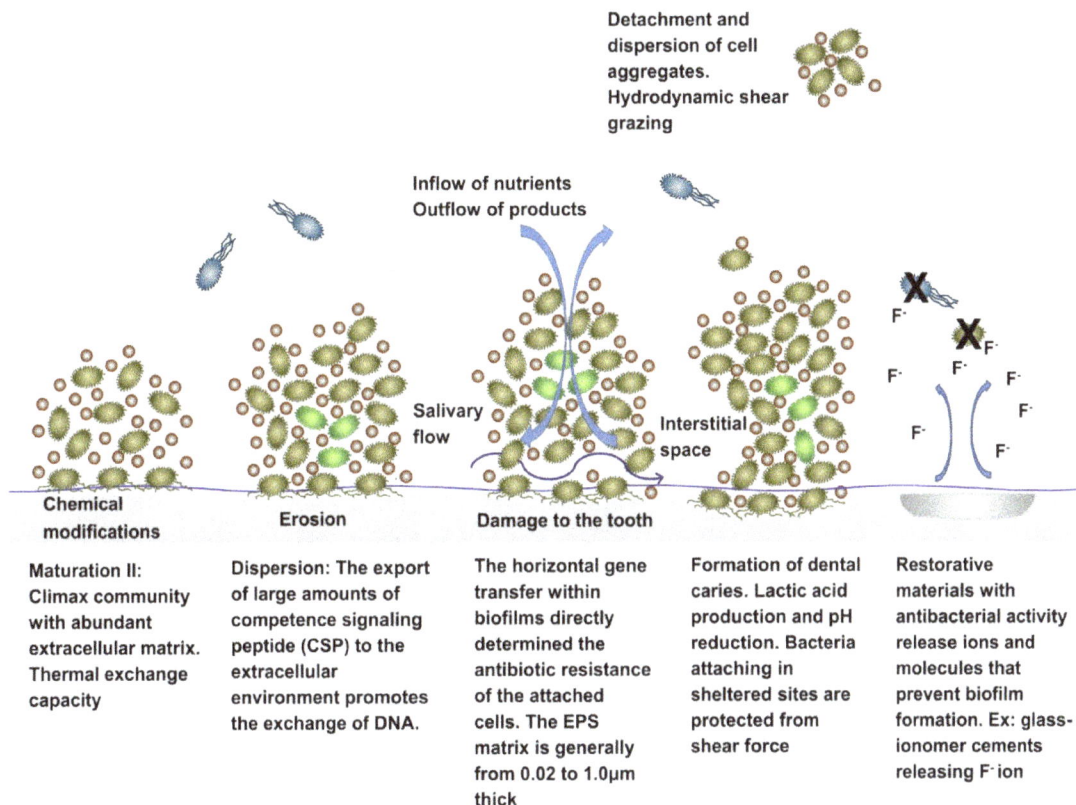

Figure 2. Schematic representation of the development of an oral biofilm and the potential of antimicrobials to interfere on this process when releasing some antimicrobial element or substance [13-18]

conditions monospecies biofilm can survive for only 72 hours in absence of sugar. The duration of survival can be extended with addition of mucin, but how close is this to the real oral mouth of a patient? [21] Another flow systems versus static models, pre-treatment of acquired pellicle or no pre-treatment at all. [22]. Finally, a crucial point is: how to validate microbial growth? BacLight staining techniques only measure the presence of intact membranes and may not correlate with the culturability or viability of bacteria from oral biofilms [23].

After all these relevant methodological points, more questions marks can be attributed on how to evaluate antimicrobial agents against biofilms. In addition to evaluate the effects in biofilms itself, one must consider the understanding of suitable methods related to the incorporation of antimicrobials into these dental restorative materials. For instance, the concentration of the antimicrobial agent, the volume or amount of material to be included and how far these substances can interfere on mechanical and esthetic features of a restoration [21-26].

Considering the presence of a mature biofilm covering a dental restoration, it must be pointed out that a major requirement of the final formulation is to deliver sufficient concentration of the inhibitor in the surroundings. Moreover, the antimicrobial effect must be kept on a prolonged time or at least for a enough period of time that will maintain an effective dose operating. This point is quite important since oral bacteria do not live as independent entities. So, as highlighted previously, a high resistance to antibiotics is likely to occur [27-30].

Along the last decades biofilms have been studied extensively because they are present in several surfaces, such as all solid surfaces in the oral cavity, in biomateriais implanted in the human body, in catheter surfaces, in water pipes [24]. After the establishment of a biofilm on dental restorations, deterioration of the outer layer surface of these materials will take place and facilitate bacteria adhesion [25]. On the other hand, the possibility that dental restoring materials can deliver antimicrobials may reduce considerably the risk of secondary caries in spite of the limitations of some dental materials.

3. Antimicrobials in dental materials: How much is enough versus how much is safe?

Oral bacteria can attach to many restorative materials like amalgam, gold, ceramics, resin composite, glass ionomer cements. In order to achieve long-term success of dental fillings there are many requirements. Some are related to the professional ability in manipulating and polishing these materials. However, some considerations rely on physical, chemical and biological characteristics of the dental material used. Surface roughness is not the focus of this review, but it may be influenced by the interplay of professionals' ability as well as dental materials features.

The incorporation of 5, 10, 15 up to 30% of antimicrobial compounds or substances into dental materials have been proposed [24-30]. However, the higher amount of antimicrobial agents, the higher is the risk to loose important features in dental restoration as biocompatibility and resistance. Hence, how much is enough and how much is safe? In the literature, addition of 1.5% can be effective if the antimicrobial is potent enough [27].

Figure 3 presents this dilemma related to the interference of "extra" substances to be incorporated into dental materials and limitations regarding the loss of important features of the material.

An interesting report showed that incorporation of 1% chlorhexidine (CHX) diacetate in GIC (glass ionomer cements) is optimal for clinical use. This is valid in terms of antimicrobial activities, CHX-release pattern, physical properties and bonding ability to tooth surfaces [28]. An additional valuable information was the conclusion that incorporation of CHX diacetate at 2% or greater values of percentage participation significantly decreased compressive strength and adversely affected bond strength to dentin.

It has been observed that some dental materials (e.g. gold and its alloys) are naturally able to kill bacteria in the adhering biofilms [29]. Glass ionomer cements (GIC) are recognized for releasing fluoride ions that can modulate biofilm formation [27,30]. The point is that this is not enough since GIC reduces its ability to release fluoride in short periods. So, it is expected that dental restoration with antimicrobial properties may have extended potential for inhibiting biofilm formation in a long-term basis.

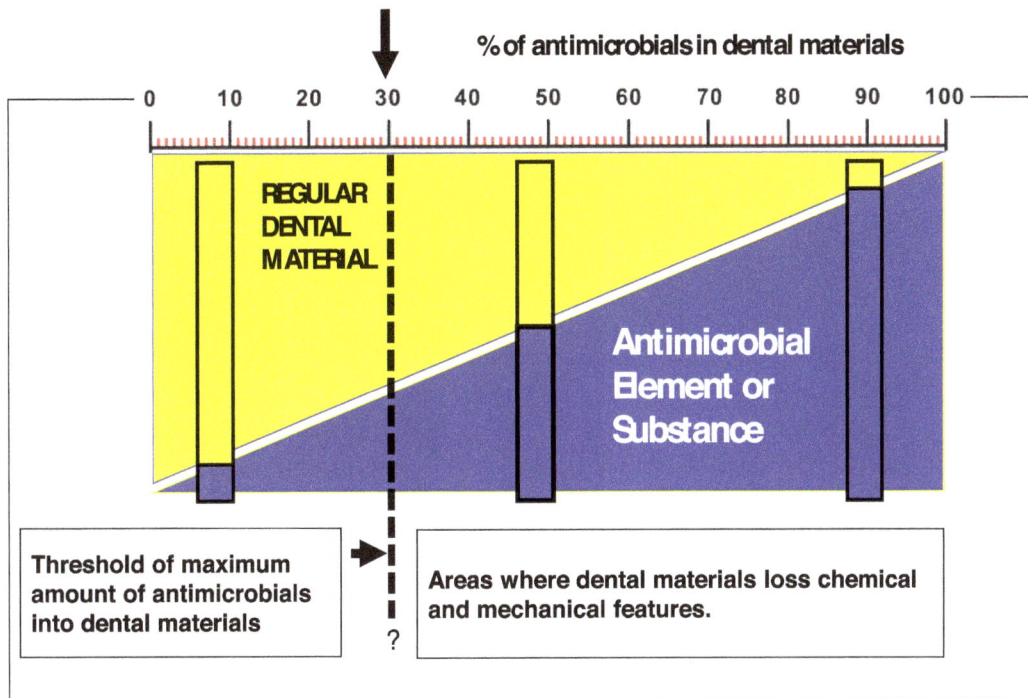

Figure 3. Schematic representation for understanding the effects of external substances and compounds when incorporated into regular dental materials.

In addition to chemical changes due to incorporation of antimicrobials into dental restorative materials, there is also the problem of chemical changes also interfere in the distribution of masticatory forces applied on a tooth. For instance, the presence of a carious lesion in molar tooth can demand fast treatment protocol for the affected area and depending on the lesion extension, it must receive a temporary filling [31-34]. In general, temporary filling materials are typically made from a combination of zinc oxide and eugenol which has good antimicrobial activity. Eugenol is also important due to its sedative properties. The zinc oxide powder is a very versatile compound that can present different properties when combined with various agents. When mixed together, the material starts off soft and in few minutes it becomes more hard and brittle. However, this mixture is not harder enough to be compared to regular dental fillings and its far from restoring tooth hardness. This material is classified as intermediate restorative material (IRM) and it is a good example that the beneficial aspects of antimicrobial and anti-inflammatory properties are achieved while mechanical properties of resistance become very low. Therefore, this material must be accepted as a temporary and not a definite filling material. Under the influence of masticatory forces, as previously mentioned, there will be a stress in the remaining parts of the dental element that will certainly compromise the longevity of the restoration as well as the whole tooth structure [31-34].

A comparative study analysing deformations done through Finite Element Method (FEM) and applying the software ANSYS shows the differences in compressive loads between sound and restored teeth with intermediate restorative materials (IRM), see figure 4A and 4B. It is shown that the restored tooth IRM (figure 4B) is deformed in a different way when compared to the sound tooth (4A). Figure 5 shows this simulation evaluating a map of tension for both conditions: A (sound tooth) and B (restored).

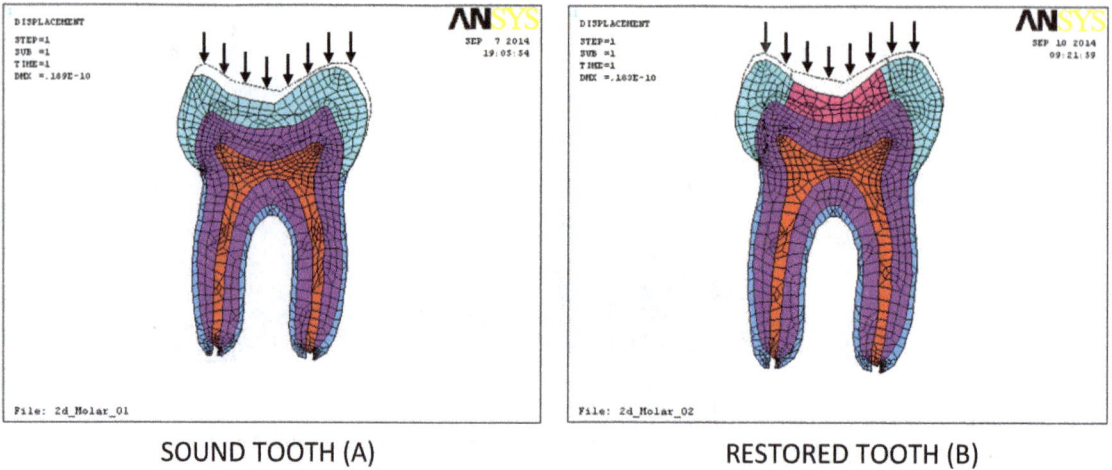

SOUND TOOTH (A)   RESTORED TOOTH (B)

Figure 4. Sites of deformations in sound and IRM restored teeth.

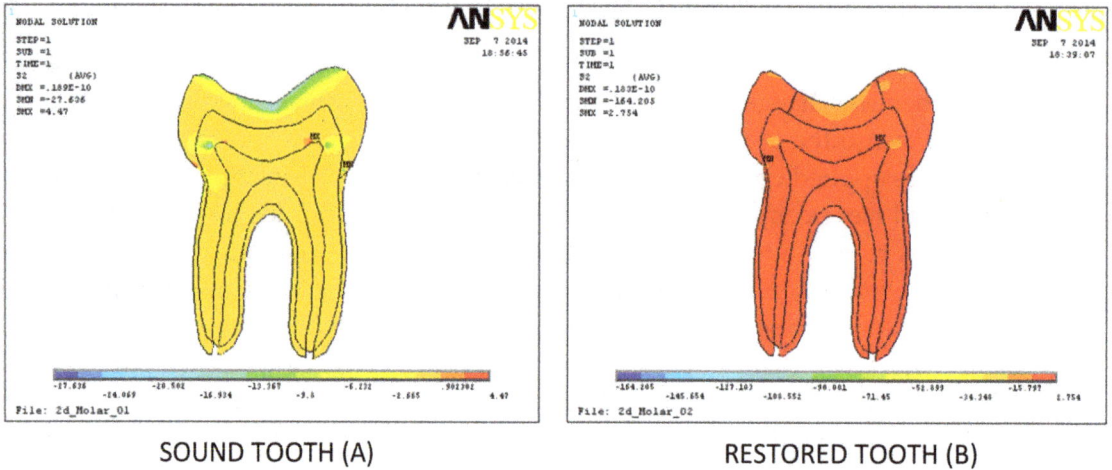

SOUND TOOTH (A)   RESTORED TOOTH (B)

Figure 5. Sites of tensions in sound and IRM restored teeth.

As expected, the analysis shows that the distribution of forces in the interior of the teeth flows in different patterns. As a result, the restored tooth experiences a higher stress in some parts. Basically, these maps show compressive forces throughout the whole sound tooth (A) whereas for restored teeth tensile stress forces are observed.

It well is established that development of a numerical model as FEM makes it possible to quantify and evaluate masticatory loads [34]. However, few studies have considered the influence of antimicrobials in dental restorations. One must bear in mind that a good balance has to be achieved between the beneficial aspects of having an "antibacterial restoration" compared do a regular one. Certainly the size and shape of the restoration are important variables but interesting results can be obtained by these simulations.

It is important to realize that the changes in the map of tensions are directly related to the changes in the physical constitution of the tooth because in this case, the dental enamel was substituted by a restorative material. This change cannot necessarily be attributed to a change of forces because the molar frequently will be constantly submitted to the same masticatory forces it was receiving before the carious lesion. As shown in figure 5, the red colour of the figure 5B indicates a significant higher tension the 5A. The structural fatigue is the main mechanism of collapse of the reminiscent dental tissue and this process can be aggravated when it is submitted to long treatment periods, particularly if IRM is used. In other words, the IRM used as temporary fillings must have a short life because they reduce the mechanical efficiency of the teeth in spite of its beneficial support to control biofilm formation.

According to Noort (2013) [35], there is a subtle distinction between safety and biocompatibility two important features of dental materials. Safety is concerned with the fact that materials when in contact with the human body should not cause any adverse effect, whereas biocompatibility is the quality of being non-destructive in the biological environment maintaining the beneficial effect to the patient. So far, few materials can be regarded as completely safe and fully biocompatible in the oral environment. Most dental materials interact with the oral environment and this interaction might be a release of components with undesirable side effects for oral tissues.

4. Dental restorative materials with antimicrobials

Dental materials must simulate dental structure and have to restore the anatomy and the function of affected dental surfaces due to dental caries or trauma. However, the desirable aesthetics and the concerns with biocompatibility have not been forgotten and this is valid for resin composite, glass ionomer cements and IRM (MJÖR et al., 1990). It must be highlighted that bone and dentin can be considered as natural composites, whose main constituents are collagen (polymer) and apatite (a ceramic) [35].

Metals have been used for centuries as antimicrobial agents and they continue to be useful at the present time. Silver, copper, gold, titanium and zinc are the most common examples in Dentistry [36]. Dioxide of titanium has been used as whitening agent. However, silver and copper has been receiving larger attention due to their antimicrobial properties. As a result, these metals are incorporate to several dental products to control halitosis and dental biofilms [5].

As for dental resins, GIC and IRM, these materials are probably the best examples of improvement of restorative materials that has contributed to the recovery of ideal anatomical form and function with less removal of tooth structure. The use of "fluoride-release" materials, "smart-materials" and "bio-active" materials are some desirable features that are becoming necessary in many clinical situations because minimally invasive treatment of carious lesions is much more acceptable nowadays. Probably, the first experiences to produce a useful "smart-material" were related to the concept that fluoride-releasing materials. Glass ionomer cements do not undergo great dimensional changes in a moist environment and exhibit noticeable shrinkage in a dry environment at temperatures higher than 50°C, which is similar to the behavior of dentin [37]. This is a good example of biocompatibility.

Attempts to improve GIC have been quite successful. There is one report indicating that zinc addition to GIC can decrease microorganisms growth and improve fluoride release, without significantly affecting the materials' flexural strength and solubility [38]. In another report, conventional glass ionomer cement (GIC) liner was mixed with different antibiotics such as metronidazole, ciprofloxacin and cefaclor to produce an antibacterial GIC. After an *in vitro* evaluation of infected dentin sealed with this product, there was a 98.6% decrease in micro-organisms, bacterial aggregates, and intertubular dentin with exposed collagen fibers and dentinal tubules [41]. When conventional GIC was added with 1.5, 3.0 and 4.5% of ciproflox-acin, metronidazole and minocycline this material was effective for inhibiting *S. mutans* and *L. casei*, and the addition of a 1.5% antibiotic mixture was optimal to provide appropriate physical and bonding properties [39]. For more than a decade, several reports in the literature has been demonstrating antibacterial activity against *S. mutans, S. oralis, S. salivarius* and Streptococcus sp when GIC are reinforced with antimicrobials or due to fluoride or pH equilibrium [7, 40-44]. It has been claimed that GIC has the ability to increase pH and this is likely to be an important mechanism of caries protection under clinical conditions since oral bacteria can produce lactic acid [43].

The resin composites have been used, frequently, as restoring material due to its great aesthetics and physiologic properties [44]. More recently, incorporation of 12-methacryloy-loxydodecylpyridinium bromide, a monomer also known as MDPB showed good results for its antibacterial activity when incorporated in bonding agents [28].

However, instead of releasing an antimicrobial substance, the strategy to incorporate them to act as part of its structure is also possible. In this perspective, nanoparticles can provide good optical properties for conventional and hybrid composites [45]. However, there is still a lack of studies in the literature showing the beneficial aspects for placing such material in a dental cavity. For instance, it is still unknown how effective these materials can inhibit caries activity close to restorations when active bioparticles are incorporated into these resins [46-48]. As a general observation, it must be highlighted that there are many in vitro studies but very few clinical trials to support their use under regular clinical activity [46].

Finally, it can be stated that two main approaches can be presented when antimicrobial bio-active materials are prepared. One approach is to prepare a substance-release material (e.g. GIC). Another perspective is to incorporate the antimicrobial to be active being part of its structure without any release of active component. Basically, this latter option is of outmost importance since the release of a substance implies in loss of matter and in theoretical basis this means some loss in mechanical properties. Taking into account that GIC acts as battery charges for fluoride, it must be pointed out that "recovery" of fluoride ions does not reach original levels [47-49]. Hence, other advantages have to be operating to consider this material as a good option for dental restorations.

Another point to be considered is the fact concentrations of substances released from some dental materials such as GIC materials were not different, regardless of the amount of antimicrobial substance incorporated. Thus, as long as the antimicrobial is not interfering in the mechanical properties, an increase in the amount of antimicrobial drug will not provide additional benefits.

5. Dental restorative materials with nanoparticles

Nanoparticles are generally defined as particles that are smaller than 100 nanometers in diameter. So, in order to provide a good perspective, it can be emphasized that nanotechnology deals with structures as small as 10^{-9} m while oral bacteria reach a size of 10^{-6} m. Although there is a large difference in size, the improvements of many technologies in the 1980s made possible the combination of these two worlds. Many researchers' points out that nanotechnology has been applied for dental materials as an innovative concept for the development of materials with better properties including the anti-caries effect [5,45,49].

It is recognized that many nanoparticles do have a great antimicrobial activity, particularly if it is a metallic nanoparticles. The antimicrobial activity of many types of nanoparticle is certainly a function of their size but other features are important such as high surface area, unusual crystal morphologies (edges and corners) and reactive sites. There is a great difference of a regular metal and a 10^{-9} m particles when incorporated into dental materials. Consequently, their properties can radically change, as hardness, area of active surface, chemical reactivity and biological activity [26].

The inverse relationship between the size of some particles and its antimicrobial activity has been demonstrated for particles of up to 10 nm were tested against *Escherichia coli* [50]. Thus, this might be valid for nanoparticles as well. The main mechanism or mechanisms behind the antimicrobial activity of nanoparticles are not fully elucidated. Hence, several studies focusing on the antimicrobial activity of different metals and metallic nanoparticles against oral microorganisms have to be performed for a clear picture on this matter. Another point to be considered is the effectiveness of these nanoparticles to control the development of a biofilm. Considering that biofilms are rather organized and can avoid the penetration of big molecules (e.g. chlorhexidine) the small size of these particles can be advantageous. However, so far these particles have been introduced into prosthetic devices coatings and oral care products. The strategy for placing them within dental materials is currently being explored in vitro and more research is needed to consider their regular use in the dental clinic.

Basically, the most promising nanoparticles are: silver, zinc oxide, calcium-phosphates [5]. Nevertheless, is must be also known that an interesting systematic map demonstrated that there is currently a limited amount of information concerning the release of nanoparticles from polymer-based dental materials. After reviewing 140 full-text articles on this matter, only 3 were regarded as methodological sound. Actually, a passive release of nanoparticles from a polymer-based dental material was not observed by the investigated reports. [51]. Table 1 summarizes some important features of these materials when present within dental materials.

Nanoparticles	Observations	References
Silver	• It may provoke structural changes and damage bacterial membranes, resulting in cell death. • Incorporated into dental adhesives could reduce *S. mutans* close to orthodontic brackets. • Concentrations of 0.5-1% provided antimicrobial activity with preservation of aesthetic and mechanical properties of dental materials (resin composites). • Future research must focus on silver-biofilm interaction and silver-polimerization processes of dental materials.	[5,26,49, 52-59]
Zinc oxide	• The mechanism of action may be attributed to oxidative stress by H_2O_2 and structural changes in cell wall. • Incorporated into dental materials ZnO may release Zn^{2+} which interferes in sucrose metabolism and magnesium depletion that is important for biofilm equilibrium. • Future research must focus on the determination of ideal concentrations of nanoparticles in order to have antimicrobial activity without compromising mechanical properties of the materials.	[5,26,49, 58, 60, 61]
Quaternary Ammonium	• This compound was selected due to its good antimicrobial activity and because it can be copolymerized with other monomers providing a strong bonding system with the material. However, difficulties in controlling the release of such agents may be a potential drawback. • The hydrophobic nature and positive charge of these nanoparticles may enhance the antimicrobial activity. • Future research must focus on kinetics to optimize the release characteristics.	[5,26,63-65]
Calcium-phosphates	• These compounds can interfere on adherence and growth of *Streptococcus mutans*. • The resin composites with these nanoparticles can increase up to four times the capacity of remineralization of the enamel in comparison with the composites with fluoride. • Hydroxyapatite nanocrystals may interact with bacterial adhesins and can reduce bacterial adherence to dental surfaces. • Future research must focus on efficacy of products that are already available in the market such as casein phosphopeptide (CPP)-amorphous and calcium phosphate (ACP) nanocomplex.	[5,26,66-71]

Table 1. Observations and conclusions related to nanoparticles incorporated into dental materials.

6. Final considerations

The oral environment imposes difficulties when it is designed a study for evaluating dental materials [3,9,10,25]. Since 1950's it is know that microbial microleakage at the cavity wall/

material interface is a problem to restoration survival. The persistence of microorganisms underneath fillings is also recognized as a serious problem in restorative dentistry. The antibacterial properties of restorative materials can substantially influence the success of a dental filling in the oral cavity. The frequent problem is that dental materials "natural" antibacterial properties are not enough to cope with the facility of biofilm formation. Thus, the incorporation of antimicrobials in restorative materials has to take into account the properties of each dental material. For instance, restorations of glass-ionomer cements are based on an acid-base reaction between a polyacrylic acid solution and fluoroaminosilicate glass particles. This reaction yields a structure that is more stable than composites. As a result, by adhering to tooth structure the glass-ionomer cements potentially reduces microleakage. This is an important property since it can enhance fluoride release. So, why not incorporating antibiotics as well? Hence, glass ionomer cements are strong candidates to have antimicrobials incorporated as long as it does not disturb the acid-base reaction. On the other hand, resin composites are much better materials considering aesthetic properties. Finally, coatings killing bacteria upon contact seems to be more promising than antimicrobial-releasing coatings. However, many in vitro studies cannot support the findings that are observed *in vivo*. This observation suggests that more clinical research is needed to clarify this issue. Hence, clinical research on this topic is of outmost relevance for minimum intervention restorative techniques in dentistry and for promoting oral health. Another point to consider is the challenge for the future dental materials with antimicrobials properties: to develop even more effective materials that are able to improve clinical antimicrobial efficacy while still preserving the benefits of the normal, resident oral microflora.

Author details

J.M.F.A. Fernandes[1], V.A. Menezes[1], A.J.R. Albuquerque[2], M.A.C. Oliveira[3], K.M.S. Meira[3], R.A. Menezes Júnior[4] and F.C. Sampaio[2,3*]

*Address all correspondence to: fcsampa@gmail.com

1 Post-graduation in Pediatric Dentistry, Faculty of Dentistry, University of Pernambuco, Camaragibe, Pernambuco, Brazil

2 RENORBIO, Northeast Network of Biotechnology, Federal University of Paraiba, Biotechnology Centre, Campus I, Joao Pessoa, Paraiba, Brazil

3 Post-graduation in Dentistry, Health Science Center, University of Paraíba, João Pessoa, Paraíba, Brazil

4 Alternative and Renewable Energy Center, Department of Renewable Energy Engineering, Federal University of Paraíba, João Pessoa, Paraíba, Brazil

References

[1] Gharechahi M, Moosavi H, Forghani M. Effect of surface roughness and materials composition on biofilm formation. JBNB 2012; 3:541-6.

[2] Marsh PD. Contemporary perspective on plaque control. Br Dent J 2012; 22:601-6

[3] Marsh PD, Martin M. Oral microbiology, 5th ed. Oxford, UK: Churchill; Livingstone; 2009.

[4] Fejerskov O, Kidd E. Dental caries: the disease and its clinical management. 2nd ed. Oxford, UK: Blackwell Munksgaard; 2011.

[5] Allaker RP. The use of nanoparticles to control oral biofilm formation. J Dent Res 2010; 89:1175–86.

[6] von der Fehr FR, Löe H, Theilade E. Experimental caries in man. Caries Res 1970; 4:131-48.

[7] Naik S, Sureshchandra B. Antimicrobial efficacy of glass ionomers, composite resin, liners & polycarboxylates against selected stock culture microorganisms: an in vitro study. Endodontology 2012; 24(2):21-8.

[8] Selwitz RH, Ismail AI, Pitts NB. Dental caries. Lancet 2007; 369:51-9.

[9] Marsh PD. Dental plaque: biological significance of a biofilm and community life-style. J Clin Periodontol 2005; 32:7–15.

[10] Fine DH, Markowitz K, Furgang D, Goldsmith D, Ricci-Nittel D, Charles CH, et al. Effect of rinsing with an essential oil-containing mouthrinse on subgingival perio-dontopathogens. J Periodontol 2007; 78:1935–42.

[11] Zobell CE. The effect of solid surfaces upon bacterial activity. J Bacteriol 1943; 46:39-56.

[12] Costerton JW, Stewart PS, Greenberg EP. Bacterial biofilms: a common cause of per-sistent infections. Science 1999; 284:1318-22.

[13] Tuson HH, Weibel DB. Bacteria–surface interactions. Soft Matter 2013; 9:4368-80.

[14] Renner LD, Weibel DB. Physicochemical regulation of biofilm formation. MRS Bull 2011 May; 36(5):347-55.

[15] Petersen FC, Tao L, Scheie AA. DNA binding-uptake system: a link between cell-to-cell communication and biofilm formation. J. Bacteriol 2005; 187:4392.

[16] Witchurch CB, Tolker-Nielsen T, Ragas PC, Mattick JS. Extracellular DNA required for bacterial biofilm formation. Science 2002; 295:1487.

[17] Bowen WH, Koo H. Biology of Streptococcus mutans-Derived Glucosyltransferases: Role in Extracellular Matrix Formation of Cariogenic Biofilms. Caries Research 2011; 45:69-86.

[18] Lembre P, Lorentz C, Di Martino P. Exopolysaccharides of the Biofilm Matrix: A Complex Biophysical World. In: Karunaratne DN. (ed). The Complex World of Polysaccharides. Rijeka: InTech; 2012. p371-392. Available from http://www.intechopen.com/books/the-complex-world-of-polysaccharides/exopolysaccharides-of-the-biofilm-matrix-a-complex-biophysical-world (accessed 27 August 2014).

[19] Palmer RJ. Oral bacterial biofilms–history in progress. Microbiology 2009; 155:2113-4.

[20] Mikkelsen H, Duck Z, Lilley KS, Welch M. Interrelationships between colonies, biofilms, and planktonic cells of *Pseudomonas aeruginosa*. J Bacteriol. 2007; 189(6): 2411-6.

[21] Renye JA, Piggot PJ, Daneo-Moore L, Buttaro BA. Persistence of Streptococcus mutans in Stationary-Phase Batch Cultures and Biofilms, Applied Environm Microbiol 2004; 70(10):6181-7.

[22] Guggenheim B, Giertsen E, Schüpbach P, Shapiro S. Validation of an *in vitro* biofilm model of supragingival plaque. J Dent Res. 2001; 80(1):363-70.

[23] Netuschil L, Auschill TM, Sculean A, Arweiler NB. Confusion over live/dead stainings for the detection of vital microorganisms in oral biofilms-which stain is suitable? BMC Oral Health 2014; 14:2.

[24] Teughels W, Van Assche N, Sliepen I, Quirynen M. Effect of material characteristics and/or surface topography on biofilm development. Clin Oral Implants Res 2006; 17(2):68-81.

[25] Busscher HJ, Rinastiti M, Siswomihardjo W, van der Mei HC. Biofilm formation on dental restorative and implant materials. J Dent Res 2010; 89(7):657-65.

[26] Allaker RP, Ren G. Potential impact of nanotechnology in the control of infectious diseases. Trans R Soc Trop Med Hyg 2008; 102:1-2.

[27] Pinheiro SL, Simionato MR, Imparato JC, Oda M. Antibacterial activity of glass-ionomer cement containing antibiotics on caries lesion. Am J Dent 2005; 18(4):261-6.

[28] Imazato S. Bio-active restorative materials with antibacterial effects: new dimension of innovation in restorative dentistry. Dental Materials J. 2009; 28(1):11-19.

[29] Auschill TM, Arweiler NB, Brecx M, Reich E, Sculean A, Netuschil L: The effect of dental restorative materials on dental biofilm. Eur J Oral Sci. 2002; 110:48-53.

[30] Chen M. Novel strategies for the prevention and treatment of biofilm related infections. Int J Mol Sci 2013; 14(9):18488-501.

[31] Lin CL, Chang CH, Wang CH, Ko CC, Lee HE. Numerical investigation of the factors affecting interfacial stresses in an MOD restored tooth by auto-meshed finite element method. J Oral Rehabil 2001; 28:517-25.

[32] Toparli M, Gokay N, Aksoy T. Analysis of a restored maxillary second premolar tooth by using three-dimensional finite element method. J Oral Rehabil 1999; 26:157-64.

[33] Farah JW, Craig RG. Finite element stress analysis of restored axisymmetric first molar. J Dent Res 1974; 53:859-66.

[34] Williams KR, Edmundson JT, Rees JS. Finite element stress analysis of restored teeth. Dent Mater 1987; 3:200-6.

[35] Noort R. Introduction to dental materials. 4th ed. Edinburgh; New York: Mosby Elsevier, 2013.

[36] Giertsen E. Effects of mouthrinses with triclosan, zinc ions, copolymer, and sodium lauryl sulphate combined with fluoride on acid formation by dental plaque in vivo. Caries Res 2004; 38(5):430-5.

[37] Khoroushi M, Keshani F. A review of glass-ionomers: From conventional glass-ionomer to bioactive glass-ionomer. Dent Res J. 2013; 10(4): 411-20.

[38] Osinaga PW, Grande RH, Ballester RY, Simionato MR, Delgado Rodrigues CR, Muench A. Zinc sulfate addition to glass-ionomer-based cements: Influence on physical and antibacterial properties, zinc and fluoride release. Dent Mater. 2003; 19:212–7

[39] Yesilyurt C, Er K, Tasdemir T, Buruk K, Celik D. Antibacterial activity and physical properties of glass-ionomer cements containing antibiotics. Oper Dent 2009; 1:18-23.

[40] Nakajo K, Imazato S, Takahashi Y, Kiba W, Ebisu S, Takahashi N. Fluoride Released from Glass-Ionomer Cement Is Responsible to Inhibit the Acid Production of Caries-Related Oral Streptococci. Dental Materials 2009; 25(6):703-8.

[41] Ferreira JMS, Pinheiro SL, Sampaio FC, Menezes VA. Use of glassionomer cement containing antibiotics to seal off infected dentin: a randomized clinical trial. Brazilian Dental Journal. 2013; 24(1):68-73.

[42] Jedrychowski JR, Caputo AA, Kerper S. Antibacterial and mechanical properties of restorative materials combined with chlorhexidines. J Oral Rehabil 1983; 10:373-381.

[43] Nicholson JW, Aggarwal A, Czarnecka B, Li-manowska-Shaw H. The rate of change of pH of lactic acid exposed to glass-ionomer dental cements. Biomaterials 2000; 21(19):1989-93.

[44] Konradsson K. Influence of a dental ceramic and a calcium aluminate cement on dental biofilm formation and gingival inflammatory response. Dissertation (Master Degree in Odontology). Umeå University, Sweden; 2007.

[45] Hamouda IM. Current perspectives of nanoparticles in medical and dental biomaterials. J Biomed Res 2012;26:143–151. http://www.readcube.com/articles/10.7555/JBR.26.20120027 (accessed 02 September 2014).

[46] Luna DMN, Andrade CAS. Nanotecnologia aplicada à odontologia. Int J Dent 2011; 10(3):161-8.

[47] Weng Y, Guo X, Gregory R, Xie D. A novel antibacterial dental glassionomer cement. Eur J Oral Sci 2010; 118:531-4.

[48] Frencken J, Pilot T, Songpaisan Y, Phantumvanit P. Atraumatic restorative treatment (ART): rationale, technique, and development. J Public Health Dent 1996; 56:135-40.

[49] Melo MAS, Guedes SFF, Xu HHK, Rodrigues LKA. Nanotechnology-based restorative materials for dental caries management. Trends Biotechnol 2013; 31(8):2-18.

[50] Verran J, Sandoval G, Allen NS, Edge M, Stratton J Variables affecting the antibacterial properties of nano and pigmentary titania particles in suspension. Dyes and Pigments. 2007; 73:298-304.

[51] Rehnman J. Release of nanoparticles from dental materials. A systematic map. Socialstyrelsen: Nordic Institute of Dental Materials. 2013.

[52] Sotiriou GA, Pratsinis SE. Antibacterial activity of nanosilver ions and particles. Environ Sci Technol 2010; 44:5649-54.

[53] Peng JJ, et al. Silver compounds used in dentistry for caries management: a review. J Dent 2012; 40:531-41.

[54] Chaloupka K, Malam Y, Seifalian AM. Nanosilver as a new generation of nanoproduct in biomedical applications. Trends Biotechnol Nov 2010; 28(11):580-8.

[55] Ahn SJ. Experimental antimicrobial orthodontic adhesives using nanofillers and silver nanoparticles. Dent Mater 2009; 25:206–13.

[56] Radzig MA, et al. Antibacterial effects of silver nanoparticles on gram-negative bacteria: Influence on the growth and biofilms formation, mechanisms of action. Colloids Surf B: Biointerfaces 2013; 102:300–6.

[57] Silver S. Bacterial silver resistance: molecular biology and uses and misuses of silver compounds. FEMS Microbiol Rev 2003; 27:341-53.

[58] Cheng L, Weir MD, Xu HH, Antonucci JM, Lin NJ, Lin-Gibson S, Xu SM, Zhou X. Effect of amorphous calcium phosphate and silver nanocomposites on dental plaque microcosm biofilms. J Biomed Mater Res B: Appl Biomater 2012; 100:1378-86.

[59] Espinosa-Cristóbal LF. Antimicrobial sensibility of Streptococcus mutans serotypes to silver nanoparticles. Mater Sci Eng C 2012; 32:896–901.

[60] Jones N, et al. Antibacterial activity of ZnO nanoparticle suspensions on a broad spectrum of microorganisms. FEMS Microbiol Lett 2008; 279:71-6.

[61] Gu H, et al. Effect of ZnCl$_2$ on plaque growth and biofilm vitality. Arch Oral Biol 2012; 57:369-75.

[62] Vaidyanathan M, et al. Antimicrobial properties of dentine bonding agents determined using *in vitro* and *ex vivo* methods. J Dent 2009; 37:514-21.

[63] Imazato S, et al. Antibacterial resin monomers based on quaternary ammonium and their benefits in restorative dentistry. Jpn Dent Sci Rev 2012; 48:115–25.

[64] Zhang K, et al. Effect of water-ageing on dentine bond strength and anti-biofilm activity of bonding agent containing new monomer dimethylaminododecyl methacrylate. J Dent 2013; 41:504-13.

[65] Cheng L, Weir MD, Xu HHK, Antonucci JM, Kraigsley AM, Lin NJ, Lin-Gibson S, Zhou X. Antibacterial amorphous calcium phosphate nanocomposites with a quaternary ammonium dimethacrylate and silver nanoparticles. Dent Mater 2012; 28:561-72.

[66] Xu HHK, Moreau JL, Sun L, Chow LC. Strength and fluoride release characteristics of a calcium fluoride based dental nanocomposite. Biomaterials Nov 2008; 9(32): 4261-7.

[67] Moreau JL, Sun L, Chow LC, Xu HHK. Mechanical and acid neutralizing properties and bacteria inhibition of amorphous calcium phosphate dental nanocomposite. J Biomed Mater Res B Appl Biomater Jul 2011; 98(1):80-8.

[68] Hannig C, Hannig M. Natural enamel wear: a physiological source of hydroxylapatite nanoparticles for biofilm management and tooth repair? Medical Hypothese. 2010; 74:670-2.

[69] Venegas SC, Palacios JM, Apella MC, Morando PJ, Blesa MA. Calcium modulates interactions between bacteria and hydroxyapatite. J Dent Res 2006; 85:1124-8.

[70] Arcís RW, López-Macipe A, Toledano M, Osorio E, Rodríguez-Clemente R, Murtra J, Fanovich MA, Pascual CD. Mechanical properties of visible light-cured resins reinforced with hydroxyapatite for dental restoration. Dent Mater Jan 2002; 18(1):49-57.

[71] Chen M. Novel strategies for the prevention and treatment of biofilm related infections. Int J Mol Sci 2013; 14(9):18488-501.

5

Evidence-Based Control of Oral Malodor

Nao Suzuki, Masahiro Yoneda and Takao Hirofuji

1. Introduction

Concern regarding halitosis is estimated to be the third most frequent reason for people to seek dental care, following tooth decay and periodontal disease [1]. Compared with tooth decay and periodontal disease, there are a diverse number of causes of halitosis. Table 1 shows a commonly used classification of halitosis [2 – 4]. Obvious bad breath is termed genuine halitosis, which is classified as physiological and pathological halitosis. Pathological halitosis is further sub-classified into halitosis as a result of oral and extra-oral causes. Physiological and oral pathological halitosis occur in the oral cavity, and comprise 85% or more of genuine halitosis [5, 6]. Physiological halitosis generally occurs at the time of waking or starving, and likely results from increased microbial metabolic activity that is aggravated by a physiological reduction in salivary flow, oral cleaning, and inadequate mouth cleaning before sleep or after eating [4]. Clinical causes of oral pathological halitosis include poor oral hygiene, tongue debris, periodontitis, inadequately fitted restorations, deep caries, endodontic lesions, ulceration, and low salivary flow [7 – 11]. The most common malodorous compounds that cause oral-derived malodor are volatile sulfur compounds (VSCs) such as hydrogen sulfide (H_2S) and methyl mercaptan (CH_3SH), which are associated with microbial amino acid metabolism [12, 13]. Halitosis derived from extra-oral causes is less common, but causes include respiratory disorders, gastrointestinal diseases, metabolic disorders, and drugs [2 – 4]. The smell of gases that have accumulated in organs during respiratory disorders and gastrointestinal diseases can be emitted directly from the oral cavity and nose. Malodorous components caused by some metabolic disorders and drugs circulate in the bloodstream and are exhaled in the breath after alveolar gas exchange. Components of extra-oral malodor include those due to disease, such as acetone in uncontrolled diabetes and trimethylamine in trimethylaminuria ("fish odor syndrome" [14]). Dimethyl sulfide (CH_3SCH_3), a VSC, is the main contributor to extra-oral or blood-borne halitosis via an as-yet-unknown metabolic disorder [15]. Some patients that complain of halitosis do not have bad breath. Although pseudo-halitosis is not diagnosed as a psychiatric disorder, some patients with this condition exhibit neurotic tendencies more frequently than do patients with genuine halitosis [6]. Halitophobia is characterized by a patient's persistent belief that he or she has halitosis, despite reassurance, treatment, and counseling. Many patients with halitophobia have slight bad breath at their first visit to a dental clinic. However, the presence of a mental condition together with bad breath has been suggested in these individuals.

Classification (treatment needs)	Description
Genuine halitosis	Obvious malodor, and of an intensity beyond the socially acceptable level is perceived.
Physiological halitosis (TN-1)	Malodor arises through putrefactive processes within the oral cavity. No specific diseases or pathological conditions that could cause halitosis are found.
Pathological halitosis	
Oral (TN-1 and TN-2)	Halitosis caused by a disease or a pathological condition that causes malfunction of the oral tissues.
Extra-oral (TN-1 and TN-3)	Malodor that originates from a respiratory system, gastrointestinal tract, metabolic disorders, or drugs.
Pseudo-halitosis (TN-1 and TN-4)	No objective evidence of malodor, although the patient thinks they have it.
Halitophobia (TN-1 and TN-5)	The patient persists in believing they have halitosis despite reassurance, treatment, and counseling.

Table 1. Classification of halitosis [2-4].

All patients that complain of halitosis should receive an explanation of halitosis and instructions for oral hygiene (TN-1; Table 2) [16]. Further professional instruction, education, and reassurance are necessary for patients with pseudo-halitosis (TN-4). Professional cleaning and treatment of oral diseases are performed in patients with oral pathological halitosis (TN-2), and treatment and control of the systemic causative disease by a physician or medical specialist is provided for patients with extra-oral pathological halitosis (TN-3). Medical treatment by a psychological specialist is required for the treatment of halitophobia, regardless of the presence of bad breath (TN-5).

Category	Treatment regimen
TN-1	Explanation of halitosis and instructions for oral hygiene.
TN-2	Oral prophylaxis, professional cleaning, and treatment for oral diseases, particularly periodontal diseases.
TN-3	Referral to a physician or medial specialist.
TN-4	Explanation of the examination data, further professional instructions, education, and reassurance.
TN-5	Referral to a clinical psychologist, psychiatrist, or other psychological specialist.

Table 2. Treatment needs (TN) for halitosis [2, 16] useful for clinical dentists.

Most genuine halitosis occurs in the oral cavity, and is known as oral-derived malodor. As mentioned above, VSCs are produced during the metabolism of the sulfur-containing amino acids cysteine and methionine by bacteria [12, 13]. Gram-negative anaerobes in the oral cavity are important producers of VSCs. Periodontopathic bacteria isolated from subgingival plaques, such as *Porphyromonas gingivalis*, *Prevotella intermedia*, *Tannerella forsythia*, and *Treponema denticola*, generate significant amounts of H_2S and CH_3SH [17]. The genera *Veillonella*, *Actinomyces* and *Prevotella* are H_2S-producing normal inhabitants of the tongue coating [18]. *Solobacterium moorei* is present in the tongue dorsa of subjects with halitosis, specifically [19]. A recent investigation of the bacterial composition of saliva reported that high proportions of the genera *Neisseria*, *Fusobacterium*, *Porphyromonas*, and SR1 were present in patients with high H_2S and low CH_3SH, whereas high proportions of the genera *Prevotella*, *Veillonella*, *Atopobium*, *Megasphaera*, and *Selenomonas* were detected in patients with high CH_3SH and low H_2S [20]. The human oral cavity contains more than 500 bacterial species that interact both with each other and host tissues, suggesting that various bacteria might play roles in malodor production. The treatment strategy for oral-derived malodor is the acquisition of a normal microbiota, as well as reducing the numbers of bacteria. The prevention and treatment of oral malodor involve primarily the removal of any causative clinical conditions, predominantly via oral hygiene instructions and the treatment of oral diseases. Persistent malodor usually originates from the posterior dorsum of the tongue and/or oral/dental diseases, including periodontal diseases. Tongue cleaning and the treatment of periodontal diseases are effective for improving oral malodor [21, 22]. In addition, many products such as mouthwash, dentifrice, gel, gum, oil, tablets, and lozenges can play supporting roles in controlling oral malodor. Such products improve oral malodor by reducing bacterial load and/or nutrient availability, exerting anti-inflammatory effects, and converting VSCs into non-volatile substances. The active ingredients used for controlling oral malodor can be separated into chemical agents and naturally derived compounds. Examples of chemical agents include chlorhexidine, cetylpyridinium chloride, zinc chloride, triclosan, stannous fluoride, hydrogen peroxide, chlorine dioxide, and sodium fluoride. Naturally derived compounds can be sub-classified into natural botanical extracts (e.g., actinidine, hinokitiol, eucalyptus-extract, green tea, magnolia bark extract, and pericarp extract of garcinia mangostana L), salivary components (lactoferrin and lactoperoxidase), and probiotic bacteria (*Lactobacillus salivarius*, *Lactobacillus reuteri*, *Weissella cibaria*, and *Streptococcus salivarius*). In this chapter, these various approaches to the prevention and treatment of oral malodor are summarized.

2. Chemical agents

Chlorhexidine (CHX), cetylpyridinium chloride (CPC), triclosan, zinc ions (Zn^{2+}), and chlorine dioxide (ClO_2) are all known to inhibit oral malodor [23, 24]. In many cases, these active ingredients have been used in mouthwashes and dentifrices, both individually and in combinations. CHX digluconate has been used most frequently to treat oral cavities as an active ingredient in mouthwash that is designed to reduce dental plaque and oral bacteria. CHX is used in mouthwashes at 0.12% or 0.2%, and a previous study revealed that these two concentrations of CHX had an identical effect on gingival inflammation [25]. Young et al. [26] evaluated the inhibitory effects of CHX, CPC, and Zn^{2+} on VSC production. Data revealed that 0.2% CHX and 1% Zn^{2+} exhibited excellent inhibitory effects, and had similar effects on VSC production; however, the two agents had different anti-VSC kinetics. Briefly, 0.2% CHX had a sustained inhibitory effect, whereas Zn^{2+} had an immediate effect. In contrast, 0.2% CPC had only a mild inhibitory effect on VSC production. These ingredients are found in commercial mouthwashes, often in combination. Roldán et al. [27] compared five commercial mouthwashes in a randomized, double-blind, crossover trial: 0.12% CHX alone, 0.12% CHX plus 5% alcohol, 0.12% CHX plus 0.05% CPC, 0.12% CHX plus sodium fluoride, and a combination of 0.05% CHX, 0.05% CPC, and 0.14% Zn^{2+}. In this study, the combination of 0.12% CHX plus 0.05% CPC resulted in the greatest reduction in oral bacterial numbers. In contrast, the combination of 0.05% CHX, 0.05% CPC and 0.14% Zn^{2+} provided the most immediate reduction in VSC levels. Zn^{2+} can be effective in reducing the activity of VSCs directly, in addition to its antimicrobial effect [28]. It has been reported that a combination of Zn^{2+} and CHX or CPC inhibited VSC formation synergistically [29]. ClO_2 and chlorite anion (ClO_2^-) also oxidize VSCs directly into non-malodorous products, which consumes the amino acids that act as precursors to VSCs [30, 31]. A randomized double-blind crossover placebo-controlled clinical trial found that mouth rinsing with ClO_2 effectively reduced morning malodor for 4 h in healthy volunteers [32]. Triclosan is a broad-spectrum antibacterial agent that blocks lipid synthesis in susceptible bacteria [33]. A double-blind, crossover, randomized study comparing the VSC-reducing effects of mouthwashes on morning bad breath in healthy subjects reported that VSC formation was inhibited by, in descending order, mouthwashes containing 0.12% CHX gluconate, 0.03% triclosan, essential oils, and 0.05% CPC [34].

However, there are concerns regarding the potential side effects of these chemical agents. The use of 0.2% CHX results in an unpleasant bitter taste, perturbs taste, causes desquamative lesions and soreness of the oral mucosa, and yellow/brown staining of the teeth and dorsum of the tongue [35]. Hypersensitivity to CHX is rare, but several immediate-type allergies such as contact urticarial, occupational asthma, and anaphylactic shock have been reported [36, 37]. In Japan, based on these reports, the concentration of CHX used near a wound is limited to 0.05%, which is lower than its effective concentration. Recently, the possibility that triclosan is hazardous to human health has been suggested. Several studies reported that triclosan might contribute to bacterial resistance to antibiotics, or interfere with endocrine functions in rats [38, 39]. The US Food and Drug Administration (FDA) named triclosan in the National Toxicology Program (NTP) for toxicological evaluation.

3. Naturally derived compounds (Table 3)

3.1. Natural botanical extracts

Due to the increase in health consciousness, many flavors and natural botanical extracts have been added to foods and medicine to reduce oral malodor. In addition, the effects of natural botanical extracts on oral malodor have been evaluated in randomized controlled trials.

Study	Conditions for the assessment (the period that avoided oral activities, mouth cleaning, etc.)	Study population (Age)	Study design	Follow-up time	Active ingredient	Study group	Sample size	Pretreatment	Vehicle	Frequency (washout period)	Malodor assessment	Results
Natural botanical extracts												
Tanaka et al [41].	4:30–6:30 pm (at least 4 h)	Volunteers with gingivitis or mild periodontitis (20–50 years)	Double-blind, randomized, placebo-controlled parallel trial	14 weeks	Eucalyptus extract	High-concentration (0.6%), low-concentration (0.4%), and placebo	32, 32, and 33, respectively	Full-mouth supragingival scaling	Chewing gum	Two tablets for 5 min, five times daily for 12 weeks	OLT score, VSCs by GC	The OLT score decreased significantly at 4, 8, 12 and 14 weeks in the 0.4%- and 0.6%-eucalyptus extract groups but not in the placebo group. The group-time interactions revealed significant reductions in the OLT score and VSCs in both experimental groups compared with the placebo group.
Rassameemasmaung et al [47].	7:00-8:30 am (at least 2 h)	Gingivitis patients (18–55 years)	Double-blind, placebo-controlled parallel trial	4 weeks	Green tea extract	Green tea and placebo	Both n = 30	None	Mouthwash	Twice daily for 4 weeks	VSCs by Halimeter	The VSC levels decreased significantly at 30 min, 3 h, and day 28 in the green tea group. On day 28 there was a significant difference between the green tea and placebo group.
Rassameemasmaung et al [49].	8:00 am (at least 2 h)	Gingivitis patients (17–37 years)	Double-blind, randomized, placebo-controlled parallel trial	8 weeks	The pericarp extract of Garcinia mangostana L.	Garcinia and placebo	Both n = 30	1) None 2) Scaling	Mouthwash	Twice daily for 2 weeks (4 weeks)	VSCs by Halimeter	1) The VSC levels decreased significantly in the Garcinia group compared with baseline and the placebo group. 2) The VSC levels in the Garcinia group was reduced significantly compared with the placebo group, but not with baseline.
Iha et al [52].	At the same time of day (at least 5 h)	Patients with oral malodor (33–71 years)	Randomized, open-label, parallel trial	4 weeks	Hinokitiol	Hinokitiol and 0.01% CPC	Both n = 9	None	Gel	Three times daily, for 4 weeks	OLT score, H_2S and CH_3SH levels using GC	The OLT score, and the levels of H_2S and CH_3SH were reduced significantly in the hinokitiol group, whereas the OLT score was improved significantly in the 0.01% CPC group.
Nohno et al [54].	Morning (at least 4 h)	Male volunteers (24–54 years)	Double-blind, randomized, placebo-controlled crossover trial	4 weeks	Actinidine	Actinidine and placebo	Both n = 14	None	Tablet	Three times daily, for a week (2 weeks)	VSCs by Oral Chroma	The VSC levels were reduced significantly in both the test and placebo groups after just taking a tablet. The VSC level was reduced significantly in the test group, but not in the placebo group, after use for 1 week.

Study	Conditions for the assessment (the period that avoided oral activities, mouth cleaning, etc.)	Study population (Age)	Follow-up time	Active ingredient	Study group	Sample size	Pretreatment	Vehicle	Frequency (washout period)	Malodor assessment	Results
Salivary components											
Shin et al [57].	Morning (from the midnight before)	Volunteers with oral malodor (26–54 years)	1 week	Double-blind, randomized, placebo-controlled crossover trial	Lactoferrin and Lactoperoxidase	Lactoferrin and Lactoperoxidase, and placebo	Both $n = 15$	None	Tablet	Twice at a 1-h interval in the morning (1 week)	H_2S, CH_3SH, and total VSCs by GC	The CH_3SH level was significantly lower in the test group compared with the placebo group 10 min after the first ingestion. The median concentration of CH_3SH in the test group was below the olfactory threshold from 10 min until 2 h, whereas the level in the placebo group remained above the threshold during the experimental period.
Probiotic bacteria											
Kang et al [58].	7:00–8:00 am (from the evening before)	Student volunteers (20–30 years)	1 day	Open label crossover trial	Weissella cibaria CMU	W. cibaria CMU, Lactobacillus casei, Weissella confusa, and distilled water	46, 10, 10, and 46, respectively	None	Solution	15 mL for 2 min, twice daily	H_2S and CH_3SH using Oral Chroma	Rinsing of the mouth with solutions containing W. cibaria CMU twice a day significantly reduced H_2S and CH_3SH the next morning; L. casei, W. confusa, and distilled water had no effect.
Burton et al [63].	Morning (from awakening)	Subjects with oral malodor (18–69 years)	1 week	Open label parallel trial	Streptococcus salivarius K12	S. salivarius K12 and placebo	13 and 10	Mechanical and chemical oral cleansing treatment	Lozenge	Day 1: at 2-h intervals over 8 h. Afterwards: twice daily for a week	VSCs by Halimeter	The VSC levels 1 week after treatment initiation was reduced significantly in the test group compared with the placebo group.
Keller et al [70].	Morning (from the evening before)	Young adult volunteers (19–25 years)	7 weeks	Double-blind, randomized, placebo-controlled crossover trial	Lactobacillus reuteri DSM 17938 and ATCC PTA 5289	L. reuteri and placebo	Both $n = 25$	None	Chewing gum	Twice daily for 2 weeks (3 weeks)	OLT, VSCs by Halimeter	The OLT score was significantly lower in the probiotic group compared with the placebo group. The VSC levels were not significantly different between groups.
Suzuki et al [76].	At the same time of day (at least 5 h)	Patients with oral malodor (22–67 years)	6 weeks	Double-blind, randomized crossover trial	Lactobacillus salivarius WB21	L. salivarius WB21 and placebo	Both $n = 23$	None	Tablet	Three daily for 2 weeks (2 weeks)	OLT, VSCs by GC	The OLT score was reduced significantly in both the probiotic and placebo periods. VSC levels were reduced significantly in the probiotic period but not in the placebo period.

OLT, organoleptic test; VSCs, volatile sulfur compounds; GC, gas chromatography; H_2S, hydrogen sulfide; CH_3SH, methyl mercaptan.

Table 3. Clinical trials to evaluate the effects of naturally derived compounds on reducing oral malodor.

Eucalyptus extract is one of the four active ingredients of Listerine® mouthwash (Pfizer Inc., Morris Plains, NJ, USA), which was created in 1879 and was formulated originally as a surgical antiseptic. It has antibacterial activity against several periodontopathic bacteria including *P. gingivalis* and *P. intermedia*, which produce VSCs [40]. The effect on oral malodor of chewing gum containing eucalyptus extract was evaluated in a double-blind randomized trial over a 12-week period [41]. Relative to baseline, organoleptic test (OLT) scores decreased significantly at 4, 8, 12, and 14 weeks in the 0.4%-and 0.6%-eucalyptus extract groups, but not in the placebo group. In addition, the group-time interactions revealed significant reductions in OLT scores, VSC levels, and tongue-coating scores in both eucalyptus concentration groups compared with the placebo group.

The catechins present in green tea have *in vitro* bactericidal activity against the odor-producing periodontal bacteria *P. gingivalis* and *Prevotella* spp. [42], inhibit the adherence of *P. gingivalis* to oral epithelial cells [43], and reduce periodontal breakdown by inhibiting the collagenase and cysteine proteinase activity of *P. gingivalis* [44, 45]. It was reported that green tea powder reduced VSC concentrations in mouth air immediately after administration [46]. A double-blind placebo-controlled clinical trial found that rinsing the mouth with green tea containing mouthwash twice per day significantly reduced VSC levels at 30 min, 3 h, and day 28, compared with baseline [47]. There was a significant difference between the green tea group and the placebo group at day 28 [47].

Pericarp extracts of *Garcinia mangostana*, which is commonly known as the mangosteen tree, exert antimicrobial activity against the oral bacteria *Streptococcus mutans* and *P. gingivalis*, and exhibit anti-inflammatory effects [48]. The use of mouthwash containing pericarp extracts of *G. mangostana* twice daily for 2 weeks reduced VSC levels significantly compared with baseline and the placebo group [49]. Furthermore, rinsing with mouthwash containing *G. mangostana* L for 2 weeks after scaling and polishing reduced VSC level significantly compared with placebo, whereas there was no significant difference between baseline and day 15 [49].

Hinokitiol (β-thujaplicin), a component of essential oils isolated from Cupressaceae, shows antibacterial activity against various bacteria, including periodontopathic bacteria and fungi [50, 51], and has been used as a therapeutic agent against periodontal disease and oral *Candida* infections. An open-label, randomized, controlled trial was performed in patients with genuine halitosis to evaluate the effects of mouth cleaning using hinokitiol-containing gels on oral malodor [52]. Mouth cleaning, including the teeth, gingiva, and tongue, was performed three times per day for 4 weeks. Organoleptic test (OLT) scores, levels of H_2S and CH_3SH, the frequency of bleeding on probing, mean probing pocket depths, and plaque indices were improved significantly in the group treated using the hinokitiol-containing gel. In contrast, only OLT scores improved significantly in the control group treated using 0.01% CPC-containing control gel.

Actidinine is a cysteine protease derived from the kiwi fruit. Tongue coating is understood to be an important factor in oral malodor and is composed of proteins [22, 53]. The effect of a tablet containing actidinine on oral malodor was evaluated in a double-blind, randomized crossover trial [54]. The subjects sucked the tablets three times per day for 1 week. VSC levels and tongue-coating ratios decreased significantly on the first day in both the test and placebo groups immediately after taking a tablet. VSC levels were significantly lower after 7 days only in the test group. There was no significant reduction in tongue-coating ratios in either group after 7 days of use.

3.2. Salivary components

Saliva contains a variety of antimicrobial proteins including lactoferrin, peroxidase, lysozyme, and secretory immunoglobulin A. Lactoferrin is an iron-binding glycoprotein that chelates two ferric ions per molecule, and decreases bacterial growth, biofilm development, iron overload, reaction oxygen formation, and inflammatory processes [55]. Salivary peroxidase, in the presence of H_2O_2 and SCN-, can reversibly inhibit bacterial enzyme and transport systems by oxidizing the sulfhydryl groups of proteins [56]. A reduction in salivary flow might inhibit antimicrobial defense systems in saliva. A relationship between low salivary flow and the generation of H_2S and CH_3SH in mouth air has been reported previously [8].

The effect of a tablet containing lactoferrin and lactoperoxidase purified from bovine milk on oral malodor was evaluated in a randomized, double-blind, crossover, placebo-controlled clinical trial [57]. According to that study, CH_3SH levels were significantly lower in the test group compared with the placebo group 10 min after taking a tablet. The median CH_3SH concentration in the test group was below the olfactory threshold between 10 min and 2 h, whereas the level in the placebo group was above the threshold throughout the experimental period.

3.3. Probiotic bacteria

The use of probiotics as preventative and therapeutic products for oral healthcare is a novel antimicrobial approach that has been proposed as an alternative to chemotherapeutics. Probiotics are defined as "live microorganisms that confer a health benefit on the host when administered in adequate amounts" by the World Health Organization and the Food and Agriculture Organization of the United States (http://www.who.int/foodsafety/fs_management/en/probiotic_guidelines.pdf). Probiotics have been used traditionally to treat diseases related to the gastrointestinal tract. Recently, the use of such probiotics to improve oral health has attracted increasing attention, although this field is still in its infancy. Nevertheless, there are several reports related to the use of probiotics to ameliorate oral malodor.

Kang et al. isolated three peroxide-generating lactobacilli, identified as *W. cibaria*, from the saliva of kindergarten children aged 4–7 years who had little supragingival plaque and no oral disease, including dental caries [58]. These isolates co-aggregated with *F. nucleatum*, inhibited VSC production by *F. nucleatum*, and prevented proliferation by *F. nucleatum in vitro*. Subsequently, the effect of *W. cibaria* CMU on morning odor was evaluated in a clinical trial of healthy volunteers. Rinsing the mouth using solutions containing *W. cibaria* CMU twice per day reduced production of H_2S and CH_3SH the next morning significantly. Conversely, use of solutions containing distilled water, *Lactobacillus casei*, and *Weissella confusa* had no effect.

Streptococcus salivarius K12 has been used to prevent the pharyngitis and tonsillitis induced by *Streptococcus pyogenes*. *S. salivarius* was selected as an oral probiotic because it is an early colonizer of oral surfaces and is the predominant member of tongue microbiota numerically in 'healthy' individuals [19, 59]. *S. salivarius* K12 produces two bacteriocins: salivaricin A and salivaricin B [60, 61]. It exerts inhibitory activities against oral malodor-related oral bacteria, such as *Atopobium parvulum*, *Eubacterium sulci*, and *S. moorei*, to varying extents [62]. According to an additional *in vitro* study, inhibitory effects were observed against *Streptococcus anginosus*, *Eubacterium saburreum*, and *Peptostreptococcus micros*, but not *P. gingivalis* and *P. intermedia* [63]. This report described the results of a preliminary clinical trial that administered lozenges containing either *S. salivarius* K12 or placebo. The subjects undertook a 3-day regimen of CHX mouth rinsing followed by the use of lozenges at specific intervals. The VSC levels 1 week after the initiation of treatment were reduced significantly in the *S. salivarius* K12 group compared with the placebo group. The salivary bacterial composition was examined using PCR-denaturing gradient gel electrophoresis, and data revealed that it changed in most subjects following K12 treatment, albeit to differing extents.

Lactobacillus reuteri is a member of the indigenous oral microbiota in humans, and it exerts antibacterial properties by converting glycerol into reuterin, a broad-spectrum antimicrobial substance [64]. Products that contain *L. reuteri* have been marketed for the prevention and treatment of gingivitis and periodontal disease [65-67]. However, data are conflicting regarding the potential of *L. reuteri* for caries management, as some studies reported useful effects whereas other did not [68, 69]. The effect of chewing gum containing two strains of probiotic lactobacilli (*L. reuteri* DSM 17938 and *L. reuteri* ATCC PTA 5289) on oral malodor was evaluated in a randomized double-blinded placebo-controlled crossover trial [70]. The study populations were healthy volunteers, and the study design included two intervention periods of 2 weeks with a 3-week washout period. The organoleptic scores were significantly lower in the probiotic group compared with the placebo group. However, there were no differences in VSC levels between the two groups, either before or after rinsing with L-cysteine. The researchers hypothesized that the probiotic gum might have affected bacteria that produce malodorous compounds other than VSCs.

Lactobacillus salivarius WB21 is an acid-tolerant lactobacillus derived from *L. salivarius* WB1004 [71], and is a potentially effective probiotic against *Helicobacter pylori*. Oral consumption of tablets containing *L. salivarius* WB21 was reported to improve periodontal conditions in healthy volunteer smokers and reduce the numbers of the periodontopathic bacterium *T. forsythia* in subgingival plaque [72, 73]. A double-blind, randomized, placebo-controlled clinical trial using oils containing *L. salivarius* WB21 in patients with periodontal disease reported reduced bleeding on probing compared with the placebo group after 2 weeks [74]. We performed an open-label pilot study previously to evaluate whether oral administration of a tablet containing *L. salivarius* WB21 altered oral malodor or clinical conditions in patients complaining of oral malodor [75]. The organoleptic scores and concentrations of H_2S and CH_3SH were reduced in patients without periodontitis after 2 weeks of treatment, and the organoleptic scores and bleeding on probing were decreased in patients with periodontitis after 4 weeks. Subsequently, we performed a 14-day, double-blind, randomized, placebo-controlled crossover trial using tablets containing *L. salivarius* WB21 or placebo taken orally by patients with oral malodor [76]. The organoleptic scores were decreased significantly in both the probiotic and placebo periods compared with the baseline scores, and there was no difference between periods. Compared with the values at baseline, the concentrations of total VSCs decreased significantly in the probiotic period but not in the placebo period, and significant differences were observed between the two periods. In addition, the mean probing pocket depth decreased significantly in the probiotic period compared with the placebo period. Quantitative analysis of the bacteria in saliva found significantly lower levels of ubiquitous bacteria and *F. nucleatum* during the probiotic period.

4. Conclusions

Chemical agents have been used widely to prevent and treat oral malodor. However, long-term use of some antiseptic agents such as CHX might result in complications such as staining of teeth and the development of microbial resistance. In addition, recent studies have raised concern regarding the potentially harmful effects of triclosan on the human body. These phenomena and consumers' increasing health consciousness have led to the development of alternative antimicrobial approaches, including herbs, natural botanical extracts, salivary components, and probiotics. Diverse natural products have been marketed as effective for preventing and treating oral malodor, and an increasingly diverse range of strategies for oral malodor is available. However, few studies have demonstrated effectiveness of new products against oral malodor clinically. Furthermore, most studies evaluated the short-term effects of products on oral malodor, either immediately or only a few weeks after taking the products. However, the products used for preventing and treating oral malodor, including mouthwash, toothpaste, tablets, and lozenges, are generally used for the long term. Therefore, the long-term effects of agents on oral malodor, as well as their safety and side effects, should be evaluated in randomized controlled trials.

Author details

Nao Suzuki*, Masahiro Yoneda and Takao Hirofuji

*Address all correspondence to: naojsz@college.fdcnet.ac.jp

Section of General Dentistry, Department of General Dentistry, Fukuoka Dental College, Japan

References

[1] Loesche WJ, Kazor C. Microbiology and treatment of halitosis. Periodontol 2000 2002;28:256–79.

[2] Yaegaki K, Coil JM. Examination, classification, and treatment of halitosis; clinical perspectives. J Can Dent Assoc 2000;66:257–61.

[3] Murata T, Yamaga T, Iida T, Miyazaki H, Yaegaki K. Classification and examination of halitosis. Int Dent J 2002;52:181–6.

[4] Scully C, Greenman J. Halitosis (breath odor). Periodontol 2000 2008;48:66–75.

[5] Delanghe G, Ghyselen J, van Steenberghe D, Feenstra L. Multidisciplinary breath-odour clinic. Lancet 1997;350:187.

[6] Suzuki N, Yoneda M, Naito T, Iwamoto T, Hirofuji T. Relationship between halitosis and psychologic status. Oral Surg Oral med Oral Pathol Oral Radiol Endod 2008;106:542–7.

[7] Morita M, Wang HL. Association between oral malodor and adult periodontitis: a review. J Clin Periodontol 2001;28:813–9.

[8] Koshimune S, Awano S, Gohara K, Kurihara E, Ansai T, Takehara T. Low salivary flow and volatile sulfur compounds in mouth air. Oral Surg Oral Med Oral Pathol Oral Radiol Endod 2003;96:38–41.

[9] Yoneda M, Naito T, Suzuki N, Yoshikane T, Hirofuji T. Oral malodor associated with internal resorption. J Oral Sci 2006;48:89–92.

[10] Garrett NR. Poor oral hygiene, wearing dentures at night, perceptions of mouth dryness and burning, and lower educational level may be related to oral malodor in denture wearers. J Evid Based Dent Pract 2010;10:67–9.

[11] Tangerman A, Winkel EG. Extra-oral halitosis: an overview. J Breath Res 2010;4:017003.

[12] Scully C, Porter S, Greenman J. What to do about halitosis. BMJ 1994;308:217–8.

[13] Tonzetich J. Production and origin of oral malodor: a review of mechanisms and methods of analysis. J Periodontol 1977;48:13–20.

[14] Whittle CL, Fakharzadeh S, Eades J, Preti G. Human breath odors and their use in diagnosis. Ann N Y Acad Sci 2007;1098:252–66.

[15] Tangerman A, Winkel EG. Intra-and extra-oral halitosis: finding of a new form of extra-oral blood-borne halitosis caused by dimethyl sulphide. J Clin Periodontol 2007;34:748–55.

[16] Coil J, Yaegaki K, Matsuo T, Miyazaki H. Treatment needs (TN) and practical remedies for halitosis. Int Dent J 2002;52:187–91.

[17] Persson S, Edlund MB, Claesson R, Carlsson J. The formation of hydrogen sulfide and methyl mercaptan by oral bacteria. Oral Microbiol Immunol 1990;5:195–201.

[18] Washio J, Sato T, Koseki T, Takahashi N. Hydrogen sulfide-producing bacteria in tongue biofilm and their relationship with oral malodour. J Med Microbiol 2005;54:889–95.

[19] Kazor CE, Mitchell PM, Lee AM, Stokes LN, Loesche WJ, Dewhirst FE, Paster BJ. Diversity of bacterial populations on the tongue dorsa of patients with halitosis and healthy patients. J Clin Microbiol 2003;41:558–63.

[20] Takeshita T, Suzuki N, Nakano Y, Yasui M, Yoneda M, Shimazaki Y, Hirofuji T, Yamashita Y. Discrimination of the oral microbiota associated with high hydrogen sulfide and methyl mercaptan production. Sci Rep 2012;2:215.

[21] Kuo YW, Yen M, Fetzer S, Lee JD. Toothbrushing versus toothbrushing plus tongue cleaning in reducing halitosis and tongue coating: a systematic review and meta-analysis. Nurs Res 2013;62:442–9.

[22] Pham TA, Ueno M, Zaitsu T, Takehara S, Shinada K, Lam PH, Kawaguchi Y. Clinical trial of oral malodor treatment in patients with periodontal diseases. J Periodontal Res 2011;46:722–9.

[23] Fedorowicz Z, Aljufairi H, Nasser M, Outhouse TL, Pedrazzi V. Mouthrinses for the treatment of halitosis. Cochrane Database Syst Rev 2008;8:CD006701.

[24] Riley P, Lamont T. Triclosan/copolymer containing toothpastes for oral health. Cochrane Database Syst Rev 2013;12:CD010514.

[25] Berchier CE, Slot DE, Van der Weijden GA. The efficacy of 0.12% chlorhexidine mouthrinse compared with 0.2% on plaque accumulation and periodontal parameters: a systematic review. J Clin Periodontol 2010;37:829–39.

[26] Young A, Jonski G, Rölla G. Inhibition of orally produced volatile sulfur compounds by zinc, chlorhexidine or cetylpyridinium chloride--effect of concentration. Eur J Oral Sci 2003;111:400–4.

[27] Roldán S, Herrera D, Santa-Cruz I, O'Connor A, González I, Sanz M. Comparative effects of different chlorhexidine mouth-rinse formulations on volatile sulphur compounds and salivary bacterial counts. J Clin Periodontol 2004;31:1128–34.

[28] Young A, Jonski G, Rölla G, Wåler SM. Effects of metal salts on the oral production of volatile sulfur-containing compounds (VSC). J Clin Periodontol 2001;28:776–81.

[29] Young A, Jonski G, Rölla G. Combined effect of zinc ions and cationinc anitibacterial agents on intraoral volatile sulphur compounds (VSC). Int Dent J 2003;53:237–42.

[30] Lynch E, Sheerin A, Claxson AW, Atherton MD, Rhodes CJ, Silwood CJ, Naughton DP, Grootveld M. Multicomponent spectroscopic investigations of salivary antioxidant consumption by an oral rinse preparation containing the stable free radical species chlorine dioxide (ClO_2). Free Radic Res 1997;26:209–34.

[31] Kim JS, Park JW, Kim DJ, Kim YK, Lee JY. Direct effect of chlorine dioxide, zinc chloride and chlorhexidine solution on the gaseous volatile sulfur compounds. Acta Odontol Scand 2014;72:645–50.

[32] Shinada K, Ueno M, Konishi C, Takehara S, Yokoyama S, Kawaguchi Y. A randomized double blind crossover placebo-controlled clinical trial to assess the effects of a mouthwash containing chlorine dioxide on oral malodor. Trials 2008;9:71.

[33] Levy CW, Roujeinikova A, Sedelnikova S, Baker PJ, Stuitje AR, Slabas AR, Rice DW, Rafferty JB. Molecular basis of triclosan activity. Nature 1999;398:383–4.

[34] Carvalho MD, Tabchoury CM, Cury JA, Toledo S, Nogueira-Filho GR. Impact of mouthrinses on morning bad breath in healthy subjects. J Clin Periodontol 2004;31:85–90.

[35] Gürgan CA, Zaim E, Bakirsoy I, Soykan E. Short-term side effects of 0.2% alcohol-free chlorhexidine mouthrinse used as an adjunct to non-surgical periodontal treatment: a double-blind clinical study. J Periodontol 2006;77:370–84.

[36] Nikaido S, Tanaka M, Yamato M, Minami T, Akatsuka M, Mori H. Anaphylactoid shock caused by chlorhexidine gluconate. Masui (Japanese) 1998;47:330–4.

[37] Krautheim AB, Jermann TH, Bircher AJ. Chlorhexidine anaphylaxis: case report and review of the literature. Contact Dermatitis 2004;50:113–6.

[38] Aiello AE, Larson EL, Levy SB. Consumer antibacterial soaps: effective of just risky? Clin Infect Dis 2007;45 Suppl 2:S137–47.

[39] Stoker TE, Gibson EK, Zorrilla LM. Triclosan exposure modulates estrogen-dependent responses in the female wistar rat. Toxicol Sci 2010;117:45–53.

[40] Nagata H, Inagaki Y, Yamamoto Y, Maeda K, Kataoka K, Osawa K, Shizukuishi S. Inhibitory effects of macrocarpals on the biological activity of *Porphyromonas gingivalis* and other periodontopathic bacteria. Oral Microbiol Immunol 2006;21:159–63.

[41] Tanaka M, Toe M, Nagata H, Ojima M, Kuboniwa M, Shimizu K, Osawa K, Shizukuishi S. Effect of eucalyptus-extract chewing gum on oral malodor: a double-masked, randomized trial. J Periodontol 2010;81:1564–71.

[42] Hirasawa M, Takada K, Makimura M, Otake S. Improvement of periodontal status by green tea catechin using a local delivery system: a clinical pilot study. J Periodontal Res 2002;37:433–8.

[43] Sakanaka S, Aizawa M, Kim M, Yamamoto T. Inhibitory effects of green tea polyphenols on growth and cellular adherence of an oral bacterium, *Porphyromonas gingivalis*. Biosci Biotechnol Biochem 1996;60:745–9.

[44] Makimura M, Hirasawa M, Kobayashi K, Indo J, Sakanaka S, Taguchi T, Otake S. Inhibitory effect of tea catechins on collagenase activity. J Periodontol 1993;64:630–6.

[45] Okamoto M, Sugimoto A, Leung KP, Nakayama K, Kamaguchi A, Maeda N. Inhibitory effect of green tea catechins on cysteine proteinases in *Porphyromonas gingivalis*. Oral Microbiol Immunol 2004;19:118–20.

[46] Lodhia P, Yaegaki K, Khakbaznejad A, Imai T, Sato T, Tanaka T, Murata T, Kamoda T. Effect of green tea on volatile sulfur compounds in mouth air. J Nutr Sci Vitaminol 2008;54:89–94.

[47] Rassameemasmaung S, Phusudsawang P, Sangalungkarn V. Effect of green tea mouthwash on oral malodor. ISRN Prev Med 2012;2013:975148.

[48] Nakatani K, Nakahata N, Arakawa T, Yasuda H, Ohizumi Y. Inhibition of cyclooxygenase and prostaglandin E2 synthesis by gamma-mangostin, a xanthone derivative in mangosteen, in C6 rat glioma cells. Biochem Pharmacol 2002;63:73–9.

[49] Rassameemasmaung S, Sirikulsathean A, Amornchat C, Hirunrat K, Rojanapanthu P, Gritsanapan W. Effects of herbal mouthwash containing the pericarp extract of *Garcinia mangostana* L on halitosis, plaque and papillary bleeding index. J Int Acad Periodontol 2007;9:19–25.

[50] Shih YH, Chang KW, Hsia SM, Yu CC, Fuh LJ, Chi TY, Shieh TM. In vitro antimicrobial and anticancer potential of hinokitiol against oral pathogens and oral cancer cell lines. Microbiol Res 2013;168:254–62.

[51] Komaki N, Watanabe T, Ogasawara A, Sato N, Mikami T, Matsumoto T. Antifungal mechanism of hinokitiol against *Candida albicans*. Biol Pharm Bull 2008;31:735–7.

[52] Iha K, Suzuki N, Yoneda M, Takeshita T, Hirofuji T. Effect of mouth cleaning with hinokitiol-containing gel on oral malodor: a randomized, open-label pilot study. Oral Surg Oral Med Oral Pathol Oral Radiol 2013;116:433–9.

[53] Yaegaki K, Sanada K. Biochemical and clinical factors influencing oral malodor in periodontal patients. J Periodontol 1992;63:783–9.

[54] Nohno K, Yamada T, Kaneko N, Miyazaki H. Tablets containing a cysteine protease, actinidine, reduce oral malodor: a crossover study. J Breath Res 2012;6:017107.

[55] Valenti P, Antonini G. Lactoferrin: an important host defence against microbial and viral attack. Cell Mol Life Sci 2005:62;2576–87.

[56] Thomas EL, Aune TM. Lactoperoxidase, peroxide, thiocyanate antimicrobial system: correlation of sulfhydryl oxidation with antimicrobial action. Infect Immun 1978;20:456–63.

[57] Shin K, Yaegaki K, Murata T, Ii H, Tanaka T, Aoyama I, Yamauchi K, Toida T, Iwatsuki K. Effects of a composition containing lactoferrin and lactoperoxidase on oral malodor and salivary bacteria: a randomized, double-blind, crossover, placebo-controlled clinical trial. Clin Oral Investig 2011;15:485–93.

[58] Kang MS, Kim BG, Chung J, Lee HC, Oh JS. Inhibitory effect of *Weissella cibaria* isolates on the production of volatile sulphur compounds. J Clin Periodontol 2006;33:226–32.

[59] Carlsson J, Grahnén H, Jonsson G, Wikner S. Early establishment of *Streptococcus salivarius* in the mouth of infants. J Dent Res 1970;49:415–8.

[60] Upton M, Tagg JR, Wescombe P, Jenkinson HF. Intra-and interspecies signaling between *Streptococcus salivarius* and *Streptococcus pyogenes* mediated by SalA and SalA1 lantibiotic peptides. J Bacteriol 2001;183:3931–8.

[61] Hyink O, Wescombe PA, Upton M, Ragland N, Burton JP, Tagg JR. Salivaricin A2 and the novel lantibiotic salivaricin B are encoded at adjacent loci on a 190-kilobase transmissible megaplasmid in the oral probiotic strain *Streptococcus salivarius* K12. Appl Environ Microbiol 2007;73:1107–13.

[62] Masdea L, Kulik EM, Hauser-Gerspach I, Ramseier AM, Filippi A, Waltimo T. Antimicrobial activity of *Streptococcus salivarius* K12 on bacteria involved in oral malodour. Arch Oral Biol 2012;57:1041–7.

[63] Burton JP, Chilcott CN, Moore CJ, Speiser G, Tagg JR. A preliminary study of the effect of probiotic *Streptococcus salivarius* K12 on oral malodour parameters. J Appl Microbiol 2006;100:754–64.

[64] Talarico TL, Casas IA, Chung TC, Dobrogosz WJ. Production and isolation of reuterin, a growth inhibitor produced by *Lactobacillus reuteri*. Antibicrob Agents Chemother 1988;32:1854–8.

[65] Teughels W, Durukan A, Ozcelik O, Pauwels M, Quirynen M, Haytac MC. Clinical and microbiological effects of *Lactobacillus reuteri* probiotics in the treatment of chronic periodontitis: a randomized placebo-controlled study. J Clin Periodontol 2013;40:1025–35.

[66] Twetman, S, Derawi B, Keller M, Ekstrand K, Yucel-Lindberg T, Stecksén-Blicks C. Short-term effect of chewing gums containing probiotic *Lactobacillus reuteri* on the levels of inflammatory mediators in gingival crevicular fluid. Acta Odontol Scand 2009;67:19–24.

[67] Vicario M, Santos A, Violant D, Nart J, Giner L. Clinical changes in periodontal subjects with the probiotc *Lactobacillus reuteri* Prodentis: a preliminary randomized clinical trial. Acta Odontol Scand 2013;71:813–9.

[68] Çaglar E, Cildir SK, Ergeneli S, Sandalli N, Twetman S. Salivary mutans streptococci and lactobacilli levels after ingestion of the probiotic bacterium *Lactobacillus reuteri* ATCC 55730 by straws or tablets. Acta Odontol Scand 2006;64:314–8.

[69] Keller MK, Hasslöf P, Dahlén G, Stecksén-Blicks C, Twetman S. Probiotic supplements (*Lactobacillus reuteri* DSM 17938 and ATCC PTA 5289) do not affect regrowth

of mutans streptococci after full-mouth disinfection with chlorhexidine: a random-ized controlled multicenter trial. Caries Res 2012;46:140–6.

[70] Keller MK, Bardow A, Jensdottir T, Lykkeaa J, Twetman S. Effect of chewing gums containing the probiotic bacterium *Lactobacillus reuteri* on oral malodour. Acta Odon-tol Scand 2012;70:246–50.

[71] Aiba Y, Suzuki N, Kabir AM, Takagi A, Koga Y. Lactic acid-mediated suppression of *Helicobacter pylori* by the oral administration of *Lactobacillus salivarius* as a probiotic in a gnotobiotic murine model. Am J Gastroenterol 1998;93:2097–101.

[72] Shimauchi H, Mayanagi G, Nakaya S, Minamibuchi M, Ito Y, Yamaki K, Hirata H. Improvement of periodontal condition by probiotics with *Lactobacillus salivarius* WB21: a randomized, double-blind, placebo-controlled study. J Clin Periodontol 2008;35:897–905.

[73] Mayanagi G, Kimura M, Nakaya S, Hirata H, Sakamoto M, Benno Y, Shimauchi H. Probiotic effects of orally administered *Lactobacillus salivarius* WB21-containing tab-lets on periodontopathic bacteria: a double-blinded, placebo-controlled, randomized clinical trial. J Clin Periodontol 2009;36:506–13.

[74] Suzuki N, Tanabe K, Takeshita T, Yoneda M, Iwamoto T, Oshiro S, Yamashita Y, Hir-ofuji T. Effects of oil drops containing *Lactobacillus salivarius* WB21 on periodontal health and oral microbiota producing volatile sulfur compounds. J Breath Res 2012;6:017106. doi:10.1088/1752-7155/6/1/017106.

[75] Iwamoto T, Suzuki N, Tanabe K, Takeshita T, Hirofuji T. Effects of probiotic *Lactoba-cillus salivarius* WB21 on halitosis and oral health: an open-label pilot trial. Oral Surg Oral Med Oral Pathol Oral Radiol Endod 2010;110:201–8.

[76] Suzuki N, Yoneda M, Tanabe K, Fujimoto A, Iha K, Seno K, Yamada K, Iwamoto T, Masuo Y, Hirofuji T. *Lactobacillus salivarius* WB21-containing tablets for the treatment of oral malodor: a double-blind, randomized, placebo-controlled crossover trial. Oral Surg Oral Med Oral Pathol Oral Radiol 2014;117:462–70.

6

Oral Fluid Biomarkers in Smoking Periodontitis Patients and Systemic Inflammation

Anna Maria Heikkinen, Päivi Mäntylä,
Jussi Leppilahti, Nilminie Rathnayake,
Jukka Meurman and Timo Sorsa

1. Introduction

Periodontitis is a chronic destructive condition caused by periodontopathogenic bacteria and inflammatory response combined with immune system effects characterized by gingival inflammation and loss of periodontal attachment and alveolar bone (Irfan et al. 2001). Host response is modified by genetic and environmental factors such as smoking (Seymour and Taylor, 2004), which has proven to be the very important risk factor for chronic periodontitis in adults (Genco and Borgnakke, 2013) as well for adolescents (Heikkinen et al. 2008, Heikkinen 2011). In periodontitis host response indeed plays an important role in the destruction of connective tissue and bone (Graves 2008). Smoking affects the immune system and impairs host response by several mechanisms both systemically and locally in saliva and gingival crevicular fluid (GCF). Systemically smoking increases the number of neutrophils in peripheral blood but their ability to migrate through capillary walls is impaired (Hind et al. 1991).

Several types of inflammatory biomarkers associating both with oral diseases and systemic diseases have been detected in saliva and GCF. These include interleukins-1β, -6 and -8 (IL-1β, -6 and -8), tumor necrosis factor-α (TNF-α) and matrix metalloproteinases (MMP)-8 and -9 (Fox 1993, Kaufman and Lamster 2000, Seymour and Gemmell 2001, Kaufman and Lamster 2002, Miller et al. 2006, Rathanayake et al. 2012 and 2013), and tissue inhibitors (TIMP)-1 of metalloproteinase (Seymour & Gemmel, 2001). Several studies have shown the association between increased MMP-8 levels and chronic periodontitis (Mäntylä et al. 2006, Kraft-Neumärker et al. 2012, Leppilahti et al. 2011). Matrix metalloproteinases (MMPs) and TIMP-1 might be candidates for monitoring periodontal status in smokers and non-smokers from oral fluids, such as GCF and saliva. GCF has a particular role in site specific diagnosis. However, saliva is easy to collect and thus more practical. Saliva is mainly composed of water (98%), and other compounds (2%) are electrolytes, glycoproteins, antibacterial compounds, and various enzymes. This unique biological fluid has multiple functions, such as rinsing, solubilisation of food substances, food and bacterial clearance, lubrication of soft tissues, bolus formation, dilution of detritus, swallowing, speech and facilitation of mastication, all of which are related to its fluid characteristics and specific components. In addition, saliva components contribute to mucosal coating, digestion and antibacterial defence (Lee & Wong, 2009).

Periodontits is a major health problem involving 10% to 60% of population depending on definition (Albandar and Rams 2002) and it is traditionally diagnosed clinically and by radiographical examinations. New methods based on oral fluid inflammatory markers have been suggested for diagnosing oral diseases and inflammation associated with systemic diseases. However, smoking has an effect on levels of several possible diagnostic biomarker candidates. Thus the aim of this chapter is to clarify the diagnostic meaning of oral fluid inflammatory biomarkers in periodontitis in smoking adolescents and adults. We also discuss systemic inflammation and possibilities to analyze it with specific biomarkers in saliva.

2. Smoking as a modifier of the host defense

Cigarette smoking is a principal modifiable environmental risk factor for periodontitis (Palmer et al. 2005). It affects the immune system by impairing host defense by inhibiting granulocyte function (Söder et al. 2002) and by neutrophil respiratory burst which causes oxidative stress in tissues (Chapple and Matthews 2007). According to previous study results by Matthews et al. (2011) cigarette smoking seems to have two-sided effect on periodontal inflammation: on one hand smoking has an effect on oxygen depletion with tissue damage and on the other hand it impairs the ability of neutrophils to response to subgingival periodontal bacteria.

Smoking decreases both the inflammatory infiltrate and number of dendritic cells (DCs) in chronic gingivitis (Souto et al., 2011). In addition it seems that smoking decreases CC chemokine ligand (CCL)3 and CXC chemokine ligand (CXCL)8, while CC chemokine ligand (CCL)5 seems to be increased in chronic periodontitis (Souto et al., 2014). Impaired neutrophil chemotaxis is observed in smokers compared to nonsmokers too (Srinivas et al. 2012). Mature DCs are involved in the production of inflammatory cytokines and Th1/Th2/Th17 immune responses in periodontal disease (Cutler and Jotwani, 2004; Allam et al., 2011). Nicotine seems to play an important role in host immune modulation. DCs differentiated in the presence of nicotine and stimulated by lipopolysaccharide induced a differentiation of naive CD4 T cells into Th2 cells. However, DCs differentiated without nicotine and stimulated by lipopolysaccharide induced Th1 immune responses (Yanagita et al. 2014).

3. Effects of smoking on oral inflammatory biomarkers

Reduced neutrophil chemotaxis and impaired phagocytosis in smokers have been shown in several studies suggesting that smokers' periodontal defence is defective compared with non-smokers (Johannsen et al. 2014). This may also be reflected in GCF and salivary content of biomarkers in smokers, which is relevant when possible point-of care diagnostic application is considered. However, the intensity and duration of smoking may also have an effect on GCF biomarker levels, but studies which take into consideration different smoking history are lacking.

In a study of Stein et al. (2006), where GCF proteins were profiled by a protein chip technology, spectral fingerprints were significantly different between smokers and non-smokers. Several spectral peaks were detected only from GCF of smokers suggesting that some proteins are there over-expressed and could potentially serve as biomarkers (Stein et al. 2006). Several studies have reported that smoking either inhibits or intensifies individual biomarkers in GCF, but contradictory findings do exist concerning some biomarkers. This underlines the effect of differences in GCF sampling and analysing methods and other study specific factors, which may lead to inter-study variation in detected biomarker levels

MMP-8, MMP-8/TIMP-1 ratio, IL-1B, myeloperoxidase (MPO), elastase, OPG and some bacterial biomarkers, so called red complex species *Tannerella forsythia, Porphyromonas gingivalis, Treponema denticola*, and *Aggregatibacter actinomycetemcomitans* have proven diagnostic properties to differentiate periodontitis from healthy sites in multiple independent studies. This has been shown both at site level in GCF samples and at patient level in saliva or mouthrinse samples (Hernandez et al. 2010, Kraft-Neumärker et al. 2012, Leppilahti et al. 2011, Leppilahti et al. 2014a,b, Mantyla et al. 2003, Nwhator et al. 2014, Ramseier et al. 2009, Rathnayake et al., 2013; Sexton et al., 2011). Analyzing of multiple biomarkers simultaneously can give even better diagnostic performance (Gursoy et al. 2011, Ramseier et al. 2009).

Nevertheless, biomarkers mentioned above have clear diagnostic properties for periodontal diseases, but many oral fluid biomarkers exhibit large variation of detected levels in both healthy and diseased sites ((Kraft-Neumärker et al 2012, Leppilahti et al. 2014, Mantyla et al. 2003, 2006). Modifying factors, such as smoking, may have an effect on the GCF biomarker levels and disturb the diagnostic interpretation, if these factors are not taken into account (Heikkinen et al. 2010, Heikkinen et al. 2012, Leppilahti et al. 2014a,b). Another reason for large variation is caused by the nature of the periodontititis itself. Progression of periodontitis is regarded to consist of quiescent periods followed by randomly occurring bursts of activity (Goodson et al. 1982, Socransky et al. 1984). Large variation of levels of inflammatory biomarkers can also be an indication of the fluctuating characteristic of peridontitis. Inflammatory GCF biomarker levels can be low in periodontitis sites during the quiet period, but levels can multiply exponentially during the burst of activity (Leppilahti et al. 2014a,b, Sorsa et al. 2010, Mäntyla et al. 2006). This means that most of GCF biomarkers do not associate with periodontitis in a linear and deterministic way, and it is the dynamics between the bursts and quiet periods that matters (Papantonopoulos et al. 2013, Papantonopoulos et al. 2014). In addition possible biomarker candidates may have a role in normal physiologic tissue regeneration. Thus, biomarkers can be used as diagnostic tool only if we can define the range of physiological levels and the cutoff for pathological bursts. One definite cutoff for a biomarker is not realistic, however, and modifying factors should be taken into account. For example, even in stable periodontitis sites after successful treatment MMP-8 levels are higher compared to healthy controls (Mäntyla et al. 200, Sorsa et al. 2010). In addition, modifying factors, such as smoking and pregnancy, has to be taken into account (Gürsoy et al. 2008, 2010, Heikkinen et al. 2010, Leppilahti et al. 2014).

Saliva would be a non-invasive sample material for oral and periodontal diagnostics. However, it is less specific than GCF and should be regarded to give a more general picture of oral health. As an example of potential diagnostic capacity of whole saliva is a study where whole saliva periodontitis associated proteome was analysed (Salazar et al. 2013). Twenty proteins were present in different abundance levels in the periodontally healthy subjects and periodontitis patients. And further, nineteen out of these 20 proteins showed higher intensities in periodontitis saliva, and eight were previously reported potential periodontitis biomarkers, among others MMP-8. Also specific protein signatures displayed characteristics of chronic periodontitis. However, effect of smoking should also be considered when salivary or oral rinse sample biomarker levels are analysed.

3.1. Matrix Metalloproteinase (MMP) -8

MMP-8 is the major collagenase in GCF, and point-of-care diagnostic tests have been developed based on analysing it (Sorsa et al. 1999; Prescher et al. 2007, Mäntylä et al. 2003, 2006, Sorsa et al. 2010). The tendency to lower MMP-8 concentrations in GCF of smokers compared to non-smokers has been observed (Persson et al. 2003) as well as lower salivary levels of MMP-8 in current smokers (Liede et al. 1999). This should be noticed when diagnostic use of MMP-8 is being considered. However, the effect of smoking on GCF MMP-8 levels seems to be two-fold. While overall MMP-8 mean level tends to be lower in GCF of smokers when compared with non-smokers, in progressing attachment loss during the maintenance phase the MMP-8 concentrations of smokers are at the same level as in non-smokers (Mäntylä et al. 2006; Leppilahti et al. 2014a). In these studies, when sites were explored in respect of repeatedly substantially elevated MMP-8 concentrations during the maintenance phase, in part of smokers' sites MMP-8 concentrations reached the highest levels of all sampled sites. Thus, lower level of MMP-8 in smokers' GCF does not relate to all sites or to all smoking periodontitis patients. For this reason when MMP-8 is considered as target for point-of-care diagnostic test different cut-off levels for MMP-8 detection should be considered for smokers and non-smokers (Leppilahti et al. 2014a). When biomarkers in saliva samples were detected and compared with periodontal health status regarding smoking as dichotomous yes-no parameter, in smokers' saliva concentration of IL-8 and MMP-8/TIMP-1 ratio were lower than in non-smokers, and salivary MMP-8 had a borderline p-value significantly lower in smokers (Rathnayake et al. 2013a). Possible explanation was considered to be the lower GCF flow of smokers, but also that the effect of smoking on periodontal inflammatory cells is reflected in saliva. In another study salivary concentration of MMP-8 differentiated periodontitis patients from controls, but in periodontitis patients who were smokers this difference was lost; however, the combination of MMP-8 and ICTP and the MMP-8/TIMP-1 ratio differentiated periodontitis cases from controls suggesting, that a combination of biomarkers could be useful when saliva is used as diagnostic sample material (Gursoy et al. 2010).

3.2. Smoking, MMP-8 and elastase levels in early periodontitis and their clinical relevance

In the study of adolescents Heikkinen et al. (2010) observed that smoking associated the lower levels of MMP-8 and PMN-leukocyte elastase (figure 1. and 2.) and the effect was strengthened by increased pack-years. However, 15% of adolescents in this birth cohort study seemed to have signs of early periodontitis (Heikkinen 2011). Salivary MMP-8 values were associated with BOP and suggestively with deep pockets in the non-smoking teenage boys. In adults MMP-8 has shown to be a key biomarker during early stages of periodontal diseases (Ramseier et al. 2009). Clinically smoking reduces the signs of gingivitis (Kumar and Faizuddin, 2011) masking periodontal diseases, and thus smokers have less observed signs of gingival inflammation, in adolescents as well as in adults, aggravating the diagnostics of periodontal disease. It is important that patients receive a proper periodontal diagnosing as part of their regular dental examination. Early diagnosis of periodontal disease could enable a successful therapeutic outcome, by reduction of etiologic factors such as smoking and by establishing periodontal therapy and maintenance protocol. Further, this might prevent the recurrence and progression of disease and reduce the incidence of tooth loss (Kumar et al. 2012). Recently Nhawator et al. (2014) demonstrated that neutrophil collagenase-2 lateral flow chair-side (point-of-care) immunoassay analysed from mouth rinse had a high sensitivity for at least two sites with BOP and two sites with periodontal pockets but a lower relationship for single-site pockets and BOP. Further studies are needed to find out the clinical relevance for this test as a screening tool in adolescents finding early periodontitis as well as for adults taking account the effect of confounders such as smoking into inflammatory biomarkers.

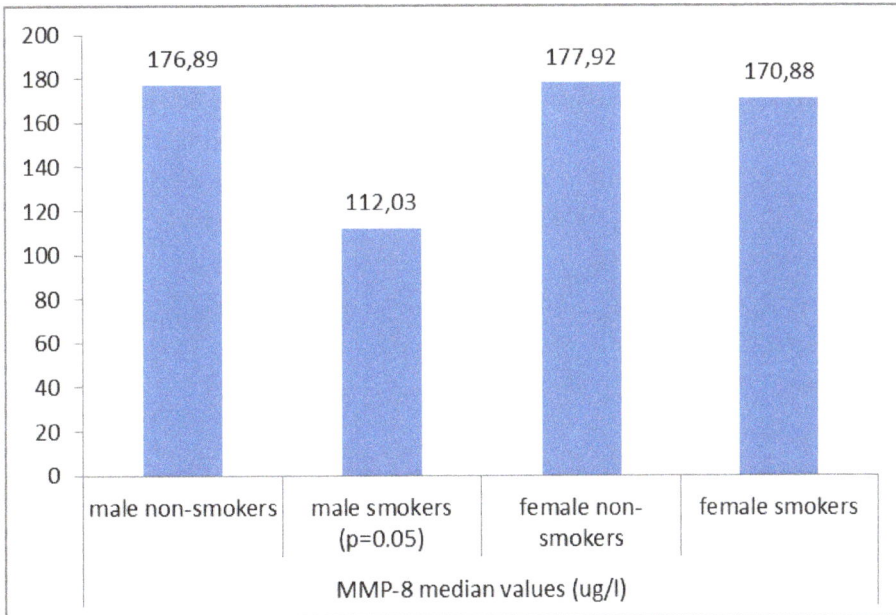

Figure 1. Salivary MMP-8 median values corresponding smoking and sex in adolescents. CI 95%s for male non-smokers, male smokers, female non-smokers and female smokers are 135.08-220.20 ug/l, 86.20-173.22 ug/l, 145.16-215.33 ug/l, 136.72-230.68 ug/l, respectively.

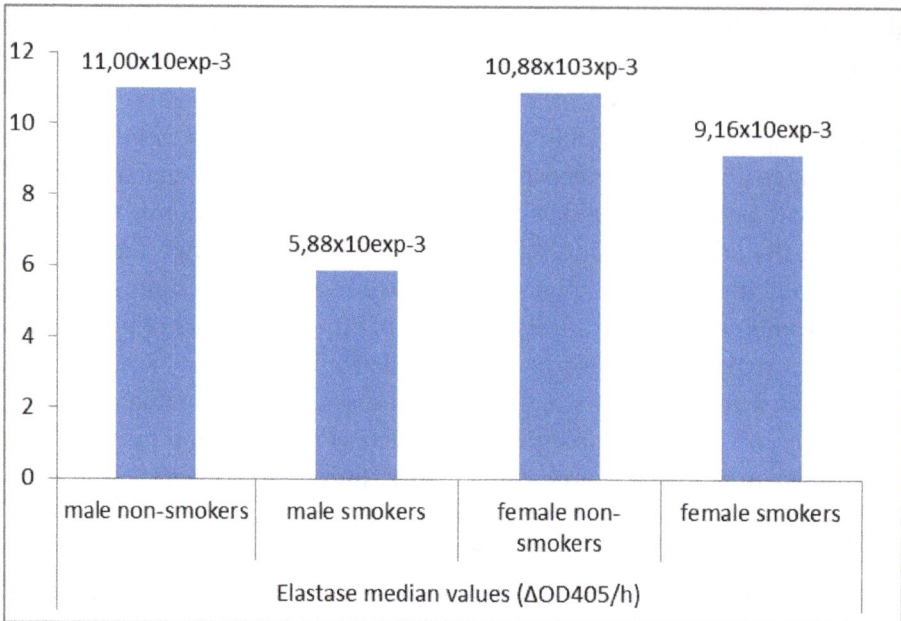

Figure 2. Salivary elastase median values corresponding smoking and sex in adolescents. CI 95%s for male non-smokers, male smokers, female non-smokers and female smokers are 8.75-13.63 x 10 exp-3 ΔOD405/h, 4.75-9.25 x 10exp-3 ΔOD405/h, 8.75-15.25 x10exp-3 ΔOD405/h, 6.63 -17.25 x10exp-3 ΔOD405/h, respectively

3.3. Predictive value of oral fluid MMP-8

It should be noted that MMP-8 levels in oral fluid possess a predictive value (Sorsa et al. 2010, Munjal et al. 2007, Prescher et al. 2007, Kraft-Neumärker et al. 2012, Leppilahti et al. 2014a,b). In this context, periodontitis patients were examined and followed over a course of 12 months at 2 month intervals. In these patients it was possible to clearly differentiate "stable sites" from "unstable" sites.

• "Stable sites": Improvement in pocket depth (PD) and attachment loss (AL) were continuously preserved after treatment, similarly the GCF MMP-8 values were and remained consistently low.

• "Unstable sites": No improvement or only temporary improvement in PD and AL were found, in parallel GCF MMP-8 values only improved shortly after treatment, followed by an immediate re-increase in the MMP-8 values.

Furthermore, Reinhardt et al. (2010) and Leppilahti et al. (2014a) demonstrated that increases in GCF MMP-8 during the periodontal maintenance are associated with increased odds of subsequent periodontal attachment loss and compromised treatment outcome. Overall, these authors concluded that elevated biomarkers of inflammation and bone resorption identify patients vulnerable to progressive periodontitis.

3.4. Elastase, protease inhibitors and sICAM-1

Elastase is another important neutrophil originating proteolytic enzyme. Contradicting findings about elastase activity in GCF of smokers compared with non-smokers with periodontitis have been reported, however: significantly higher mean levels of neutrophil elastase activity in smokers' than non-smokers' sites with matching PD has been detected (Söder 1999), but on the other hand lower concentrations of functional elastase in smokers' than in non-smokers' GCF has also been found (Alavi et al. 1995). This finding led Alavi et al. (1995) to the hypothesis that smokers' neutrophils may release elastase prior to reaching the periodontal tissues for example during passing through the lungs, or possibly a greater proportion of the elastase is bound to substrate and remains undetected which may complicate the diagnostic value of GCF elastase in smokers.

Smoking possibly intervenes in the levels of protease inhibitors α2-macroglobulin (α2-MG) and α1-antitrypsin (α1-AT), which may be one mechanism by which smoking can affect the inflammatory process. In severe periodontal lesions of smokers significantly lower concentrations and total amounts of GCF α2-MG as well as significantly lower total amounts of α1-AT were found. These findings lead to conclusion that decreased local levels of these inhibitors may result in increased tissue damage due to increased activity of elastase and collagenase (Persson et al. 2001).

A soluble form of intercellular molecule-1 (sICAM-1) is known to be elevated in smokers' blood compared with non-smokers (Koundouros et al. 1996). Conversely, in smokers with periodontitis GCF sICAM-1 is significantly lower compared with non-smokers (Fraser et al. 2001). Based on this finding Fraser et al. (2001) hypothesised that sICAM-1 molecules possibly bind to sequestrated neutrophils in periodontal microvasculature and provoke an inappropriate endogenous protease release contributing to periodontal destruction in the vicinity of the gingival microvasculature.

3.5. Cytokines

Bacterial products stimulate monocytes, macrophages and lymphocytes as well as resident fibroblasts and endothelial cells to secrete pro-inflammatory and immunoregulatory cytokines, which control cell growth and differentiation. Bacteria further stimulate chemokines and pro-inflammatory cytokines or subdue with anti-inflammatory cytokines and interferons the inflammation and regulate the development of the antimicrobial immunity in cooperation with antigen presenting cells (Julkunen et al. 2003). Smoking appears to affect normal balance of several cytokines, which are described as local hormones or cell-to-cell messengers. Especially the reduction of chemokines in smokers has been regarded to contribute to weakened neutrophil chemotaxis and migration to the site of inflammation in spite of the existing leukocytosis (Palmer et al. 2005).

In earlier studies increased levels of tumour necrosis factor (TNF) -α but decreased levels of IL-6 and IL-1β were detected in GCF of smoking periodontitis patients compared with non-smokers especially with tendency towards higher TNF-α levels in sites with an inferior treatment outcome (Boström et al. 1998a, 1999, 2000). Former smokers have also been reported to exhibit significantly higher GCF levels of TNF-α than non-smokers (Boström et al. 1998b). Parallel effect of smoking has been detected on GCF IL-10 both prior to as well as after periodontal treatment compared with non-smokers (Goutoudi et al. 2004).

Smoking seems to decrease the mean levels of GCF IL-1α concentrations significantly but does not affect mean total protein concentration (Petropoulos et al. 2004). In this study by Pertropulos et al. (2004) neutrophil numbers were not significantly different between smokers and non-smokers suggesting that the reduced IL-1α concentration of smokers may be independent of any effect of smoking on neutrophil chemotaxis, and smoking may directly inhibit IL-1α production. Thus GCF IL-1α may be derived from the inflamed tissues rather than being locally produced by neutrophils in pocket.

Recently multiplex immunoassays have been used to analyse simultaneously multiple GCF cytokines. A comprehensive investigation by a multi-bead array assay facilitated the characterization of 22 GCF cytokines, which were studied with respect to possible alterations in host response caused by smoking (Tymkiw et al. 2011). Quantities of pro-inflammatory cytokines, chemokines and regulators of T-cells and NK cells were found to be affected by smoking. Healthy sites of smoking periodontitis patients showed significantly less IL-6 and IL-12 than similar sites of non-smoking patients. In addition to these, smokers' periodontitis sites showed also significantly lower quantity of IL-1α. Of chemokines IL-8, IL-10, monocyte chemoattractant protein (MCP)-1, macrophage inflammatory protein (MIP) -1α and RANTES were detected in lower amounts both from healthy and diseased sites of smoking periodontitis patients compared with similar sites in non-smokers suggesting that low chemokine response leads to inability to recruit inflammatory and immune cells and further to ineffective defence. This may have a major role in the pathogenesis of periodontitis in smokers. Also IL-7 and IL-15, regulators of T-cells and NK cells, showed a decrease in smokers compared with non-smokers (Tymkiw et al. 2011).

However, another study also utilizing a multiplex immunoassay concluded that there were no correlations between GCF levels of MIP-1α and RANTES and the smoking status suggesting that at the local level smoking is not a major determinant of the CC group chemokine concentrations in GCF, and that the determinant is the level of local inflammation (Haytural et al. 2014). Another contradicting finding was detected by analysing MCP-1 with enzyme linked immunosorbent assay (ELISA), where MCP levels in GCF were highest in smokers with periodontitis when compared with non-smoking periodontitis patients and healthy controls (Anil et al. 2013), showing the possible effect of the analyse method on the results.

3.6. sRANKL and OPG

Soluble receptor activator of nuclear factor κ B ligand (sRANKL), its cellular receptor RANK and osteoprotegerin (OPG), a protein, which binds to RANKL blocking its interaction with RANK, are the regulators of bone formation and resorption (Tang et al. 2009). Periodontitis patients compared with healthy controls exhibit higher expression of RANKL in gingival tissues and GCF, which associates especially with active sites (Vernal et al. 2004). RANKL:OPG ratios may be increased in GCF of periodontitis patients (Bostanci et al. 2007). In current and former smoking periodontitis patients GCF OPG concentrations were lower compared with never smokers, and finding was opposite concerning the sRANKL concentration (Tang et al. 2009). Consequently, the sRANKL:OPG ratio also appeared to be higher in current and former smokers but the finding was not statistically significant. Interestingly, when pack-years were included in the analysis, OPG concentration decreased with increasing pack years and also the sRANKL:OPG ratio was significantly higher in the high pack-years group being significant also in the multivariate analysis (Tang et al. 2009). An increased lifetime exposure above a minimum threshold of cigarette smoking was required for this pattern. This finding is supported by earlier results where the combination of lipopolysaccharide and nicotine were shown to decrease OPG production in osteoblasts in a dose dependent manner (Tanaka et al. 2006) and where periodontal ligament fibroblasts and epithelial cells directly exposed to nicotine decreased their overall protein synthesis (Giannopoulou et al. 2001; Chang et al. 2002). This may lead to increased sRANKL:OPG ratio in smokers and further cause imbalanced tissue homeostasis and consequent tissue degradation (Tang et al. 2009).

4. Systemic inflammation and salivary biomarkers

Analyzing and utilization of inflammatory and disease specific biomarkers in saliva could offer an attractive solution for the diagnosis of different systemic diseases (Rathanayake et al. 2013b). The composition of saliva mainly originates from blood but in the salivary glands active transport and secretion mechanisms may change the saliva composition as the organic components of glandular specific saliva are derived from protein synthesis and are stored within the acinar cells (Kaufman & Lamster (2002), Malamud 1992). Nevertheless, saliva could be an alternative to blood as a biological fluid for analysis in diagnostic and prognosis purposes since the collection of saliva is non-invasive and is a plausible method. Systemic inflammation leads to the relief of pro-inflammatory mediators from immune cells, and the activation of the innate immune system. An increasing number of specific molecular markers for different conditions, such as cancer, cardiovascular disease (CVD), rheumatoid arthritis (RA), diabetes and human immunodeficiency virus has been identified (Boyle et al. 1994, Hu et al. 2008, Zhang et al. 2010).

4.1. Cardiovascular disease

High sensitive methods for biomarker detection have been developed since year 2000. There are certain biomarkers released due to a myocardial injury caused by myocardial ischemia- and necrosis, such as cardiac troponins I (TnI) and T (TnT), creatine kinase-MB (CK-MB), total creatine kinase, myoglobin, and lactate dehydrogenase (Mueller et al. 2013, Tiwari et al. 2012). Analysis of cardiac TnI and TnT are considered as the golden standard for diagnosis of acute myocardial infarction (AMI) as they are tissue specific for the myocardium (Tiwari et al. 2012). There are few earlier publications that have revealed correlations between serum and salivary biomarkers of CVD (Mirzaii-Dizgah et al. 2012, Quellet-Morin et al. 2011). The Tn I levels reaches its peak within 10–14 hours followed to an AMI, and according to the previous studies Tn I levels could be detected in saliva within 24 hours of onset of AMI (Mirzaii-Dizgah & Riahi 2013). A bedside saliva-based Nano-Biochip test together with electrocardiogram could provide prompt screening method for AMI patients in prehospital stage and the investigators of this study were able to detect elevated salivary levels of creatine kinase-MB, myoglobin, TnI and TnT, C-reactive proteins (CRP), TNF-α, MMP-9 and myeloperoxidase from AMI patients (Floriano et al. 2009).

In the study of Palm et al. (2013) on patients with acute ischemic stroke, systemic and local inflammatory markers were analysed of patients saliva. In this study, controls had enhanced levels of salivary MMP-8, MPO and IL-1β compared to the patients, since the control group was suffering from ongoing periodontal disease and the patients more often had evidence of end-stage periodontitis with edentulism and missing teeth. They also had higher levels of serum MMP-8 and MPO. Additional longitudinal studies are needed, however, to check the potential of salivary biomarkers associated in ischemic stroke.

4.2. Diabetes

There are a few studies concerning the detection of inflammatory biomarkers in saliva of patients with diabetes. Goodson and co-authors reported that in a child population unstimulated saliva samples were analysed and the salivary levels of CRP, insulin and leptin were remarkably higher in obese children compared with healthy normal weight children (Goodson et al. 2014). In a cross sectional study on 451 patients elevated salivary levels of MMP-8 were found among diabetes patients (Rathnayake et al. 2013). Salivary N-acetyl-β-D-hexosaminidase (HEX) which is associated with type I diabetes was found to be significantly increased in children with type 1 diabetes compared with healthy children (Zalewska-Szajda et al. 2013a).

4.3. Rheumatoid arthritis

The disease pattern of RA is similar to periodontal disease. Systemic inflammatory biomarkers from different chronic inflammatory conditions, such as RA could thus appear in saliva. There are few studies in this area, but when conducting an exploration of inflammatory biomarkers in RA patients, the periodontal status and the anti-TNF-α therapy taken by these patients need to take in to consideration. Salivary IL-1β was found to be significantly higher in the RA patients who were not on anti-TNF-α therapy compared with RA patients receiving anti-TNF-α therapy (Zalewska-Szajda et al. 2013b). Salivary exoglycosidases for detection of salivary gland involvement in RA patients were studied, in xerostomic RA group salivary β-glucuronidase was found to be significantly higher compared with healthy controls but the activity of salivary N-acetyl-β-hexosaminidase and β-glucuronidase was significantly lower than in xerostomic hyposalivary RA patients (Zalewska-Szajda et al. 2013b).

4.4. Cancer

To use salivary biomarkers to detect on / monitor all types of cancer is a growing research field in salivary diagnostics. The most common malignant neoplasm of the oral cavity is oral squamous cell carcinoma (OSCC). Patients with OSCC indicated that a specific marker of oxidative stress, malondialdehyde (MDA) in saliva was a better diagnostic tool as MDA in blood (Rasool et al. 2014). Salivary IL-8 levels seem to be higher in patients who had experienced tumour diseases (Rathnayake et al. 2013a,b). To detect head and neck squamous cell carcinoma (HNSCC) microRNAs (miRNAs) of saliva was used, and the results showed that miR-9, miR-134 and miR-191 were differentially expressed between saliva from HNSCC patients and healthy controls. Additionally, the authors suggested that these saliva-derived miRNAs may serve as novel biomarkers to reliably detect HNSCC (Salazar et al. 2014).

There are number of cytokines and chemokins involved in the cancer progression, such as interferon-gamma (IFN-γ), TNF-α, IL-1β, transforming growth factor-beta-1 (TGF-β1), epidermal growth factor (EGF), IL-6 and -8, vascular endothelial growth factor (VEGF), interleukins-4 and -10, tumour necrosis factor (TNF) and endothelin. Saliva based testing of these biomarkers is promising depending on the methods of analysis (Prasad & McCullough 2013). About 5 % of all cancers of the head and neck are salivary gland carcinomas (SGCs). Thus there is a need to develop new molecular biomarkers for early diagnosis and to improve the diagnosis of SGCs. Further research in this is required.

To identify disease specific molecular biomarkers in whole saliva is challenging. There are certain biomarkers found in saliva of high sensitivity and specificity, particularly in oral diseases, such as periodontal disease and oral cancer. There are factors that have an influence for the expression and release of biomarkers, such as their intracellular location, the size of the proteins, and the characteristics of the local biological fluid flow. The type of saliva used for diagnostic purpose to detect systemic conditions has an impact. In this regard unstimulated saliva reveals more information than stimulated saliva since unstimulated saliva contains higher concentrations of diagnostic biomarkers. High sensitivity and sophisticated methods and techniques are required for valuable outcome of the analyses of saliva samples.

5. Conclusion remarks

Inflammatory saliva and GCF biomarkers can be used as an aid in periodontal diagnostics, but there is a need to define the range of physiological levels and cutoff for pathological bursts of periodontitis progression. However, using just one definite cutoff point or merely one biomarker is not rational for adults or adolescents. Adolescence might have certain character-istics with different cutoff points compared to adults. The clinical use of salivary biomarkers to identify systemic conditions is another interesting area for developing non-invasive screening and diagnostic procedure. This might be the main goal for saliva research but in this regard it is important to consider the influence of oral health conditions which may confound the utility of the biomarkers. Modifying factors, such as smoking and pregnancy also should be taken into account when interpreting the results of the oral fluid inflammatory biomarkers.

Acknowledgements

This work was supported by grant from the National Fund for Scientific and Technological Development, Chilean Government (1120138), the Finnish Dental Society Apollonia and the

Research Foundation of Helsinki University Central Hospital. The authors declare that they have no competing interests. Timo Sorsa is an inventor of US-patents 5652227, 5736341, 5866432 and 6143476.

Author details

Anna Maria Heikkinen[1], Päivi Mäntylä[1], Jussi Leppilahti[1], Nilminie Rathnayake[3], Jukka Meurman[1,2] and Timo Sorsa[1,2,3]

1 Institute of Dentistry, Helsinki University, Central Hospital Helsinki, Finland

2 Departments of Oral and Maxillofacial Diseases and Periodontology, Helsinki University, Central Hospital Helsinki, Finland

3 Division of Periodontology, Department of Dental Medicine, Karolinska Institutet, Huddinge, Sweden

References

[1] Alavi, A.L., R.M Palmer, E.W. Odell, P.Y. Coward, and R.F. Wilson. Elastase in gingival crevicular fluid from smokers and non-smokers with chronic inflammatory periodontal disease. Oral Dis 1995; 1: 110-4.

[2] Albandar, J.M., and T.E. Rams. Global epidemiology of periodontal diseases: an overview. J Periodontology 2000 2002; 29:7-10.

[3] Allam, J.P., Y. Duan, F. Heinemann, J. Winter, W. Gotz W, J. Deschner, M. Wenghoefer, T. Bieber, S. Jepsen, and N. Novak. IL-23-producing CD68(+) macrophage-like likecells predominate within an IL-17-polarized infiltrate in chronic periodontitislesions. J. Clin. Periodontol. 2011; 38, 879–886.

[4] Anil, S., R.S. Preethanath, M. Alasqah, S.A. Mokeem, and P.S. AnandS. Increased levels of serum and gingival crevicular fluid monocyte chemoattractant protein-1 in smokers with periodontitis. J Periodontol 2013; 84: e23-8.

[5] Bostanci, N., T. Ilgenli, G.Emingil, B. Afacan, B. Han, H. Töz H., G. Atilla, F.J. Hughes, and G.N. Belibasakis. Gingival crevicular fluid levels of RANKL and OPG in periodontal diseases: implications of their relative ratio. J Clin Periodontol 2007; 34: 370-6.

[6] Boström, L., L.E. Linder, and J. Bergström. Clinical expression of TNF-alpha in smoking-associated periodontal disease. J Clin Periodontol 1998; 25: 767-73.

[7] Boström, L., LE. Linder, and J. Bergström. Smoking and cervicular fluid levels of IL-6 and TNF-alpha in periodontal disease.J Clin Periodontol 1999; 26: 352-7.

[8] Boström, L., L.E. Linder, and J. Bergström. Smoking and GCF levels of IL-1beta and IL-1ra in periodontal disease. J Clin Periodontol 2000; 27: 250-5.

[9] Boström, L., L.E. Linder, and J. Bergström. Influence of smoking on the outcome of periodontal surgery. A 5-year follow-up. J Clin Periodontol 1998; 25: 194-201.

[10] Boyle, J.O., L. Mao, J.A Brennan, W.M. Koch, D.W. Eisele, J.R. Saunders, and D. Sidransky. Gene mutations in saliva as molecular markers for head and neck squamous cell carcinomas. Am J Surg 1994;168: 429–432.

[11] Fox, P.C. Salivary monitoring in oral diseases. Ann N Y Acad Sci 1993; 694: 234–237.

[12] Chang, Y.C., F.M Huang, K.W Tai, L.C. Yang, and M.Y Chou. Mechanisms of cytotoxicity of nicotine in human periodontal ligament fibroblast cultures in vitro. J Periodontal Res 2002; 37: 279-85.

[13] Chapple, I.L.C., and J.B. Matthews. The role of reactive oxygen and antioxidant species in periodontal tissue destruction. Periodontology 2000 2007;2:160-232.

[14] Cutler, C.W., and R. Jotwani. Antigen-presentation and the role of dendritic cells in periodontitis. Periodontology 2000 2004; 35, 135–157.

[15] Genco, R.J., and W.S. Borgnakke. Risk factors for periodontal disease. Periodontology 2000 2013; 62, 59–94.

[16] Goodson, J.M., A.C. Tanner, A.D. Haffajee, G.C. Sornberger, and S.S. Socransky. Patterns of progression and regression of advanced destructive periodontal disease. J Clin Periodontol 1982; 9,472-481.

[17] Goodson, J.M., A. Kantarci, M.L. Hartman, G.V. Denis, D. Stephens, H. Hasturk, T. Yaskell, J. Vargas, X. Wang, M. Cugini, R. Barake, O. Alsmadi, S. Al-Mutawa, J. Ariga, P. Soparkar, J. Behbehani, K. Behbehani, and F. Welty. Metabolic disease risk in children by salivary biomarker analysis. PLoS One 2014; 10: 9: e98799.

[18] Floriano, P.N., N. Christodoulides, C.S Miller, J.L. Ebersole, J. Spertus, B.G. Rose,D.F. Kinane, M.J Novak, S. Steinhubl, S. Acosta, S. Mohanty, P. Dharshan, C.K. Yeh, S. Redding, W. Furmaga W, and J.T. McDevitt. Use of saliva-based nano-biochip tests for acute myocardial infarction at the point of care: a feasibility study. Clin Chem 2009; 55: 1530–1538.

[19] Fraser, H.S., R.M. Palmer, R.F. Wilson, P.Y. Coward, and D.A. Scott. Elevated systemic concentrations of soluble ICAM-1 (sICAM) are not reflected in the gingival crevicular fluid of smokers with periodontitis. J Dent Res 2001; 80: 1643-7.

[20] Giannopoulou, C., N. Roehrich, and A. Mombelli. Effect of nicotine-treated epithelial cells on the proliferation and collagen production of gingival fibroblasts. J Clin Periodontol 2001; 28: 769-75.

[21] Goutoudi, P., E. Diza, and M. Arvanitidou. Effect of periodontal therapy on crevicular fluid interleukin-1beta and interleukin-10 levels in chronic periodontitis. J Dent 2004; 32: 511-20.

[22] Graves, D. Cytokines that promote periodontal tissue destruction. J Periodontol 2008; 79, 1585–1591.

[23] Gursoy, M., E. Kononen, T. Tervahartiala, U.K. Gursoy, R. Pajukanta, and T. Sorsa. Longitudinal study of salivary proteinases during pregnancy and postpartum. J Periodontal Res 2010; 45,496-503.

[24] Gursoy, M., R. Pajukanta, T. Sorsa, and E. Kononen E. Clinical changes in periodontium during pregnancy and post-partum. J Clin Periodontol 2008; 35, 576-583.

[25] Gursoy, U.K., E. Könönen, P. Pradhan-Palikhe, T. Tervahartiala, P.J. Pussinen, L. Suominen-Taipale, and T. Sorsa. Salivary MMP-8, TIMP-1, and ICTP as markers of advanced periodontitis. J Clin Periodontol 2010; 37: 487-93.

[26] Gürsoy U.K., E. Könönen, P.J. Pussinen, T. Tervahartiala, K. Hyvärinen, A.L. Suominen, V.J. Uitto, and S. Paju. Use of host- and bacteria-derived salivary markers in detection of periodontitis: A cumulative approach. Dis Markers 2011; 30, 299-305.

[27] Haytural, O., D.,Yaman, E.C. Ural, A. Kantarci, and K. Demirel. Impact of periodontitis on chemokines in smokers. Clin Oral Investig 2014; Sep 6.

[28] Heikkinen, A.M., R. Pajukanta, J. Pitkäniemi, U. Broms, T. Sorsa, M. Koskenvuo, and J.H.

[29] Meurman. The effect of smoking on periodontal health of 15- to 16-year-old adolescents J Periodontol 2008; 79: 2042-2047.

[30] Heikkinen, A.M., T. Sorsa, J. Pitkäniemi, T. Tervahartiala, K. Kari, U. Broms,

[31] M. Koskenvuo, and J.H. Meurman. Smoking affects diagnostic salivary periodontal disease biomarker levels in adolescents. J Periodontol 2010; 81: 1299-1307.

[32] Heikkinen, A.M. (2011). Oral health, smoking and adolescence. University of Helsinki, Faculty of Medicine, Institute of Dentistry. http://urn.fi/URN:ISBN: 978-952-10-7250-5.

[33] Hernandez, M., J. Gamonal, T. Tervahartiala, P. Mantyla, O. Rivera, A. Dezereg,

[34] N. Dutzan, and T. Sorsa. Associations between matrix metalloproteinase-8 and-14 and myeloperoxidase in gingival crevicular fluid from subjects with progressive chronic periodontitis: A longitudinal study. J Periodontol 2010; 81, 1644-1652.

[35] Hind, C.R., H. Joyce, G.A. Tennent, M.B. Pepys,and N.M.Pride. Plasma leukocyte elastase concentrations in smokers. JClin Pathol 1991; 44: 232-235.

[36] Hu, S. and M. Arellano, P. Boontheung, J. Wang, H. Zhou, J. Jiang, D. Elashoff, R. Wei,

[37] J.A. Loo, and D.T. Wong. Salivary proteomics for oral cancer biomarker discovery. Clin Cancer Res 2008; 14: 6246–6252.

[38] Irfan, U.M., D.V. Dawson, and N.F. Bissada. Epidemiology of periodontal disease: a review and clinical perspectives. J Int Acad Periodontol 2001; 3: 14-21.

[39] Johannsen, A., C. Susin, and A. Gustafsson A. Smoking and inflammation: evidence for a synergistic role in chronic disease. Periodontol 2000 2014; 64: 111-126.

[40] Julkunen, I., O. Silvennoinen and M. Hurme. Sytokiinit, niiden toiminta ja kliininen merkitys. In book: Huovinen, P., S. Meri, H. Peltola, M. Vaara, A. Vaheri and V. Valtonen (eds.). Mikrobiologia ja infektiosairaudet, book I. Kustannut Oy Duodecim. Gummerus Kirjapaino Oy. Jyväskylä 2003; 734-747.

[41] Kaufman, E., and I.B. Lamster. Analysis of saliva for periodontal diagnosis–a review. J Clin Periodontol 2000; 27: 453–465.

[42] Kaufman, E.,and I.B. Lamster. The diagnostic applications of saliva-a review. Crit Rev Oral Biol Med 2002; 13: 197–212.

[43] Kumar, A., S.S. Masamatti, and M.S. Virdi. Periodontal diseases in children and adolescents: a clinician's perspective part 2. Dent Update 2012; 39:639-642, 645-646, 649-652.

[44] Kraft-Neumärker, M., K. Lorenz, R. Koch, T. Hoffmann, P. Mäntylä, T. Sorsa, and L. Netuschil. Full-mouth profile of active MMP-8 in periodontitis patients. J Periodontal Res 2012; 47: 121-8.

[45] Koundouros, E., E. Odell, P. Coward, R. Wilson, and R.M. Palmer. Soluble adhesion molecules in serum of smokers and non-smokers, with and without periodontitis. J Periodontal Res 1996; 31: 596-599.

[46] Lee, Y.H., and D.T. Wong. Saliva: an emerging biofluid for early detection of diseases. Am J Dent 2009; 22, 241–248.

[47] Leppilahti, J.M., M. Ahonen, M. Hernández, S. Munjal, L. NetuschilL, V. Uitto, T. Sorsa, and P. Mäntylä. Oral rinse MMP-8 point-of-care immuno test identifies patients with strong periodontal inflammatory burden. Oral Diseases 2011; 17, 115-122.

[48] Leppilahti, J.M., M.A. Kallio, T. Tervahartiala, T. Sorsa, and P. Mäntylä. Gingival crevicular fluid matrix metalloproteinase-8 levels predict treatment outcome among smokers with chronic periodontitis. J Periodontol 2014a; 85: 250-260.

[49] Leppilahti, J.M., P.A. Hernández-Ríos, J.A. Gamonal, T. Tervahartiala, R. Brignardello-Petersen, P. Mantyla, T. Sorsa and M. Hernández. Matrix metalloproteinases and myeloperoxidase in gingival crevicular fluid provide site-specific diagnostic value for chronic periodontitis. J Clin Periodontol 2014b; 41: 348-356.

[50] Liede, K.E., J.K. Haukka, J.H. Hietanen, M.H. Mattila, H. Rönkä H, and T. Sorsa. The association between smoking cessation and periodontal status and salivary proteinase levels. J Periodontol 1999; 70: 1361-8.

[51] Malamud, D. Saliva as a diagnostic fluid. BMJ 1992; 305: 207–208.

[52] Matthews, J.B., F.M. Chen, M.R. Milward, M.R Ling, and I.L.C.Chapple. Neutrophil superoxide production in the presence of cigarette smoke extract, nicotine and cotinine. J Periodontol 2012; 39; 626-634.

[53] Miller,C.S., C.P. King, M.C. Langub, R.J. Kryscio, and M.V. Thomas. Salivary biomarkers of existing periodontal disease: a cross-sectional study. J Am Dent Assoc 2006; 137: 322–329.

[54] Mirrielees, J., L.I. Crofford, Y. Lin Y., R.J. Kryscio, D.R. 3 rd. Dawson, J.L. and Ebersole, and C.S. Miller. Rheumatoid arthritis and salivary biomarkers of periodontal disease. J Clin Periodontol 2010; 37: 1068-1074.

[55] Mirzaii-Dizgah, I., and E. Riahi. Salivary troponin I as an indicator of myocardial infarction. Indian J Med Res 2013; 138: 861–865.

[56] Mirzaii–Dizgah, I., S.F. Hejazi, E. Riahi, and M.M. Salehi MM. Saliva-based creatine kinase MB measurement as a potential point-of-care testing for detection of myocardial infarction. Clin Oral Invest 2012; 16: 775–779.

[57] Mueller,M., M. Vafaie, M. Biener, E. Giannitsis, and H.A. Katus. Cardiac troponin T: from diagnosis of myocardial infarction to cardiovascular risk prediction. Circ J 2013; 77: 1653-1661.

[58] Mäntyla, P., M. Stenman, D.F., Kinane, S. Tikanoja, H. Luoto, T. Salo, and T. Sorsa. Gingival crevicular fluid collagenase-2 (MMP-8) test stick for chair-side monitoring of periodontitis. J Periodontal Res 2003;38, 436-439.

[59] Mäntylä, P., M. Stenman, D.F. Kinane, T. Salo, K. Suomalainen, S. Tikanoja, and T. Sorsa. Monitoring periodontal disease status in smokers and nonsmokers using a gingival crevicular fluid matrix metalloproteinase-8-specific chair-side test. J Periodontal Res 2006; 41: 503-512.

[60] Nwhator, S.O., P.O. Ayanbadejo, K.A. Umeizudike, O.I. Opeodu, G.A. Agbelusi, J.A. Olamijulo, M.O. Arowojolu, T. Sorsa, B.S. Babajide, and D.O. Opedun. Clinical correlates of a lateral-flow immunoassay oral risk indicator. J Periodontol 2014; 85: 188-94.

[61] Palm, F., L. Lahdentausta, T. Sorsa, T. Tervahartiala, P. Gokel, F. Buggle, A. Safer, H. Becher, A.J. Grau, and P. Pussinen. Biomarkers of periodontitis and inflammation in ischemic stroke: A case-control study. Innate Immun 2013; 17; 20: 511-518.

[62] Palmer, R.M., R.F. Wilson, A.S. Hasan, and D.A. Scott. Mechanisms of action of environmental factors--tobacco smoking. J Clin Periodontol 2005; 32: 180-95.

[63] Papantonopoulos, G., K. Takahashi, T. Bountis, and B.G. Loos. Mathematical modeling suggests that periodontitis behaves as a non-linear chaotic dynamical process. J Periodontol 2013; 84,e29-39.

[64] Papantonopoulos, G., K. Takahashi, T. Bountis, and B.G. Loos Artificial neural networks for the diagnosis of aggressive periodontitis trained by immunologic parameters. PloS One 2014;9, e89757.

[65] Persson, L., J. Bergström, and A. Gustafsson A. Effect of tobacco smoking on neutrophil activity following periodontal surgery. J Periodontol 2003; 74: 1475-1482.

[66] Persson, L., J. Bergström, H. Ito, and A. Gustafsson. Tobacco smoking and neutrophil activity in patients with periodontal disease. J Periodontol 2001; 72: 90-95.

[67] Petropoulos, G., I.J. McKay, and F.J. Hughes. The association between neutrophil numbers and interleukin-1alpha concentrations in gingival crevicular fluid of smokers and non-smokers with periodontal disease. J Clin Periodontol 2004; 31: 390-395.

[68] Prasad, G., and M. McCullough. Chemokines and cytokines as salivary biomarkers for the early diagnosis of oral cancer. Int J Dent 2013; 2013: 813756.

[69] Prescher, N., K. Maier, S.K. Munjal, T. Sorsa, C.D. Bauermeister, F. Struck, and L. Netuschil. Rapid quantitative chairside test for active MMP-8 in gingival crevicular fluid: first clinical data. Ann N Y Acad Sci 2007; 1098: 493-495.

[70] Ouellet-Morin, I., A. Danese, B. Williams, and L. Arseneault. Validation of a high-sensitivity assay for C-reactive protein in human saliva. Brain Behav Immun 2011; 25: 640–646.

[71] Ramseier, C.A., J.S. Kinney, A.E. Herr, T. Braun, J.V. Sugai, C.A. Shelburne, L.A. Rayburn, H.M. Tran, A.K. Singh, and W.V. Giannobile.Identification of pathogen and host-response markers correlated with periodontal disease. J Periodontol 2009; 80, 436-446.

[72] Rasool, M., S.R. Khan, A. Malik, K.M.4. Khan, S. Zahid, A. Manan, M.H. Qazi, and M.I. Naseer. Comparative Studies of Salivary and Blood Sialic Acid, Lipid Peroxidation and Antioxidative Status in Oral Squamous Cell Carcinoma (OSCC). Pak J Med Sci 2014; 30: 466-471.

[73] Rathnayake, N., S. Akerman, B. Klinge, N. Lundegren, H. Jansson H, Y. Tryselius, T. Sorsa, and A. Gustafsson. Salivary biomarkers of oral health: a cross-sectional study. J Clin Periodontol 2013a; 40: 140-147.

[74] Rathnayake, N., S. Akerman, B. Klinge, N. Lundegren, H. Jansson, Y. Tryselius, T. Sorsa, A. Gustafsson. Salivary biomarkers for detection of systemic diseases. PLoS One. 2013b; 24; 8: e61356.

[75] Salazar, M.G., N. Jehmlich, A. Murr, V.M. Dhople, B. Holtfreter, E. Hammer, U. Völker, and T. Kocher. Identification of periodontitis associated changes in the pro-

teome of whole human saliva by mass spectrometric analysis. J Clin Periodontol 2013 ; 40: 825-832.

[76] Salazar, C., R. Nagadia, P. Pandit, J. Cooper-White, N. Banerjee, N. Dimitrova, W.B Coman, and C. Punyadeera. A novel saliva-based microRNA biomarker panel to detect head and neck cancers. Cell Oncol 2014; 37: 331-338.

[77] Seymour, G.J.,and E. Gemmell. Cytokines in periodontal disease: where to from here? Acta Odontol Scand 2001; 59: 167–173.

[78] Seymour, G.J.,and J.J Taylor. Shouts and whispers: an introduction to immunoregulation in periodontal disease. Periodontology 2000 2004; 35, 9–13.

[79] Sexton, W. M., Y. Lin, R.J. Kryscio, D.R.3rd. Dawson, J.L. Ebersole, and C.S. Miller. Salivary biomarkers of periodontal disease in response to treatment. J Clin Periodontol 2011; 38, 434-441.

[80] Socransky, S.S., A.D. Haffajee, J.M. Goodson, and J. Lindhe. New concepts of destructive periodontal disease. J Clin Periodontol 1984; 11, 21-32.

[81] Sorsa, T., P. Mäntylä, H. Rönkä, P. Kallio, G.B. Kallis, C. Lundqvist, D.F. Kinane, T. Salo, L.M. Golub, O. Teronen, and S. Tikanoja. Scientific basis of a matrix metalloproteinase-8 specific chair-side test for monitoring periodontal and peri-implant health and disease. Ann N Y Acad Sci 1999; 878: 130-40.

[82] Sorsa, T., M. Hernández, J. Leppilahti, S. Munjal, L. Netuschil, and P. Mäntylä. Detection of gingival crevicular fluid MMP-8 levels with different laboratory and chairside methods. Oral Diseases 2010; 16, 39-45.

[83] Souto, G.R., T.K. Segundo, F.O. Costa, M.C. Aguiar, and R.A. Mesquita. Effect of smoking on Langerhans and dendritic cells in patients with chronic gingivitis. J.Periodontol 2011; 82, 619–625.

[84] Souto, G.R., C.M. Queiroz-Junior, F.O. Costa, and R.A. Mesquita. Smoking effect on chemokines of the human chronic periodontitis. Immunobiology 2014; 219, 633–636.

[85] Srinivas, M., K.C. Chethana, R. Padma, G. Suragimath, M. Ani, B.S. Pai, and A. Walvekar. A study to assess and compare the peripheral blood neutrophil chemotaxisin smokers and non-smokers with healthy periodontium, gingivitis, and chronicperiodontitis. J. Ind. Soc. Periodontol 2012; 16, 54–58.

[86] Stein, S.H., K.J. Wendell, M. Pabst, and M. Scarbecz. Profiling gingival crevicular fluid from smoking and non-smoking chronic periodontitis patients. J Tenn Dent Assoc 2006; 86: 20-4.

[87] Söder, B. Neutrophil elastase activity, levels of prostaglandin E2, and matrix metalloproteinase-8 in refractory periodontitis sites in smokers and non-smokers. Acta Odontol Scand 1999; 57: 77-82.

[88]   Söder, B., L.I. Jin, and S. Wickholm. Granulocyte elastase, matrix metalloproteinase-8 and prostaglandin E2 in gingival crevicular fluid in matched clinical sites in smokers and non-smokers with persistent periodontitis. J Clin Periodontol 2002; 29:384-91.

[89]   Tanaka, H., N. Tanabe, M. Shoji, N. Suzuki, T. Katono, S. Sato, M. Motohashi, and M. Maeno M. Nicotine and lipopolysaccharide stimulate the formation of osteoclast-like cells by increasing macrophage colony-stimulating factor and prostaglandin E2 production by osteoblasts. Life Sci 2006; 78: 1733-1740.

[90]   Tang, T.H., T.R. Fitzsimmons, and P.M. Bartold. Effect of smoking on concentrations of receptor activator of nuclear factor kappa B ligand and osteoprotegerin in human gingival crevicular fluid. J Clin Periodontol 2009; 36: 713-8.

[91]   Tiwari, R.P., A. Jain, Z. Khan, V. Kohil, R.N. Bharmal, S. Kartikeyan, and P.S. Bisen. Cardiac Troponin I and T: Molecular markers for early diagnosis, prognosis, and accurate triaging of patients with acute myocardial infarction. Mol Diagn Ther 2012; 16: 371–381.

[92]   Tymkiw, K.D., D.H. Thunell, G.K. Johnson, S. Joly, K.K. Burnell, J.E. Cavanaugh, K.A. Brogden, and J.M. Guthmiller. Influence of smoking on gingival crevicular fluid cytokines in severe chronic periodontitis. J Clin Periodontol 2011; 38: 219-28.

[93]   Vernal, R., A. Chaparro, R. Graumann, J. Puente, M.A. Valenzuela, and J. Gamonal. Levels of cytokine receptor activator of nuclear factor kappaB ligand in gingival crevicular fluid in untreated chronic periodontitis patients. J Periodontol 2004; 75: 1586-1591.

[94]   Yanagita, M., K. Mori, R. Kobayashi, Y. Kojima, M. Kubota, K. Miki, S. Yamada, M. Kitamura, and S. Murakami. Immunomodulation of dendritic cellsdifferentiated in the presence of nicotine with lipopolysaccharide from Porphy-romonas gingivalis. Eur. J. Oral. Sci. 2012b; 120, 408–414.

[95]   Zalewska-Szajda, B., S. Dariusz Szajda, N. Waszkiewicz, S. Chojnowska, E. Gościk, U. Łebkowska, A. Kępka, A. Bossowski, A. Zalewska, J. Janica, K. Zwierz, J.R. Ładny, and D. Waszkiel D. Activity of N-acetyl-β-D-hexosaminidase in the saliva of children with type 1 diabetes. Postepy Hig Med Dosw 2013a; 67: 996-999.

[96]   Zalewska, A., J. Szulimowska, N. Waszkiewicz, D. Waszkiel, K. Zwierz, and M. Knaś. Salivary exoglycosidases in the detection of early onset of salivary gland involvement in rheumatoid arthritis. Postepy Hig Med Dosw 2013b; 3; 1182-1188.

[97]   Zhang, L., H. Xiao, S.K. Karlan, H. Zhou, and J. Gros. Salivary Transcriptomic and Proteomic Biomarkers for Breast Cancer Detection 2010; 5: 1–7.

7

Herbal Dentifrices for Children

Marisa Alves Nogueira Diaz,
Isabela de Oliveira Carvalho and Gaspar Diaz

1. Introduction

The use of plant extracts as antimicrobial agents has been increasing every daily. Currently, these applications are mainly found in dentistry with the increased use of plant extracts in toothpastes for both adults and children. This finding results from the fact that the oral cavity is considered a favorable environment for the colonization and growth of a wide range of microorganisms, bacteria being the most common [1, 2]. One of the core arguments for the pharmaceutical industry to use toothpastes made from plant extracts is that they can act as antibiotics, analgesics, sedatives, and anti-inflammatories, in addition to being less likely to cause side effects. In the case of toothpastes for children's use where the presence of fluoride can lead to fluorosis, the presence of extracts with antimicrobial activity is quite interesting, given that these combat microorganisms by preventing the formation of biofilms [3].

The presence of microorganisms in the physiology of the oral cavity is essential for normal development, since most species are commensal microorganisms. In some cases, these microorganisms contribute to preventing the establishment of pathogenic microorganisms [4]. However, some of these microorganisms are considered to be opportunistic pathogens that play an important role in the etiology of periodontitis and dental caries, which are believed to be the most prevalent diseases in the world [5]. These microorganisms have also regularly been involved in the etiology of a number of systemic diseases, such as respiratory infections, infective endocarditis, and cardiovascular diseases [6, 7].

Dental caries is a complex oral disease, caused mainly by dental plaque. Dental plaque has been described as an ordered structure in which the primary colonizers are *Actinomyces* and *Streptococci*. These microorganisms bind tightly to one another, in addition to the solid tooth surface, by means of an extracellular matrix consisting of polymers of both host and microbial origin [8-10]. The formation of dental plaque includes a series of steps that begins with the initial colonization of the pellicle and ends with the complex formation of a mature biofilm. Additionally, through the growth process of the biofilm, the microbial composition changes from one that is primarily Gram-positive and *Streptococcus*-rich to a structure filled with Gram-negative anaerobes in its more mature state [11]. It is widely accepted that the accumulation of microorganisms plays a key role in the initiation and progression of gingivitis and other oral diseases [12].

Gram-positive bacteria, such as *Lactobacilli* and the *Streptococci* species are associated with the formation of dental caries. As a result, strategies for treating this disease must concentrate on controlling the growth of these bacteria [13-15].

According to data from the World Health Organization (WHO), the prevalence of caries in schoolchildren is 60-90%, while among adults it is universal in most countries [16]. Biofilm formation is a natural process in the oral environment, and its control should be done through chemical and mechanical means. Brushing is a preventive measure considered essential for the prevention of caries and periodontal diseases, and can be effectively increased by using the toothpaste formulations containing antimicrobial agents [17-19].

1.1. Dental fluorosis

Dental fluorosis is the exposure of the tooth germ during its formation process at high concentrations of fluoride, resulting in defects of enamel mineralization with severity directly linked to the amount ingested. Clinically, the formation of opaque spots on the enamel of homologous teeth turning to a yellow or brown color, can be observed in more severe cases. In addition to the high dosage of fluoride, other factors contribute to the onset of fluorosis: low body weight, nutritional status, rate of skeletal growth and bone remodeling periods. In this sense, dental fluorosis is a more common disease in teeth of late mineralization (permanent teeth) in children with a low weight or poor nutritional state, occurring mainly at the ages of the first to second stages of childhood where there is a high incidence of systemic fluoride intake and subsequent harmful effects [20].

The decrease in the prevalence of dental caries has been attributed in large part to the use of fluoride toothpastes when brushing, one of the most accepted measures for the control of dental caries [21, 22]. By contrast, the prevalence of dental fluorosis has increased worldwide. The use of fluoride toothpaste before 6 years of age has been identified as one of the main risk factors for dental fluorosis [23]. However, other factors have also been found to cause fluorosis, especially commercially sold drinks, such as mineral water and soft drinks, among others, a fact that has increased the incidence of fluorosis in both places with fluoridated water consumption as well as in areas with non-fluoridated water consumption. This finding indicates that there is an intake of fluoride from other sources as well, in addition to the public water supply. Several studies have been conducted in many countries to determine the amount of fluoride in mineral waters, especially in soft drinks. The values obtained range from 0.007 mg/L to more than 4.1 mg/L for mineral waters and from 0.02 to 1.28 ppm, an average level of 0.72 ppm, for soft drinks, with no significant difference when the tastes of diet sodas are compared [24].

Depending on its severity, dental fluorosis may not only have aesthetic consequences, but it may also cause pain and affect masticatory efficiency [25]. Due to these facts, it is necessary to develop alternative formulations of toothpaste based on plant extracts with proven antimicrobial activity for use in children's dentistry to minimize the risk of dental fluorosis in infants and children from 1 to 6 years of age. Thus, many plant extracts with antimicrobial activity have been incorporated into toothpastes to prevent oral diseases. The plant extracts of the *Chordata macleya* and *Prunella vulgaris* species are examples of plants with an anti-inflammatory activity used in the international toothpaste market [26].

2. Toothpastes and antimicrobial agents

Common antimicrobial compounds added to toothpastes include: triclosan, stannous fluoride, and chlorhexidine. Nevertheless, despite the effectiveness of many formulations of toothpaste with antibacterial properties, the search for natural products with these properties has been increasing. Thus, plant extracts are being investigated as potential sources of new antibacterial compounds [27-29]. Dental plaque is considered an essential factor linked to the onset of caries, thus justifying the measures taken to control it. It is well-known that many metabolites produced by plants, such as tannins, terpenoids, flavonoids, and alkaloids, may represent a new source of antimicrobial substances [30, 31].

Natural toothpastes are considered to be those that do not incorporate the antimicrobial triclosan and fluoride. These toothpastes contain natural ingredients, such as the salts of sodium fluoride and sodium chloride and plant extracts, such as lemon, eucalyptus, rosemary, chamomile, sage, and myrrh [32]. Chamomile extract, for example, exhibits anti-inflammatory properties. By contrast, salvia extract decreases the tissue bleeding, whereas the extract of myrrhis, a natural antiseptic and extract of mentha, presents antiseptic, anti-inflammatory, and antimicrobial activities [33, 34]. Terpenoid compounds derived from medicinal plants and natural products, such as ursolic acid (UA) and oleanolic acid (OA), inhibited the growth of cariogenic microorganisms in a study conducted by Zhou and co-workers [35], suggesting that both compounds have the potential for use as antibacterial agents in the prevention of dental caries. Oral care products that are incorporated together with plant extracts are widely used due to their low toxicity, as compared to oral care products that contain antimicrobials, such as triclosan, cetyl pyridinium chloride, chlorhexidine, and fluoride [36, 37].

Toothpastes for children's use have had their contents changed in the name of progress and development in dentistry. In the past, toothpastes consisted of creams with a high fluorine content, masked by packaging illustrated with children's themes and flavored goodies that attracted children to the product. Nowadays, the cosmetics industry has reduced the fluorine content in these toothpastes to minimize the risk of fluorosis in children of less than 5 years of age, where fluorosis primarily affects the aesthetic appearance of their teeth [38].

3. Medicinal plants with antibacterial activity used in dentistry

The use of medicinal plants for the treatment of dental problems has widely been discussed by many researchers. Many cultures still use medicinal plants for the treatment of oral diseases, including caries for the cleaning and brushing of teeth, especially in rural areas of underdeveloped countries where people still brush their teeth without toothpaste [39]. The scientific field that uses the knowledge of medicinal plants for use in oral health is called Ethno-dentistry, which combines the knowledge of plants used by rural populations, indigenous populations, and communities in general. A brief description of some of the most common plants used in oral health was compiled, as described below.

3.1. *Myristica fragrans*

Myristica fragrans (Myristicaceae) is grown to be used as a spice and for medicinal purposes [40]. Its main constituents include alkylbenzenes (myristicin, elemicin, safrole, etc.); terpenes (α-pinene, β-pinene, myristic acid, trimyristin); and neolignans (myrislignan and macelignan) [41-43]. Its seed (known as nutmeg) is widely used in traditional medicine as an antithrombotic and antifungal drug, for the treatment of nausea and dyspepsia, and as an anti-inflammatory drug [44-46].

Studies have shown that *M. fragrans* has a great potential benefit in the field of dentistry, as its ethanol extract has proven to provide antibacterial activity against cariogenic bacteria [47]. According to Chung [42], the macelignan, an active compound isolated from *M. fragrans*, also presents an antibacterial activity against *Streptococcus mutans* and other oral microorganisms, such as *Streptococcus sobrinus*, *Streptococcus salivarius*, *Streptococcus sanguinis*, *Lactobacillus acidophilus*, and *Lactobacillus casei*, which indicates that it can be used as a natural antibacterial agent in oral hygiene products.

3.2. Propolis

Propolis, a natural antibiotic, is a resinous yellowish-brown to dark-brown substance collected by bees (*Apis mellifera*) from tree buds and is mixed with secreted beeswax. Bees use propolis as a glue to seal the opening of the hives protecting it from outside contaminants, which features over 300 compounds in its composition [48]. Among these constituents, one can find: flavonoids, steroids, sugars, and amino acids. The composition depends on the vegetation of the place from which it was collected and the season [48-50]. Thus, its biological activity is related to the plant ecology of the region visited by bees [51, 52]. Propolis has been outstanding for its anesthetic anti-inflammatory, healing, anti-trypanosome, and anti-cariogenic activities [53-56]. Brazilian propolis is one of the most active resinous substance, whose major components include diterpenes, lignans, *p*-coumaric acid, and flavonoids. A flavonoid is a compound with a wide range of biological activities, mainly antioxidant, anti-inflammatory, and antimicrobial activities [57, 58, 49].

Ikeno *et al.* [59] and Park *et al.* [60], respectively, have shown that propolis has *in vitro* effects on bacterial growth as well as on the activity of the glucosyltransferase enzyme (GTF), responsible for the formation of *S. sobrinus*, *S. mutans*, and *S. cricetus* biofilms in caries developed in rats. These studies demonstrate that propolis may well become a promising alternative for the prevention of caries and other oral diseases [61-63].

3.3. Chitosan

Chitin and chitosan are copolymers consisting of *N*-acetyl-D-glucosamine and D-glucosamine units in varying proportions. Chitin is the second most abundant polysaccharide in nature and is the main component of the exoskeleton of crustaceans and insects, but can also be found in nematodes, fungal cell walls, and yeasts. Chitosan has interesting medicinal properties, especially the antimicrobial activity *in vitro* against oral biofilm formations. This finding was reported in studies conducted by Verkaik *et al.* [64-66], who found that chitosan-based toothpaste, when compared with chlorhexidine-based toothpaste, traditionally used as an antimicrobial agent in toothpastes, may be equally as effective.

Chitosan showed a significant action in reducing dental plaque and presented antimicrobial activity *in vitro* against several pathogens in the oral cavity associated with the formation of dental plaque and periodontal disease, such as *Actinobacillus*, *S. mutans*, and *P. gingivalis* [67, 68]. Tarsie *et al.* [69] demonstrated that chitosan could influence the adherence of *S. mutans* to tooth surfaces, thus confirming the possibility of using this polysaccharide as a preventive agent in the formation of biofilms. According to the literature [70, 71], chitosan mouthwash was quite effective in reducing plaque that adheres to the teeth and reducing the count of *S. mutans* in saliva.

According to Mohiree Yadav [72], the addition of chitosan to toothpastes reduced plaque levels by 70% and caries caused by bacteria by 85%, respectively. Thus, toothpastes containing plant extracts and chitosan present an antibacterial efficacy comparable to those containing chlorhexidine [65]. The proven antimicrobial, anti-inflammatory, and healing effects of chitosan, coupled with their ability to inhibit the formation of biofilms, may well represent a formidable advantage in the treatment of diseases associated with the oral cavity [73].

3.4. *Punica granatum* Linn.

Punica granatum Linn. (Punicaceae), known in Brazil as "romã", is a small shrub cultivated worldwide in tropical and subtropical climates, has been used in traditional medicine as an astringent, hemostatic agent, and in the control of diabetes [74]. It is also commonly used to treat throat infections, cough and fever due to its anti-inflammatory and antimicrobial potential [75]. The antibiotic activity of the *P. granatum* extract is associated with its chemical constituents, including tannins and alkaloids found in the leaves, roots, stems and fruits [76, 77]. The alcoholic extract obtained from the fruit of *P. granatum* has shown effective antimicrobial activity against cariogenic bacteria, such as *S. mitis*, *S. mutans*, *S. sanguinis*, *S. sobrinus*, and *L. casei* [78, 79]. Toothpaste obtained from the alcoholic extract of *P. granatum* showed activity against cariogenic *S. mutans*, *S. sanguinis*, and *S. mitis* bacteria, demonstrating its antibacterial effect, suggesting the effective use of this herbal agent in the control of the adherence of different microorganisms within the oral cavity [80].

3.5. *Lentinus edodes* and *Cichorium intybus*

Lentinula edodes is the second most cultivated species of edible mushroom in the world, behind only champignon (*Agaricus bisporus*) [81]. It can be grown on tree trunks or on prepared substrates, and has attracted the interest of researchers, as it presents scientifically proven nutritional and therapeutic qualities [82].

Cichorium intybus (Compositae) has been used by humans as food since the dawn of civilization. It is a native plant of Europe that can be grown virtually everywhere [83, 84]. Studies have shown that various plant foods contain components with antibacterial and anti-dental plaque activity [85], including the alcoholic extracts of edible mushrooms, namely *L. edodes* and *C. intybus*, which can be used in products formulated for daily oral hygiene, such as mouthwashes and toothpastes [86-88].

3.6. *Copaifera officinalis* L.

Copaifera officinalis L. (Fabaceae) is a tree found mainly in Latin America and West Africa, also known as "Copaiba", copaiba balsam, Jesuit's balsam, copal, and capivi [89-91]. The copaiba oil has been documented to contain antibacterial activity. It corresponds to an excretion product, whose purpose is most likely to protect the plant against animals, fungi, and bacteria [92]. It is a liquid of varying viscosity and color, which can vary from yellow to brown [93, 94]. The extracted oil can vary in relation to its concentration of diterpenes and sesquiterpenes [95]. It is popularly used as an anti-inflammatory and healing agent whose actions are related to the presence of diterpenes within its composition [96]. Pieri *et al.* [97] studied the antimicrobial activity of copaiba oil on plaque-forming bacteria in dogs. The results showed that the oil was active against cariogenic bacteria, presenting an inhibitory effect on the adhesion of plaque-forming bacteria.

3.7. *Rosmarinus officinalis* Linn.

Rosmarinus officinalis Linn. (Labiatae) is a small shrub whose leaves have small glands containing essential oils. Tests performed *in vitro* with the essential oil showed an inhibitory effect on the adherence of *S. mutans* and the inhibitory growth activity of Gram-negative bacteria [98-100]. This plant has great potential in inhibiting bacterial growth and in the synthesis of glucan, suggesting its potential use in the control of cariogenic bacteria, whose activities were observed when its hydro-alcoholic extract showed significant activity on the glucosyltransferase enzyme produced by *S. mutans* [101-103]. It could also be observed that the alcoholic extract proved to be efficient in inhibiting the adherence of *S. mitis*, *S. mutans* and *S. sobrinus*, which suggests that it contains compounds with antibacterial activity against oral bacteria [104].

3.8. *Lippia sidoides* Cham.

Lippia sidoides Cham. (Verbenaceae) is a shrub originating from northeastern Brazil, popularly known as "alecrim pimenta". It is used in the treatment of allergic rhinitis, sore throat, gum inflammation, and the treating of skin wounds and cuts [105, 106]. *L. sidoides* contains an essential oil rich in thymol, which contains bactericidal properties [107, 108]. Tests performed *in vivo* have proven the effectiveness of a mouthwash and toothpaste-based essential oil of *L. sidoides*. An inhibition of approximately 12% of the microorganisms could be observed, with a 6% of reduction in the biofilm formation rate, thus demonstrating the efficiency of this essential oil in oral-based hygiene products [109, 110].

3.9. *Calendula officinalis* L.

Calendula officinalis L. (Asteraceae) is an herbaceous plant that is widely cultivated in many parts of the world for ornamental, medicinal, and cosmetic purposes [111]. In the dental field, this plant has been tested as regards its capacity to control the growth of biofilm-forming bacteria. Tests performed *in vivo* have demonstrated the effect of a 10% tincture of *C. officinalis* against chronic gingivitis, presenting significant improvement in the gingival tissues, with no apparent side effects [112, 19]. From these results, a toothpaste and a mouthwash containing 10% tincture of *C. officinalis* was developed. Tests performed *in vivo* using the type of toothpaste have demonstrated the effectiveness of this dental cream on gingival inflammation and the reduction of biofilm formation caused by *S. mutans* [113, 103]. Tests performed *in vivo* using a mouthwash containing 10% tincture of *C. officinalis* verified its efficiency in improving periodontal health, concluding that the performance was similar to mouthwashes prepared with 0.12% chlorhexidine in most evaluated parameters [114]. Another test performed *in vivo* using a toothpaste containing hydroalcoholic extracts of *C. officinalis* and *C. sylvestris* also showed bacteriostatic and fungistatic actions against microorganisms, such as *S. aureus, S. mutans*, and *C. albicans*, showing the associated therapeutic properties of these extracts [115].

3.10. *Schinus terebinthifolius* Raddi and *Myracrodruon urundeuva* Fr. All.

Schinus terebinthifolius Raddi and *Myracrodruon urundeuva* Fr. All. (Anacardiaceae), known in Brazil as "aroeira da praia" and "aroeira do sertão", respectively, are plants that are commonly found in South America. These plants are still used in traditional medicine in the northeastern regions of Brazil [116-119]. A 10% tincture of *S. terebinthifolius* showed efficacy in controlling biofilms formed by *S. mutans*, with a significant reduction in colony-forming units, as well as in the treatment of chronic gingivitis, presenting similar results when compared to 0.12% chlorhexidine-based toothpastes. This tincture also showed anti-inflammatory and antifungal activities against *Candida albicans*, suggesting its potential as an antibacterial agent, especially in the prevention oral cavity disease [120-123]. By contrast, the alcoholic extract of *M. urundeuva* also showed significant antimicrobial and anti-adherent activities against microorganisms that form biofilms [124].

3.11. *Matricaria recutita* Linn.

Matricaria recutita Linn. (Compositae) is a native plant of Europe and western Asia and is known for its variety of active flavonoids as well as for its essential oil, which is rich in terpenoids and is responsible for its anti-inflammatory and antibacterial activities [125, 126]. This plant has been widely used in inflammatory and infectious processes of the oral cavity [127]. Costa *et al.* [128] found that the alcoholic extract of *M. recutita* has antibacterial and anti-adherent activities against cariogenic bacteria *S. mutans, S. sanguinis* and *L. casei* [129]. According to studies performed by Lins *et al.* [130], a simple application of a mouthwash based on the hydroalcoholic extract of *M. recutita* proved effective in controlling biofilm formations caused by microorganisms, such as *S. mutans* and *S. sanguinis*, found in the oral cavity. In addition, this plant has been used in commercial toothpastes formulations for adults and children.

3.12. *Eugenia uniflora* L.

Eugenia uniflora L. (Myrtaceae), popularly known as "pitangueira", is a fruitful plant that is native to Brazil but can also be found in northern Argentina and Uruguay. [131]. Its leaves have been related to the treatment of various ailments, including fever, stomach ailments, hypertension, and obesity [132]. Antimicrobial activity was observed in this plant's leaves and cherries against *S. mutans, S. sanguinis, S. salivarius, S. mitis,* and *S. oralis* bacteria. Toothpastes containing the alcoholic extract of the ripe fruit of *E. uniflora* showed a similar efficacy to the Colgate Total 12 toothpaste, used as controlling agents in tests performed *in vivo* by Jovito *et al.* [133]. Castro *et al.* [134] demonstrated that hydroalcoholic extracts of *E. uniflora* showed antibacterial activity against *L. casei.*

3.13. *Myrciaria cauliflora* (Mart.) O. Berg.

Myrciaria cauliflora (Mart.) O. Berg. (Myrtaceae) is a native plant from Brazil and can be found throughout the country [135]. Tests performed *in vitro* using the alcoholic extract of this plant's leaves against *S. mutans* demonstrated that this extract acts on biofilm formation and could be an alternative for use in toothpastes [136, 137].

3.14. *Syzygium aromaticum*

Syzygium aromaticum (Myrtaceae), an aromatic flower bud of a tree that is native to the Maluku Islands in Indonesia, is commonly used as a spice. Cloves are commercially harvested primarily in Indonesia, India, Madagascar, Zanzibar, Pakistan, and Sri Lanka. The essential oil of *S. aromaticum* is used for flavoring and as a natural food preservative, as it presents antifungal and antibacterial activities [138, 139]. Its essential oil is rich in the compound eugenol, which is the most abundant substance in the tree's bark and is widely used in dentistry as an anesthetic in dental hygiene and to relieve toothaches [140]. This tree's branches contain a predominance of α and β-pinene, α-phellandrene, *p*-cymene, limonene, linalool, α-sequiterpenes copaene, β-caryophyllene, caryophyllene oxide, alilbenzenos ϵ-cinnamaldehyde, and aceto of ϵ-cinnamyl monoterpenes [141]. Tests performed *in vitro* demonstrated that the essential oil of *S. aromaticum*, when pure and incorporated into a toothpaste, presented antibacterial activity against *S. mutans* [142].

3.15. *Cinnamomum zeylanicum*

Cinnamomum zeylanicum (Lauraceae), native to Sri Lanka in South Asia, is a small or medium sized tree, commonly reaching 20 to 40 ft. in height. *C. zeylanicum* was widely used in ancient times as a spice. It is currently used as a flavoring in cooking food as well as in medicine as an antimicrobial agent. The essential oil extracted from its leaves contain a greater quantity of an aldehyde called cinnamaldehyde. Oliveira *et al.* [142] evaluated the essential oil of this plant against *S. mutans* and *L. casei*. These authors observed that the essential oil of *C. zeylanicum* showed inhibition zones of close to or above those of standard chlorhexidine, which was the same result observed for toothpastes formulated with the oil. Other studies have demonstrated the action of this essential oil on yeasts, such as *C. albicans* and *C. tropicalis*, which produce oral candidiasis in denture users [143].

3.16. *Cymbopogon citratus*

Cymbopogon citratus (Poaceae) is a herbaceous plant that is, native to the tropical regions of Asia, especially India. Also known as *Cymbopogon (nardus)* or by synonyms, such as *Andropogon citratus ceriferus, Andropogon citratus, Andropogon citriodorum, Andropogon nardus ceriferus, Andropogon roxburghiie,* and *Andropogon schoenanthus*. The essential oil extracted from this plant's leaves contains the main components of citral, geraniol, methyleugenol, myrcene, and citronellal [144]. Oliveira *et al.* [142] evaluated this plant's essential oil against *S. mutans* and *L. casei* and noted that it presented inhibition zones of close to those of standard chlorhexidine against the microorganism *S. mutans*. However, when analyzing the formulation of toothpastes containing the essential oil, it was found that this oil proved ineffective in the concentration tested to inhibit the growth of microorganisms. Perazzo *et al.* [145] also evaluated the essential oil of *C. citratus* on bacterial biofilm formation, especially in strains of *S. mutans* (ATCC 25175), *S. salivarius* (ATCC7073), and *S. oralis* (ATCC1055) and observed that this essential oil was more effective against *S. mutans*.

3.17. *Malva sylvestris*

Malva sylvestris (Malvaceae) is a biennial or perennial erect herbaceous species that is native to Europe and is widely known for its anti-inflammatory and antimicrobial properties [146]. Its phytochemical composition includes tannins, glycolipids, and flavonoids, which were tested as regards their capacity to control the growth of bacteria and biofilm formation [147, 18]. *M. sylvestris* has proven to be so effective that it already exists on the commercial market, called Malvatricin®, which is widely used as an antimicrobial agent against cariogenic bacteria. This effect is most likely due to the action of quinosol, a substance present in its composition [148].

3.18. *Nasturtium officinale*

Nasturtium officinale (Cruciferaceae) is a native plant of Europe and Asia that has many uses in medicine and pharmacology [149]. It is rich in vitamins and active substances, and is most commonly used in the treatment of urinary tract infections in children [150]. Tests performed *in vitro* with a mouthwash containing 10% hydroalcoholic extract of *N. officinale* was effective in controlling the growth of the microorganisms present in the oral cavity and dental plaque [151].

3.19. *Aloe vera*

Aloe vera (L.) Burm and *Aloe barbadensis* Miller (Asphodelaceae), popularly known as "aloe", are native from Africa and are widely used in traditional medicine. The gel of this plant contains healing, antibacterial, and antifungal activities due to the presence of anthraquinones, such as aloenin, barbaloin, and isobarbaloin in its chemical composition [152-155]. Studies have demonstrated the antimicrobial activity of toothpastes containing *A. vera* on oral microorganisms, such as *S. mutans*, *S. sanguis*, *A. viscosus*, and *C. albicans* [27].

3.20. *Magnolia officinalis*

Magnolia officinalis (Magnoliaceae) is a native plant of the mountains and valleys of China at altitudes of 300-1500 meters. The highly aromatic bark is stripped from the stems, branches, and roots, and is used in traditional Chinese medicine, where it is known as "hou po" [156]. The traditional use indications are to eliminate the dampness and phlegm, and relieve the distension. Huang *et al.* [157] have shown that the magnolol isolated from this plant was able to inhibit the growth of cariogenic bacteria.

Plants	Pharmaceutical form	Use
Salvia officinalis	mouthwash	plaque and bleeding on probing
Plantago psyllium L	mouthwash	periodontitis
Punica granatum Linn. and *Centella asiatica*	mouthwash	periodontitis
Aloe ferox Mill	mouthwash	gingivitis
Calendula officinalis L	mouthwash	Gengivite and periodontitis
Lippia sidoides Cham	mouthwash	plaque and bleeding on probing
Punica granatum Linn.	toothpaste	gingivitis
M. recutita L./Enchinacea angustifólia/ Krameria triandria Ruíze Pavon	toothpaste	gingivitis
Calendula officinalis L	toothpaste	gingivitis
Punica granatum Linn.	Gel	candidiasis, plaque and gingivitis

Table 1. Medicinal plants use in the treatment of oral diseases clinical studies.

3.21. *Salvia officinallis*

Salvia officinallis (Labiatae) is plant that is native to the Mediterranean region, though it has been naturalized in many places throughout the world. It is a perennial, evergreen subshrub that has a long history of medicinal and culinary uses. Its essential oil contains cineole, borneol, and thujone. Sage leaf contains tannic acid, oleic acid, ursonic acid, ursolic acid, carnosol, carnosic acid, fumaric acid, chlorogenic acid, caffeic acid, niacin, nicotinamide, flavones, flavonoid glycosides, and estrogenic substances [158]. Tests performed *in vivo* by Celeste *et al.* [159] have shown that a mouthwash containing a 10% alcoholic extract of *S. officinalis* reduced the visible plaque index (VPI) of the volunteers in 15.3% and the gingival index (GI) in 9.3% when compared to the chlorhexidine control.

3.22. *Azadirachta indica*

Azadirachta indica (Meliaceae) is native plant of India and the Indian subcontinent including Nepal, Pakistan, Bangladesh, and Sri Lanka. The tree can reach a height of 15 to 20 m (49 to 66 ft.). It has been used in India for decades in the treatment of several diseases in medicine and dentistry. Chatterjee *et al.* [160] evaluated a 0.19% *A. indica* mouthwash in tests performed *in vivo* and observed that the *A. indica* mouthwash is as effective in reducing periodontal indices as is chlorhexidine, which was used as the control, showing a significant reduction in gingival bleeding, and plaque indices.

4. Conclusion

The decrease in the amount of fluoride associated with the presence of plant extracts with proven antimicrobial activity is a positive factor for the reduction of fluorosis. For babies, we recommend the use of toothpastes containing only plant extracts, with no fluoride, since there is no risk of caries at this age. In such cases, these toothpastes can be used to adapt the babies to a proper hygiene of their oral cavity as well as maintain their beneficial microbiota.

Acknowledgements

The authors are grateful to CNPq, CAPES and FAPEMIG for their financial support.

Author details

Marisa Alves Nogueira Diaz[1*], Isabela de Oliveira Carvalho[1] and Gaspar Diaz[2]

*Address all correspondence to: marisanogueira@ufv.br

1 Departament of Biochemistry and Molecular Biology, Federal University of Viçosa, Viçosa, Minas Gerais, Brazil

2 Departament of Chemistry, Federal University of Minas Gerais, Belo Horizonte, Minas Gerais, Brazil

References

[1] Aas JA, Paster BJ, Stokes LN, Olsen I, Dewhirst FE. Defining the normal bacterial flora of the oral cavity. Journal of Clinical Microbiology 2005;43(5) 721–732.

[2] Zaura E, Keijser BJ, Huse SM, Crielaard W. Defining the healthy "core microbiome" of oral microbial communities. BMC Microbiology 2009;9(1) 259-271.

[3] Groppo FC, Bergamaschi CC, Cogo K, Franz-Montan M, Motta RHL, Andrade ED. Use of Phytotherapy in Dentistry. Phytotherapy Research 2008; 22 993–998.

[4] Marsh PD, Moter A, Devine DA. Dental plaque biofilms: communities, conflict and control. Periodontology 2011;53(1) 16-35.

[5] Meyer DH, Fives-Taylor PM. Oral pathogens: from dental plaque to cardiac disease. Current Opinion in Microbiology 1998;1(1) 88-95.

[6] Barrau K, Boulamery A, Imbert G, Casalta JP, Habib G, Messana T, Bonnet JL, Rubinstein E, Raoult D. Causative organisms of infective endocarditis according to host status. Clinical Microbiology and Infection 2004;10(4) 302-308.

[7] Okuda K, Kato T, Ishihara K. Involvement of periodontopathic biofilm in vascular diseases. Oral Diseases 2004;10(1) 5-12.

[8] Kolenbrander PE. Intergeneric coaggregation among human oral bacteria and ecology of dental plaque. Annual Review of Microbiology 1988;42(1) 627-656.

[9] Bowenand WH, Koo H. Biology of *Streptococcus mutans* derived glucosyltransferases: role in extracellular matrix formation of cariogenic biofilms. Caries Research, 2011;45(1) 69-86.

[10] Bradshaw DJ, Marsh PD, Watson GK, Allison C. Role of *Fusobacterium nucleatumand* coaggregation in anaerobe survival in planktonic and biofilm oral communities during aeration. Infection and Immunity 1998;66(10) 4729-4732.

[11] Marsh PD. Dental plaque as a biofilm and a microbial community-implications for health and disease. BMC Oral Health 2006;6(suppl 1) S14.

[12] Socransky SS, Haffajee AD. Periodontal microbial ecology. Periodontol 2000. 2005;38(1) 135-187.

[13] Thibodeau EA, O'Sullivan DM. Salivary *mutans* streptococci and caries development in the primary and mixed dentitions of children. Community Dentistry and Oral Epidemiology 1999;27(6) 406-412.

[14] Loesche W. Dental caries and periodontitis: contrasting two infections that have medical implications. Infectious Disease Clinics of North America 2007;21(2) 471-502.

[15] Featherstone JDB. Dental caries: a dynamic disease process. Australian Dental Journal 2008;53(3) 286-291.

[16] Petersen PE, Bourgeois D, Ogawa H, Estupinan-Day S, Ndiaye C. The global burden of oral disease and risks to oral health. Bulletin of the World Health Organization 2005;83(9) 661-669.

[17] Long SR, Santos AS, Nascimento CMO. Avaliação da contaminação de escovas dentais por enterobactérias. Revista de Odontologia da Universidade de Santo Amaro 2000;5(1) 21-25.

[18] Buffon MCM, Lima MLC, Galarda L, Cogo L. Avaliação da eficácia dos extratos de *Malva sylvestris, Calendula officinalis, Plantago major* e *Curcuma zedoarea* no controle do crescimento das bactérias da placa dentária. Estudo *"in vitro"*. Revista Visão Acadêmica 2001;2(1) 31-38.

[19] Van Rijkom HM, Truin GJ, Van't Hof MA. A meta-analysis of clinical studies on the caries-inhibiting effect of chlorhexidine treatment. Journal of Dental Research 1996;75(2) 790-795.

[20] Cangussu MCT, Narvai PC, Castellanos Fernandez R, Djehizian V. A fluorose dentária no Brasil: uma revisão crítica. Cadernos de Saúde Pública 2002;18(1) 7-15.

[21] Cury JA, Tenuta LMA, Ribeiro CCC, Paes Leme AF. The importance of fluoride dentifrices to the current dental caries prevalence in Brazil. Brazilian Dental Journal 2004;5(3) 167-174.

[22] Ricomini Filho AP, Tenuta LMA, Fernandes, FSF, Calvo SCK, Cury JA. Fluoride concentration in the top-selling Brazilian toothpastes purchased at different regions. Brazilian Dental Journal 2012;23(1) 45-48.

[23] Mascarenhas AK. Risk factors for dental fluorosis: A review of the recent literature. Pediatric dentistry 2000;22(4) 269-277.

[24] Moysés SJ, Moysés ST, Allegretti AC, Argenta M, Werneck R. Dental fluorosis: epidemiological fiction?. Revista Panamericana de Salud Pública 2002;12(5) 339-346.

[25] National Research Council. Fluoride in drinking water: a scientific review of EPA's standards. The National Academies Press, 2006.

[26] Adamkova H, Vicar J, Palasova J, Ulrichova J, Simanek V. Macleya cordata and Prunella vulgaris in oral hygiene products – their efficacy in the control of gingivitis. Biomed Pap Med Fac Univ Palacky Olomouc Czech Repub. 2004;148(1) 103-105.

[27] Lee SS, Zhang W, Li Y. The antimicrobial potential of 14 natural herbal dentifrices: results of anin vitro diffusion method study. The Journal of the American Dental Association 2004;135(8) 1133-1141.

[28] Gunsolley JC. A meta-analysis of six-month studies of antiplaque and antigingivitis agents. The Journal of the American Dental Association 2006;137(12) 1649-1657.

[29] Allaker RP, Douglas CW. Novel anti-microbial therapies for dental plaque-related diseases. International Journal of Antimicrobial Agents 2009;33(1) 8-13.

[30] DenBesten P, Berkowitz RJ. Early childhood caries: an overvview with reference to our experience in California. Journal of California Dental Association 2003;31(1) 139-143.

[31] Agarwala M, Yadav RNS. Phytochemical analysis of some medicinal plants. Journal of Phytology 2011;3(12) 10-14.

[32] Okpalugo J, Ibrahim K, Inyang US. Toothpaste formulation efficacy in reducing oral flora. Tropical Journal of Pharmaceutical Research 2009;8(1) 71-77.

[33] Pistorius A, Willershausen B, Steinmeier EM, Kreislert M. Efficacy of subgingival irrigation using herbal extracts on gingival inflammation. Journal of Periodontology 2003;7 4616–622.

[34] Pannuti CM, Mattos JP, Ranoya PN, Jesus AM, Lotufo RF, Romito GA. Clinical effect of a herbal dentifrice on the control of plaque and gingivitis: a double-blind study. Pesquisa Odontológica Brasileira 2003;17(4) 314-318.

[35] Zhou L, Ding Y, Chen W, Zhang P, Chen Y, Lv X. Thein vitro study of ursolic acid and oleanolic acid inhibiting cariogenic microorganisms as well as biofilm. Oral Diseases 2013;19(5) 494-500.

[36] Knoll-Kohler E, Stiebel J. Amine fluoride gel affects the viability and the generation of superoxide anions in human polymorphonuclear leukocytes: an in vitro study. European Journal of Oral Sciences 2002;110(4) 296-301.

[37] Neumegen RA, Fernández-Alba AR, Chisti Y. Toxicities of triclosan, phenol, and copper sulfate in activated sludge. Environmental Toxicology 2005;20(2) 160-164.

[38] Vieira MD, Hirata Júnior R, Barbosa ARS. Avaliação antimicrobiana de três dentifrícios para uso infantil: estudo in vitro. Revista Brasileira de Odontologia 2008;65(1) 52-56.

[39] Jose M, Deepa KC, Prabhu V. Ethnomedicinal Practices for Oral health and hygiene of Tribal population of Wayanad Kerala. In International Journal of Research in Ayurveda & pharmacy (IJRAP) 2011;2(4) 1246-1250.

[40] Jaiswal P, Kumar P, Singh VK., Singh D.K. Biological effects of *Myristica fragrans.* Annual Review of Biomedical Sciences 2009;11(1) 21-29.

[41] Qiu Q, Zhang G, Sun X, Liu X. Study on chemical constituents of the essential oil from *Myristica fragrans* Houtt. by supercritical fluid extraction and steam distillation. Journal of Chinese Medicinal Materials 2004; 27(11) 823-826.

[42] Chung JY, Choo JH, Lee MH, Hwang JK. Anticariogenic activity of macelignan isolated from *Myristica fragrans* (nutmeg) against *Streptococcus mutans*. Phytomedicine 2006;13(4) 261-266.

[43] Yang XW, Huang X, Ahmat M. "New neolignan from seed of *Myristica fragrans*," Zhongguo Zhongyao Zazhi 2008;33(4) 397-402.

[44] Sonavane GS, Sarveiya VP, Kasture VS, Kasture SB. Anxiogenic activity of *Myristica fragrans* seeds. Pharmacology Biochemistry and Behavior 2002;71(1-2) 239-244.

[45] Zaidi SFH, Yamada K, Kadowaki M, Usmanghani K, Sugiyama T. Bactericidal activity of medicinal plants, employed for the treatment of gastrointestinal ailments, against *Helicobacter pylori*. Journal of Ethnopharmacology 2009;121(2) 286-291.

[46] Ozaki Y, Soedigdo S, Wattimena YR, Suganda AG. Anti-inflammatory effect of Mace, aril of *Myristica fragrans* Houtt. and its active principles. Japanese Journal of Pharmacology 1989;49(2) 155-163.

[47] Shafiei Z, Shuhairi NN, Yap NMFS, Sibungkil C-AH, Hindawi JL. Antibacterial activity of *Myristica fragrans* against oral pathogens.vol. 2012, Article ID 825362, 7 pages, 2012. doi:10.1155/2012/825362.

[48] Burdock GA. Review of the biological properties and toxicity of bee propolis (propolis). Food and Chemical Toxicology 1998;36(4) 347-363.

[49] Tosi EA, Ré E, Ortega ME, Cazzoli AF. Food preservative based on propolis: bacteriostatic activity of propolis polyphenols and flavonoids upon *Escherichia coli*. Food Chemistry 2007;104(3) 1025-1029.

[50] Valencia D, Alday E, Robles-Zepeda R, Garibay-Escobar A, Galvez-Ruiz JC, Salas-Reyes M, Jiménez-Estrada M, Velázquez-Contreras E, Hernández J, Velázquez C. Seasonal effect on chemical composition and biological activities of Sonoran propolis. Food Chemistry 2012;131(2) 645-651.

[51] Park YK, Ikegaki M, Alencar SM, Moura FF. Evaluation of brazilian propolis by both physicochemical methods and biological activity. Honeybee Science 2000;21(2) 85-90.

[52] Marcucci MC, Ferreres F, Custódio AR, Ferreira MMC, Bankova VS, García-Viguera C, Bretz WA. Evaluation of phenolic compounds in Brazilian propolis from different geographic regions. Zeistchrift fur Naturforschung, 2000;55(1/2) 76-81.

[53] Cunha IBDS, Salomao K, Shimizu M, Bankova VS, Custodio AR, De Castro SL, Marcucci MC. Anti-trypanosomal activity of Brazilian propolis from *Apis mellifera*. Chemical & pharmaceutical Bulletin 2004;52(5) 602-604.

[54] Koo H, Rosalen PL, Cury JA, Park YK, Ikegaki M, Sattler A. Effect of *Apis mellifera* propolis from two Brazilian regions on caries development in desalivated rats. Caries Research 1999;33(5) 393-400.

[55] Koo H, Rosalen PL, Cury JA, Ambrosano GMAB, Murata RM, Yatsuda R, Ikegaki M, Alencar SM, Park YK. Effect of a new variety of *Apis mellifera* propolis on mutans Streptococci. Current Microbiology 2000;41(3) 192-196.

[56] Duarte S, Rosalen PL, Hayacibara MF, Cury JA, Bowen WH, Marquis RE, Rehder VLG, Sartoratto A, Ikegaki M, Koo H. The influence of a novel propolis on mutans

streptococci biofilms and caries development in rats. Archives of Oral Biology 2006;51(1) 15-22.

[57] Bankova V. Chemical diversity of propolis and the problem of standardization. Journal of Ethnopharmacology 2005;100(1-2) 114-117.

[58] Piccinelli AL, Fernández MC, Cuesta-Rubio O, Hernández IM, De Simone F, Rastrelli L. Isoflavonoids isolated from Cuban propolis. Journal of Agricultural and Food Chemistry 2005;53(23) 9010-9016.

[59] Ikeno K, Ikeno T, Miyazawa C. Effects of propolis on dental caries in rats. Caries Research 1991;25(5) 347-351.

[60] Park YK, Koo MH, Abreu JA, Ikegaki M, Cury JA, Rosalen PL. Antimicrobial activity of propolis on oral microorganisms. Current Microbiology 1998;36(1) 24-28.

[61] Duailibe SA, Gonçalves AG, Ahid FJ. Effect of a propolis extract on *Streptococcus mutans* counts *in vivo*. Journal of Applied Oral Science 2000;15(5) 420-423.

[62] Arslan S, Silici S, Perçin D, Ko AN, Er Ö. Antimicrobial activity of poplar propolis on mutans streptococci and caries development in rats. Turkish Journal of Biology 2012;36(1) 65-73.

[63] Barrientos L, Herrera CL, Montenegro G, Ortega X, Veloz J, Alvear M, Cuevas A, Saavedra N, Salazar LA. Chemical and botanical characterization of Chilean propolis and biological activity on cariogenic bacteria *Streptococcus mutans* and *Streptococcus sobrinus*. Brazilian Journal of Microbiology 2013;44(2) 577-585.

[64] Kubota N, Tastumoto N, Sano T, Toya K. A simple preparation of half N-acetylated chitosan highly soluble in water and aqueous organic solvents. Carbohydrate Research 2000;324(4) 268-274.

[65] Kittur FS, Kumar ABV, Varadaraj MC, Tharanathan RN. Chitooligosaccharides-preparation with the aid of pectinase isozyme from *Aspergillus nigerand* their antibacterial activity. Carbohydrate Research 2005;340(6) 1239-1245.

[66] Verkaik MJ, Busscher HJ, Jager D, Slomp AM, Abbas F, van der Mei HC. Efficacy of natural antimicrobials in toothpaste formulations against oral biofilms *in vitro*. Journal of dentistry 2011;39(3) 218-224.

[67] Choi BK, Kim KY, Yoo YJ, Oh SJ, Choi JH, Kim CY.*in vitro* antimicrobial activity of a chitooligosaccharide mixture against *Actinobacillus actinomycete comitans* and *Streptococcus mutans*. International Journal of Antimicrobial Agents 2001;18(6) 553-557.

[68] İkinci G, Şenel S, Akıncıbay H, Kaş S, Erciş S, Wilson CG, Hıncal AA. Effect of chitosan on a periodontal pathogen *Porphyromonas gingivalis*. International Journal of Phamaceutics 2002; 235(1/2) 121-127.

[69] Tarsi R, Muzzarelli R, Guzmàn C, Pruzzo C. Inhibition of *Streptococcus mutans* adsorption to hydroxyapatite by low-molecular-weigth chitosans. Journal of Dental Research 1997;76(2) 665-672.

[70] Sano H, Shibasaki KI, Matsukubo T, Takaesu Y. Effect of chitosan rinsing on reduction of dental plaque formation. The Bulletin of Tokyo Dental College 2003;44(1) 9-16.

[71] Decker EM, von Ohle C, Weiger R, Wiech I, Brecx M. A synergistic chlorhexidine/chitosan combination for improved antiplaque strategies. Journal of Periodontal Research 2005;40(5) 373-377.

[72] Mohire NC, Yadav AV. Chitosan-based polyherbal toothpaste: As novel oral hygiene product. Indian Journal of Dental Research 2010;21(3) 380-384.

[73] Tavaria FK, Costa EM, Pina-Vaz L, Carvalho MF, Pintado MM. A quitosana como biomaterial odontológico: estado da arte. Brazilian Journal of Biomedical Engineering 2013;29(1) 110-120.

[74] Ross RG, Selvasubramanian S, Jayasundar S. Immunomodulatory activity of *Punica granatum* in rabbits-a preliminary study. Journal of Ethnopharmacology 2001;78(1) 85-87.

[75] Machado TB, Pinto MCFR, Leal LCR, Silva MG, Amaral ACF, Kuster RM, Netto-Dos-Santos KR. In vitro activity of Brazilian medicinal plants, naturally occurring naphthoquinones and their analogues, against methicillin-resistant *Staphylococcus aureus*. International Journal of Antimicrobial Agents 2003;21(3) 279-284.

[76] Nawwar MAM, Hussein SAM, Merfort L. Leaf phenolics of *Punica granatum*. Phytochemistry 1994;37(4) 1175-1177.

[77] Machado TB, Leal LCR, Amaral ACF, Santos KRN, Silva MG, Kuster RM. Antimicrobial ellagitannin of *Punica granatum* fruits. Journal of the Brazilian Chemical Society 2002;13(5) 606-610.

[78] Pereira JV, Pereira MSV, Higino JS, Sampaio FC, Alves PM, Araújo CRF. Estudos com o extrato da *Punica granatum* Linn. (romã): efeito antimicrobiano in vitro e avaliação clínica de um dentifrício sobre microrganismos do biofilme dental. Revista Odonto Ciência 2005;20(49) 262-269.

[79] Pereira JV, Pereira MSV, Sampaio FC, Correia MC, Alves PM, Araújo CRF, Higino JS. Efeito antibacteriano e antiaderente *in vitro* do extrato da *Punica granatum* Linn.sobre microrganismos do biofilme dental. Revista Brasileira de Farmacognosia 2006;16(1) 88-93.

[80] Vasconcelos LCS, Sampaio FC, Sampaio MCC, Pereira MSV, Higino JS, Peixoto MHP. Minimum inhibitory concentration of adherence of *Punica granatum* Linn (pomegranate) gel against *S. mutans, S. mitis* and *C. albicans*. Brazilian Dental Journal 2006;17(3) 223-227.

[81] Chang ST, Kwan HS, Kang YN. Collection, characterization and utilization of germ plasm of *Lentinula edodes*. Canadian Journal of Botany 1995;73(1) 955-961.

[82] Eira AF, Kaneno R, Rodrigues Filho E, Barbisan LF, Pascholati SF, Di Piero RM, Salvadori DMF, Lima PLA, Ribeiro LR. Farming technology, biochemistry characterization, and protective effects of culinary-medicinal mushrooms *Agaricus brasiliensis* and *Lentinus edodes*: five years of research in Brazil. International Journal of Medicinal Mushrooms 2005;7(1/2) 281-300.

[83] Galvão G. Almeirão. Natureza 1995;8(7) 53-55.

[84] Van Lo J, Coussement P, Leenheer L, Hoebregs H, Smits G. On the presence of inulin and oligofructose as natural ingredients in the western diet. Critical Reviews in Food Science and Nutrition 1995;35(6) 525-552.

[85] Signoretto C, Canepari P, Pruzzo C, Gazzani G. Anticaries and antiadhesive properties of food constituents and plant extracts and implications for oral health. In: Wilson M. (ed) Food constituents and oral health: current status and future prospects. Cambridge: Woodhead Publishing Limited; 2009.

[86] Daglia, M, Papetti A,Mascherpa D,Grisoli P, Giusto G, Lingström P, Pratten J, Signoretto C, Spratt DA, Wilson M, Zaura E, Gazzan G. Plant and fungal food components with potential activity on the development of microbial oral diseases. Journal of Biomedicine and Biotechnology 2011;1-9.

[87] Spratt DA, Daglia M, Papetti A, Stauder M, Donnell DO, Ciric L, Tymon A, Repetto B, Signoretto C, Houri-Haddad Y, Feldman M, Steinberg D, Lawton S, Lingström P, PrattenJ, Zaura E,Gazzani G,Pruzzo C,Wilson M. Evaluation of plant and fungal extracts for their potential antigingivitis and anticaries activity. Journal of Biomedicine and Biotechnology 2012;1-12.

[88] Signoretto AM, Bertoncelli A, Burlacchini G, Tessarolo F, Caola L, Pezzati E, Zaura E, Papetti A, Lingstrom P, Pratten J, Spratt DA, Wilson M, Canepari P. Effects of mushroom and chicory extracts on the physiology and shape of *Prevotella intermedia*, a periodonto pathogenic bacterium. Journal of Biomedicine and Biotechnology 2011;1-8.

[89] Veiga Junior VF, Pinto AC, Calixto JB, Zunino L, Patitucci ML. Phytochemical and antiedematogenic studies of commercial copaíba oils available in Brazil. Phytotherapy Research 2001;15(6) 476-480.

[90] Lima SRM, Veiga Junior VF, Christo HB, Pinto AC, Fernandes PD. *In vivo* and *in vitro* studies on the anticancer activity of *Copaifera multijuga* Hayne and its fractions. Phytotherapy Research 2003;17(9) 1048-1053.

[91] Francisco SG. Uso do óleo de copaíba (*Copaifera officinalis*) em inflamação ginecológica. Femina 2005;33(2) 89-93.

[92] Pontes AB, Correia DZ, Coutinho MS, Mothé CG. Emulsão dermatológica a base de copaíba. Revista Analytica 2003; 7(7) 36-42

[93] Cascon V, Gilbert B. Characterization of the chemical composition of oleoresins of *Copaifera guianensis* Desf.,*Copaifera duckei* Dwyer and *Copaifera multijuga* Hayne. Phytochemistry 2000;55(7) 773-778.

[94] Pinto AC, Braga WF, Rezende CM, Garrido FMS, Veiga Júnior VF, Bergyer L, Patitucci ML, Antunes AC. Separation of acid diterpenes of *Copaifera cearenses* Huber ex Duke by flash chromatography using potassium hydroxide impregnated silica gel. Journal of the Brazilian Chemical Society 2000;11(4) 355-360.

[95] Veiga Junior VF, Pinto AC, Maciel MAM. Plantas medicinais: cura segura?. Química nova 2005;28(3) 519-528.

[96] Brito MVH, Oliveira RVB, Reis JMC. Estudo macroscópico do estômago de ratos após administração do óleo de Copaíba. Revista Paraense de Medicina 2000;14:(3) 29-33.

[97] Pieri FA, Mussi MC, Fiorini JE, Schneedorf JM. Efeitos clínicos e microbiológicos do óleo de copaíba (*Copaifera officinalis*) sobre bactérias formadoras de placa dental em cães. Arquivo Brasileiro de Medicina Veterinária e Zootecnia 2010;62(3) 578-585.

[98] Al-Sereiti MR, Abu-Amer KM, Sen P. Pharmacology of rosemary (*Rosmarinus offi cinalis* Linn.) and its therapeutic potentials. Indian Journal of Experimental Biology 1999;37(2) 124-130.

[99] Newall CA, Anderson LA, Phillipson JD. Plantas Medicinais: guia para profissional de saúde. São Paulo: Premier 2002.

[100] Takarada K, Kimizuka R, Takahashi N, Honma K, Okuda K, Kato T. A comparison of the antibacterial efficacies of essential oils against oral pathogens. Oral Microbiology and Immunology 2004;19(1) 61-64.

[101] Alves MP, Pereira VJ, Higino JS, Pereira MSV, Queiroz, MG. Atividade antimicrobiana e antiaderente in vitro do extrato de *Rosmarinus officinalis* Linn. (alecrim) sobre microrganismos cariogênicos. Arquivos em Odontologia 2008;44(2) 5-10.

[102] Battagin J. Cinética enzimática e efeito de extratos naturais na atividade da enzima glicosiltransferase de *Streptococcus mutans*. Master thesis. Universidade São Francisco; 2010.

[103] Pinheiro, MA, Brito DBA, Almeida LFD, Cavalcanti YW, Padilha WWN. Efeito antimicrobiano de tinturas de produtos naturais sobre bactérias da cárie dentária. Revista Brasileira em Promoção da Saúde, 2012;25(2) 197-201.

[104] Silva MSA, Silva MAR, Higino JS, Pereira MSV, Carvalho AAT. Atividade antimicrobiana e antiaderente in vitro do extrato de *Rosmarinus officinalis* Linn. sobre bactérias orais planctônicas. Revista Brasileira de Farmacognosia 2008;18(2) 236-240.

[105] Lemos TL, Craveiro AA, Alencar JW, Matos FJ, Clarck AM, Macchesney JD. Antimicrobial activity of essential oil of Brazilian plants. Phytotherapy Research 1990;4(2) 82-84.

[106] Nunes RS. Desenvolvimento galënico de produtos de uso odontologico (creme dental e enxaguatorio bucal) a base de *Lippia sidoides* Cham (verbenaceae) Master thesis. Universidade Federal de Pernambuco; 1999.

[107] Girão VCC, Nunes-Pinheiro DCS, Morais SM, Sequeira JL, Gioso MA. A clinical trial of the effect of a mouthrinse prepared with *Lippia sidoides* Cham essential oil in dogs with mild gingival disease. Preventive Veterinary Medicine 2003;59(1/2) 95-102.

[108] Cavalcanti ESB, Morais SM, Lima MA, Santana EWP. Larvicidal activity of essential oils from Brazilian plants against *Aedes aegypti* L. Memórias do Instituto Oswaldo Cruz 2004;99(5) 541-544.

[109] Sobreira FFE, Morais SM, Fonseca SGC, Mota OML. Preparation and clinical evaluation of an antiseptic mouthrinse using *Lippia sidoides* Cham (Alecrim pimenta) essencial oil. Revista ABO Nacional 1998;6(5) 323-325.

[110] Nunes RS, Lira AAM, Lacerda CM, Silva, DOB, Silva JA, Santana DP. Obtenção e avaliação clínica de dentifrícios à base do extrato hidroalcoólico da *Lippia sidoides* Cham (Verbenaceae) sobre o biofilme dentário Revista de Odontologia 2006;35(4) 275-283.

[111] Ramos A, Edreira A, Vizoso A, Betancourt J, López M, Décalo M. Genotoxicity of extract of *Calendula officinalis* L. Journal of Ethnopharmacology 1998;61(1) 49-55.

[112] Lorenzo MRO, Madrigal RG, Pineda PJ. Efectos de la tintura de calendula al 10 por ciento en adolescentes afectados por gingivitis crónica. Mediciego 1997;3(2) 33-36.

[113] Amoian B, Moghadamnia AA, Mazandarani M. The effect of calendula extract toothpaste on the plaque index and bleeding in gingivitis. Research Journal of Medicinal Plant 2010;4(3) 132-140.

[114] Vinagre NPL, Farias CG, Araújo RJG, Vieira JMS, Silva Júnior JOC, Corrêa AM. Clinical efficacy of a phytotherapic mouthrinse with standardized tincture of *Calendula officinalis* in the maintenance of periodontal health. Revista de Odontologia da UNESP 2011;40(1) 30-35.

[115] Arantes AB, Luz MMS, Santos CAM, Sato MEO. Desenvolvimento de dentifrícios com extratos fluídos de *Calendula officinalis* L. (Asteraceae) e *Casearia sylvestris* Sw. (Flacourtiaceae) destinado ao combate à placa bacteriana. Revista Brasileira de Farmacognosia 2005;86(2) 61-64.

[116] Kato ETM, Akisue G. Estudo farmacognóstico de cascas *Myracrodruon urundeuva* Fr. All. Revista Lecta 2002;20(1) 69-76.

[117] Santin DA, Leitão HF. Restabelecimento e revisão taxonômica do gênero *Myracrodruon* Freire Allemão (Anacardiacea). Revista Brasileira de Botânica 1991;14(2) 133-145.

[118] Deharo E, Baelmans R, Gimenez A, Quenevo C, Bourdy G. *In vitro* immunomodulatory activity of plants used by the *Tacana* ethnic group in Bolívia. Phytomedicine 2004;11(6) 516-522.

[119] Biavatti M, Marensi V, Leite SN, Reis A. Ethnopharmacognostic survey on botanical compendia for potential cosmeceutic species from Atlantic Forest. Revista Brasileira de Farmacognosia 2007;17(4) 640-653.

[120] Brandão EHS, Oliveira LD, Landucci LF, Koga-Ito CY, Cardoso JAO. Antimicrobial activity of coffee based solutions and their effects on *Streptococcus mutans* adherence. Brazilian Journal of Oral Science 2006;6(20) 1274-1277.

[121] Soares DGS, Oliveira CB, Leali C, Drumond MRS, Padilha WWN.Atividade antibacteriana *in vitro* da tintura de aroeira (*Schinus terebinthifolius*) na descontaminação de escovas dentais contaminadas pelo *S. mutans*. Odontologia Clínico-Científica 2007;7(3) 253-257.

[122] Freires IA, Alves LA, Jovito VC, Almeida LFD, Castro RD, Padilha WWN. Atividades antibacteriana e antiaderente *in vitro* de tinturas de *Schinus terebinthinfolius* (Aroeira) e *Solidago microglossa* (Arnica) frente a bactérias formadoras do biofilme dentário. Odontologia Clínico-Científica 2010;9(2) 139-143.

[123] Lins R, Vasconcelos FHP, Leite RB, Coelho-Soares RS, Barbosa DN. Avaliação clínica de bochechos com extratos de Aroeira (*Schinus terebinthifolius*) e Camomila (*Matricaria recutita* L.) sobre a placa bacteriana e a gengivite. Revista Brasileira de Plantas Medicinais 2013;15(1) 112-120.

[124] Alves PM, Queiroz LMG, Pereira JV, Pereira MSV. Atividade antimicrobiana, antiaderente e antifúngica *in vitro* de plantas medicinais brasileiras sobre microrganismos do biofilme dental e cepas do gênero *Candida*. Revista da Sociedade Brasileira de Medicina Tropical 2009;42(2) 222-224.

[125] Mulinacci N, Romani A, Pinelli P, Vincieri FF, Prucher D. Characterization of *Matricaria recutita* L. flower extracts by HPLC-MS and HPLC-DAD analysis. Chromatography 2000;51(5/6) 301-307.

[126] McKay DL, Blumberg JBA. Review of the bioactivity and potential health benefits of chamomile tea (*Matricaria recutita* L.). Phytotherapy Research 2006;20(7) 519-530.

[127] Paixão CCB, Santos AA, Oliveira CCC, Silva LG, Nunes MAR. Uso de plantas medicinais em pacientes portadores de afecções bucais. Odontologia Clinica Científica, 2002;1(1) 23-27.

[128] Costa MR, Albuquerque AC, Pereira L, Vieira A, Diniz DN, Pereira MSV, Pereira JV, Trevisan LFA. Efeito antimicrobiano do extrato da *Myrciaria cauliflora* Berg e *Matrica-*

ria recutita Linn. sobre microrganismos do biofilme dental. Revista de Biologia e Farmácia 2010;4(1) 19-25.

[129] Albuquerque ACL, Pereira MSV, Pereira JV, Pereira LF, Silva DF, Macedo-Costa MR, Higino JS. Efeito antiaderente do extrato da *Matricaria recutita* Linn. sobre microrganismos do biofilme dental. Revista de Odontologia da UNESP 2010; 39(1) 21-25.

[130] Lins R, Vasconcelos FHP, Leite RB, Coelho-Soares RS, Barbosa DN. Avaliação clínica de bochechos com extratos de Aroeira (*Schinus terebinthifolius*) e Camomila (*Matricaria recutita* L.) sobre a placa bacteriana e a gengivite. Revista Brasileira de Plantas Medicinais 2013;15(1) 112-120.

[131] Bezerra JEF, Lederman IE, Silva Júnior JF, Alves MA. Comportamento da pitangueira (*Eugenia uniflora*) sob Irrigação na Região do Vale do Rio Moxotó, Pernambuco. Revista Brasileira de Fruticultura 2004;26(1) 177-179.

[132] Schmeda-Hirschmann G, Theoduloz C, Franco L, Ferro E, Arias AR. Preliminary pharmacological studies on *Eugenia uniflora* leaves: xanthine oxidase inhibitory activity. Journal of Ethnopharmacology 1987;21(2) 183-186.

[133] Jovito VC, Almeida LFD, Ferreira DAH, Moura D, Paulo MQ, Padilha WWN. Avaliação *in vivo* de dentifrício contendo extrato da *Eugenia uniflora* L. (Pitanga) sobre Indicadores de saúde bucal. Pesquisa Brasileira em Odontopediatria e Clínica Integrada 2009;9(1) 81-86.

[134] Castro RD, Freires IA, Ferreira DAH, Jovito VC, Paulo, MQ. Atividade antibacteriana *in vitro* de produtos naturais sobre *Lactobacillus casei.* International Journal of Dentistry 2010;9(2) 74-77.

[135] Agra MF, França PF, Barbosa-Filho JM. Synopsis of the plants known as medicinal and poisonous in Northeast of Brazil. Revista Brasileira de Farmacognosia 2007;17(1) 114-140.

[136] Carvalho CM, Macedo-Costa MR, Pereira MSV, Higino JS, Carvalho LFPC, Costa, LJ. Efeito antimicrobiano in vitro do extrato de jabuticaba (*Myrciaria cauliflora* (Mart.) O. Berg.) sobre *Streptococcus* da cavidade oral. Revista Brasileira de Plantas Medicinais 2009;11(1) 79-83.

[137] Costa, MR, Diniz, DN, Carvalho, CM, Pereira MSV, Pereira JV, Higino JS. Eficácia do extrato de *Myrciaria cauliflora* (Mart.) O. Berg. (jabuticabeira) sobre bactérias orais. Revista Brasileira de Farmacognosia 2009;19(2B) 565-571.

[138] Lima IO, Oliveira RAG, Lima EO, Farias NMP, Souza EL. Antifungal activity from essential oils on Candida species. Revista Brasileira de Farmacognosia 2006;16(2) 197-201.

[139] Matan N, Rimkeeree H, Mawson AJ, Chompreeda P, Haruthaithanasan V, Parker M. Antimicrobial activity of cinnamon and clove oils under modified atmosphere conditions. International Journal of Food Microbiology 2006;107(2) 180-185.

[140] Chong BS, Ford TRP, Kariyawasam SP. Short-term tissue response to potential root-end filling materials in infected root canals. International Endodontic Journal 1997;30(4) 240-249.

[141] Lima MP, Zoghbi MGB, Andrade EHA, Silva TMD. Fernandes CS. Constituintes voláteis das folhas e dos galhos de *Cinnamonum zeylanicum* Blume (Lauraceae). Acta Amazônica 2005;35(3) 363-366.

[142] Oliveira SMM, Lorscheider JA, Nogueira MA. Avaliação da ação *in vitro* de gel dentifrício contendo óleos essenciais sobre bactérias cariogênicas. Latin American Journal of Pharmacy 2008;27(2) 266-269.

[143] Castro RD, Lima EO. Screening of essential oils antifungal activity on candida Strains. Pesquisa Brasileira em Odontopediatria e Clínica Integrada 2011;11(3) 341-345.

[144] Brito ES, Garruti DS, Alves PB, Blank AF.Caracterização odorífera dos componentes do óleo essencial de capim-Santo (*Cymbopogon citratus* (DC.) Stapf., Poaceae) por cromatografia gasosa (CG) – Olfatometria. Fortaleza: Empresa Brasileira de Pesquisa Agropecuária; 2011.

[145] Perazzo MF, Costa Neta MC, Cavalcanti YW, Xavier AFC, Cavalcanti AL. Antimicrobial effect of *Cymbopogon citratus* essential oil on dental biofilm-forming bacteria. Revista Brasileira de Ciências da Saúde 2012;16(4) 553-558.

[146] Alzugaray D, Alzugaray C. Plantas que curam. São Paulo: Três; 1996.

[147] Torres CRG, Cubo CH, Anido AA, Rodrigues JR. Agentes antimicrobianos e seu potencial de uso na odontologia. Revista da Faculdade de Odontologia de São José dos Campos 2000;3(2) 43-52.

[148] Moreira MJS, Ferreira MBC, Hashizume LN. Avaliação in vitro da atividade antimicrobiana dos componentes de um enxaguatório bucal contendo malva. Pesquisa Brasileira em Odontopediatria e Clínica Integrada 2012;12(4) 505-509.

[149] Carvalho JLS. Contribuição ao estudo fitoquímico e analítico no *Nasturtium officinale* R. Br., Brasicaceae. Master thesis. Universidade Federal do Paraná; 2001.

[150] Blumenthal M, Goldberg A, Brinckmaann J. Herbal medicine In: Hardcover (ed) Integrative Medicine Communications.2000. p 404-407.

[151] Cordeiro CHG, Sacramento LVS, Corrêa MA, Pizzolitto AC, Bauab TM. Análise farmacognóstica e atividade antibacteriana de extratos vegetais empregados em formulação para a higiene bucal. Revista Brasileira de Ciências Farmacêuticas 2006;42(3) 395-404.

[152] Schimid R. An old medicinal plant: *Aloe vera*. Parfümerie und kosmetik 1991;72(3) 146-150.

[153] Okamura N, Asai M, Hine N, Yagi A. High-performance liquid chromatographic determination of phenolic compounds in Aloe species. Journal of Chromatography 1996;746(2) 225-231.

[154] Kuzuya H, Tamai I, Beppu H, Shimpo K, Chihara T. Determination of aloenin, barbaloin and isobarbaloin in Aloe species by micellar electrokinetic chromatography. Journal of Chromatography 2001;752(1) 91-97.

[155] Steinert J, Khalaj S, Rimpler M. High-performance liquid chromatographic separation of some naturally occurring naphthoquinones and anthraquinones. Journal of Chromatograhy A 1996;723(1/2) 206-209.

[156] Ho KY, Tsai CC, Chen CP, Huang JS, Lin CC. Antimicrobial activity of honokiol and magnolol isolated from *Magnolia officinalis*. Phytotherapy Research 2001;15(2) 139-141.

[157] Huang BB, Fan MW, Wang SL, Huang YB, Zhou J, Wang Q. Inhibitory effect of *Magnolia officinalis* extract on growth of *Streptococcus mutans*. The Chinese Journal of Dental Research 2004;7(2) 15-9.

[158] Oliveira FQ, Gobira B, Guimarães C, Batista J, Barreto M, Souza M. Espécies vegetais indicadas na odontologia. Revista Brasileira de Farmacognosia 2007;17(3) 466-476.

[159] Celeste RK, Slavutzky SMB, Van PGL. Ação preventiva do bochecho de sálvia: efeitos sobre placa dental e gengivite. Revista Gaúcha de Odontologia 1998;46(2) 97-99.

[160] Chatterjee A, Saluja M, Singh N, Kandwal A. To evaluate the antigingivitis and antiplaque effect of an Azadirachta indica (neem) mouthrinse on plaque induced gingivitis: A double-blind, randomized, controlled trial. Journal of Indian Society of Periodontology 2011;15(4) 398–401.

Assorted Errands in Prevention of Children's Oral Diseases and Conditions

H.S. Mbawala, F.M. Machibya and F.K. Kahabuka

1. Introduction

Children are young human beings; they are vulnerable to various ailments including oral diseases and conditions. In order to prevent the various oral diseases and conditions in children, all people responsible in looking after the children have a role to play so as to protect them from acquiring oral diseases or receive appropriate prompt management. This chapter presents responsibilities of various stakeholders in prevention of children's oral diseases and conditions. The impact of oral diseases in children's general health, growth and development is presented. The various oral diseases and conditions and the significance of their prevention is described. Finally, responsible stake holders and their various errands are elucidated.

2. Prevention of children's oral diseases and conditions

The word *prevent* comes from the Latin *"praeventus"*, which means anticipate or hinder. Prevention literally implies the act of putting a stop to something from happening. It refers to measures taken to make the occurrence of something from none existence or not progressing to a worse situation [1]. Subsequently, prevention of diseases is actions aimed at eradicating, eliminating or minimizing the impact of disease and disability, or if none of these are feasible, retarding the progress of the disease and disability. Prevention of oral diseases and conditions, therefore means to put a stop or to avoid the oral diseases and or conditions from occurring, control the already existing condition or disease not to progress further or take charge such that the impact of the condition or diseases is handled to improve quality of life of the affected individual. Disease preventive strategies are acting on the chain of disease causation where individuals who are at risk or have higher possibilities of contracting the disease or having the stated condition are made less likely to contract the disease by decreasing their susceptibility, for example action of fluoridated dentifrices on strengthening the teeth to prevent dental caries.

3. Essence of prevention of children's oral diseases and conditions

The rationale behind prevention of oral diseases in children lays back to the sense of widespread of the common oral diseases (dental caries and periodontal conditions) among them, where about 60-90% of children worldwide are affected [2].

Unfortunately, these oral diseases and conditions tend to create socio-demographic gradients [3]; where regardless of knowledge and scientific based evidence advances and achievement for the control and treatment, globally oral diseases have tended to accumulate in the most disadvantaged populations. In these populations the affected child usually have severe and multiple conditions or diseases. It is reported that about 50 million school hours are lost annually in USA due to dental pain as a result of dental caries and that dental pain is the second common condition at medical emergencies, hence oral diseases in children are a public health problem as they impact children's socio and psychological well being as well as restrict school activity [4]. Table 1 summarizes a range of research findings showing the socio-psychological impact of oral diseases to children. In most developing countries, the cost of treating dental caries among children alone will require their total health care budget [5]. Furthermore the clinical approach to dental treatment has proved to be an economic burden in industrialized countries where expenditure on oral health is about 3%-12% of total health expenditures.

Country	Age (yrs)	Dental pain prevalence (%)	Socio-psychological impact
South Australia [6]	5-15	31.8	Disturbed sleep and schoolwork
England [7]	8	47.5	Crying disturbed sleep, play, schoolwork, eating
Tanzania [8]	10-19	36.4	Disturbed eating, smiling, study and socializing
Thailand [10]	11-12	25.1	Disturbed eating, smiling, study and socializing
Uganda [11]	10-14.	42.1	Caries, subjective oral health indicators, dental attendance
Kerala, India [12]	12	68.0	Dissatisfaction with oral status and dental appearance

Table 1. Socio-psychological impacts of dental caries

4. Benefits of prevention of children's oral diseases and conditions

Children are young human beings who are dependent on adults to take care of their health issues both socially and economically. They are more vulnerable to diseases, and once sick it is their parents or guardians who decide and act for their health care. On the other hand, prevention of oral diseases through instituting most oral health related-behaviours like tooth brushing and use of fluoridated toothpaste are determined by the family. Likewise, associated expenses are to be incurred by a family earner.

Oral health is an integral part of overall well-being and essential for eating, growth, speech, social development, learning capacity and quality of life and tooth decay has been reported to have negative impact on childhood nutrition, growth and weight gain [13]. Additionally; World Federation of Public Health Associations [14] admits that oral health problems in children can impact on many aspects of their general health and development, causing substantial pain and disruption to their lives and often altering their behaviour.

Prevention of oral diseases is relatively less costly compared to curative dental services, therefore it is considered beneficial. For example, water fluoridation may appear expensive, but because of its wider coverage and its easy application versus dental treatment for a decayed tooth in an individual, it remains a better choice. Prevention of oral diseases is cost effective particularly in middle and low income countries where resources necessary for conventional dental treatment are scarce and a substantial proportion of their financial resources for health is directed to address infectious diseases.

Another benefit of preventing oral diseases in children is to minimize pain, discomfort and suffering; enable them to eat and socialize well, avoid loss of school hours ultimately contribute into their growth and development.

5. Levels of disease prevention

The concept of prevention is conveniently defined at four levels, namely primordial, primary, secondary and tertiary prevention though in reality the stages blur one into the next.

5.1. Primordial prevention

This is a relatively recent classification of disease prevention. It seeks to prevent at a very early stage, often before the risk factor is present in the particular context, the activities which encourage the emergence of lifestyles, behaviours and exposure patterns that contribute to increased risk of disease. Or it is actions and measures that inhibit the emergence of risk factors in the form of environmental, economic, social, and behavioral conditions and cultural patterns of living. In primordial prevention, efforts are directed towards discouraging children from adopting harmful lifestyles, the main intervention being through individual and mass education. According to Porta [15], primordial prevention consists of conditions, actions, and measures that minimize hazards to health and hence inhibit the emergence and establishment of processes and factors (environmental, economic, social, behavioral, cultural) known to increase the risk of diseases. Furthermore, Porta [15] states that primordial prevention is accomplished through many public and private healthy public policies and intersectoral action and that it may be seen as a form of primary prevention. Primordial prevention addresses broad health determinants rather than preventing personal exposure to risk factors, which is the goal of primary prevention. For instance, outlawing alcohol would represent primordial prevention, whereas a campaign against drinking would be an example of primary prevention. In dentistry primordial prevention will include enforcing a law on fluoride levels in various products and education on causes and prevention of oral diseases and conditions to individuals and to the community.

5.2. Primary prevention

Primary prevention can be defined in several ways. One of these definitions states that primary prevention is the action taken prior to the onset of disease, which removes the possibility that the disease will occur. It also can be defined as the first level of health care, designed to prevent the occurrence of disease and promote health, or as prevention of disease through the control of exposure to risk factors. Approaches for primary prevention include population-wide strategies and high-risk strategies focusing on population sub-groups. It may be accomplished by measures of "Health promotion" and "specific protection" that is; measures designed to promote general health and well-being, and quality of life of people or by specific protective measures. Examples of primary prevention in dentistry include fluoridation of public water, oral evaluation, dental prophylaxis, Fluoride use as preventive agent, fissure sealants, use of Xylitol, mouth guards, regular dental examinations and self-care such as tooth brushing, flossing, use of dental rinses and medicinal mouthwashes.

5.3. Secondary prevention

Is defined as the application of available measures to detect early departures from health and to introduce appropriate treatment and interventions. Others define secondary prevention as the second level of health care, based on the earliest possible identification of disease so that it can be more readily treated or managed and adverse sequelae can be prevented. This level of prevention is also defined as action which halts the progress of a disease at its incipient stage and prevents complications. Screening is a major component of secondary prevention. Examples of secondary prevention in dentistry are Fluoride use on incipient caries, dental restorations, periodontal debridement, root canal treatments, serial extraction, fixed and removable appliances, installation of caps and crowns. Removal of broken or impacted teeth, especially the third molars is also a type of secondary preventive dentistry.

5.4. Tertiary prevention

Is the application of measures to reduce or eliminate long-term impairments and disabilities, minimising suffering caused by existing departures from good health and to promote the patient's adjustments to his/her condition. In other words, it is the third phase or level of health care, concerned with promotion of independent function and prevention of further disease-related deterioration. It also can be defined as all the measures available to reduce or limit impairments and disabilities, and to promote the patients' adjustment to irremediable conditions. Examples of tertiary prevention in dentistry include; denture fabrication, bridges, implants, oro-maxillofacial surgery, periodontal surgery, fixed prosthodontics and space maintainers. Most dental procedures aiming at children fall under the first three levels of prevention.

6. Rationale of oral disease prevention in children

Although dental diseases are not among the feared killer diseases like ebola and malaria, their high prevalence inflict heavy pain in the community in terms of treatment cost, physical and physiological incapacitation and rarely death. Oral health is part and parcel of the general health in such a way that severe illness on orofacial region can lead to systemic problems like malnutrition, immunosupresion, septicaemia etc.

The rationale for preventing oral diseases and especially in children can be viewed under three areas; the disease burden inflicted by oral diseases to the community, the common risk factors shared by oral diseases and other chronic diseases and the lifelong effects to be gained if efforts for prevention are directed to children.

6.1. Disease burden

Despite great improvements in the oral health of populations in several countries, globally, oral health problems still persist [16]. Traditional treatment of oral diseases is extremely costly; it is the fourth most expensive disease to treat in most industrialized countries where 5–10% of public health expenditure relates to oral health [17, 18]. In most developing countries resources are primarily allocated to emergency oral care and pain relief; it is estimated that, if treatment were available in these countries, the costs of dental caries in children alone would exceed the total health care budget for children [5].

6.2. Relation to general health

There is a group of risk factors common to many chronic diseases and oral diseases. They include tobacco and alcohol use, frequent consumption of sugars and inadequate physical activity, especially when coupled with consumption of excess calories, [19-23]. Hence, addressing these factors will ultimately prevent other systemic diseases. The four most prominent non-communicable diseases sharing risk factors with oral diseases are cardiovascular diseases, diabetes, cancer and chronic obstructive pulmonary diseases; the factors are preventable and relate to lifestyles.

6.3. Lifelong effect in children

Children are young, easy to learn and usually what they learn at early age is retained for life. Therefore, efforts for directing disease prevention to children who are likely to practice preventive measures and maintain good oral health throughout adulthood are justified.

7. Oral diseases and conditions that affect children

There are many oral diseases affecting children. They may be congenitally transmitted or acquired through environmental interaction. The chapter describes some of the common oral diseases and conditions in children

7.1. Dental caries

Dental caries or tooth decay is the disease which causes destruction of tooth material, which includes: enamel, dentin, root and pulp. It is one of the most prevalent chronic diseases worldwide [16]. Dental caries forms over time through interaction between cariogenic bacteria and fermentable carbohydrates or cariogenic food particles left on the surface of the tooth. When bacteria feed on the sugars in the food they produce acids responsible for tooth demineralization. All people carry bacteria in their mouth which make them susceptible to tooth decay. In particular, risks for caries development include physical, biological, environmental, behavioural, and lifestyle-related factors such as poor oral hygiene, inappropriate methods of feeding infants, diet high in sugars, high numbers of bacteria, and frequent use of medications containing sugar or causing dry mouth, insufficient fluoride, malnutrition including vitamin and mineral deficiencies and some medical conditions, such as Sjogren's syndrome, that decreases the flow of saliva in the mouth. The teeth are susceptible to caries throughout lifetime, though host factors including tooth structure and saliva modify the progression of the disease. Children are susceptible to aggressive tooth decay of primary teeth known as early childhood caries.

Treatment of dental caries: Some initial dental caries process may stop if prevention actions (like oral hygiene improvement) are put in place. Nevertheless, treatment options for more severe caries include dental fillings. When decay reaches the dentin but not yet in the pulp, it can be treated by removing the decay using rotary or hand instruments; the cavity is then cleaned and filled with dental materials of choice. When the lesion extends into the pulp and/or root canal of the tooth, it is treated by root canal treatment procedure. The procedure involves preparation of an access cavity followed by removal of dead tissue, blood vessels and nerves from the canal and finally cleaning of the root canal(s). Biocompatible materials are filled in the cavity and the canals. When indicated, a crown is placed on the tooth to strengthen the restored tooth crown.

Tooth Extraction: Removal of the tooth is opted if the extent of tooth decay and/or tooth infection is beyond repair with filling or root canal treatment. When the tooth is extracted, it can be replaced with dental implant, partial bridge or denture.

7.2. Periodontal diseases

Periodontal disease refers to gingivitis (an inflammatory condition of the soft tissues surrounding a tooth or the gingiva) and periodontitis (involving the destruction of tooth supporting structures such as the periodontal ligament, bone, cementum and soft tissues). Periodontal disease is initiated by a complex of bacterial species, mainly composed of Gram-negative, anaerobic bacteria growing in subgingival areas. The persistent inflammation due to host response to pathogens causes the destruction of periodontal tissues, leading to clinical manifestations of the disease [24]. In general, most children and adolescents worldwide have signs of gingivitis. An aggressive periodontitis affects about 2% of young individuals during puberty and may lead to premature tooth loss.

Causes of periodontal diseases: Periodontal diseases are caused by bacteria in dental plaque-a sticky substance that forms on tooth surface, but other factors influence the disease progression. In reaction to bacterial invasion, the body immune system releases substances that inflame and damage the connective tissues of the gingiva, periodontal ligament or even the alveolar bone. This leads to swollen, bleeding gums which are signs of gingivitis. Further damage involving cementum, alveolar bone with periodontal pockets indicates severe form of periodontal disease. Some genetic and environmental factors put the host susceptible to periodontal diseases. Rare syndromes affecting phagocytes, the structure of the epithelia, connective tissue, or teeth, could have severe periodontal manifestations. For some disorders, the responsible gene or tissue defect has been identified.

Haim-Munk and Papillon-Lefèvre syndromes are rare autosomal recessive disorders associated with periodontitis onset at childhood and early loss of both deciduous and permanent teeth [25, 26].

Tobacco and alcohol use: Tobacco use is clearly a risk factor for periodontal disease. In contrast, a small but significant association exists between alcohol consumption and loss of periodontal support [27].

Infection like HIV and AIDS: An infection process impairs the immune response thereby lowering the gingival protection from local infection.

Nutrition: Historically, specific, overt nutritional deficiencies have been associated with periodontal disease. Vitamin C deficiency leads to scurvy with decreased formation and maintenance of collagen, increased periodontal inflammation, haemorrhage, and tooth loss.

Diabetes: The relation between periodontal health and diabetes has been described as bidirectional; although periodontitis is a potential complication of diabetes, evidence suggests that treatment of periodontal infections in diabetics could improve glycaemic control [28].

Stress: Emotional and psychosocial stresses clearly are factors in periodontal disease, but their precise role in the pathogenesis of this disease is unknown [29].

Impaired immune response: Severe periodontal disease and loss of tooth-supporting tissues often occurs if the individual's host response or immune function is impaired. Various systemic diseases such as leukaemia and thrombocytopenia could be associated with increased severity of periodontal disease.

Treatment for periodontal diseases: The foundation of periodontal therapy is anti-infective non-surgical treatment aimed at controlling the bacterial plaque and other prominent risk factors. Proper tooth brushing can prevent and treat initial stages of bacterial induced gingivitis. However, scaling and root planning is indicated for treating advanced periodontal disease.

Dental plaque and calculus can be removed from tooth-crown and root surfaces (scaling and root planing) by use of various manual or powered instruments. Special attention is devoted to biofilm debridement in periodontal pockets combined with improved personal oral hygiene. Additional use of local antibiotics, local antiseptic drugs, and systemic antibiotics provides some extra benefit compared with debridement alone.

7.3. Dental trauma

Dental trauma is any injury to the mouth, including teeth, lips, gums, tongue, and jawbones. About one third of 5 years old children have sustained traumatic dental injuries involving primary teeth mostly tooth luxation: boys have slightly higher frequency than girls. A prevalence of 5–12% has been found in children aged 6–12 years in the Middle East. A significant proportion of dental trauma relates to falls, sports, unsafe playgrounds or schools, road accidents and violence [30].

An important predisposing factor for dental trauma is large maxillary overjet and incomplete lip closure. Other risk factors associated with incisors injury in elementary school children are playing without mouthguard and/or faceguard and sociobehavour factors including gender (Male>Female) and increased participation in sport activities [31, 32].

Treatment of dental trauma varies according to the type or extent of injury like fracture, avulsion and luxation (tooth displacement). Tetanus booster and antibiotics should be administered whenever a dental injury is at risk for infection. Arrangements should be made for prompt follow-up with a dentist or an oral and maxillofacial surgeon [33, 34]. Specific procedural details of each type of fracture is beyond the scope of this chapter

7.4. Dental malocclusion

Malocclusion is not a disease but rather a set of dental deviations which in some cases can influence quality of life and interfere with oral functions. The prevalence of different traits of malocclusions varies with age, ethnicity and geographical location. The reported incidence ranges from 32 to 93 percent [35].

The causes of malocclusion include hereditary transmission, oral habits such as thumb sucking, tongue thrusting, pacifier use, prolonged use of a bottle early loss of teeth, impacted teeth, or abnormally shaped teeth, misalignment of jaws due to fractures after a severe injury, tumours of the mouth and jaw, congenital and acquired jaw deformities and abnormal orofacial muscle function.

Treatment: Every dentist who treats children practices orthodontics, whether knowingly or not. It is not enough to think of orthodontics as being solely concerned with appliances.

Orthodontics is the longitudinal care of the developing occlusion and any problems associated with it. All qualified dental practitioners should be encouraged to consider the orthodontic requirements of their patients. Orthodontic treatments include the uses of fixed and removable appliances, tooth extraction for space gain and surgery to correct dental and jaws relation [36].

7.5. Oral mucosal lesions

There are many mucosa lesions occurring in the mouth. Some are local due to local derangement, while others occur in the mouth manifesting systemic diseases like HIV/AIDS. Of the oral mucosa lesions, Leukoplakia is the most frequent form of oral precancer and appears in the oral cavity as a white patch that cannot be rubbed off [37]. Oral lesions may be in form of a swelling, blisters, cyst, ulcers and mucosa coulour change or mucosa plaque.

Oral manifestations of systemic diseases: Many systemic disease manifests with oral signs and symptoms, hence, the mouth is considered as the mirror of the general body health. Some oral lesions (e.g. Koplik's sport) are very specific thus are used in confirming diagnosis of some diseases. Some lesions appear at the initial stage of systemic diseases that should alert clinician to speculate and work for early diagnosis of particular systemic conditions. Before the introduction of Highly Active Antiretroviral Therapy (HAART), approximately 40–50% of people who were HIV-positive had oral disease caused by fungal, bacterial or viral infections that often occur early in the course of the disease [38]. The common systemic diseases with oral lesions include; HIV, Sickle cell anaemia, Hodgkin's lymphoma, Sjögren's syndrome, drugs side effects, Herpes simplex, Varicella-zoster, measles, oral hairy leukoplakia and syphilis.

Congenital anomalies: There are many orofacial conditions occurring congenitally. Of the developmental disorders, congenital diseases of the enamel or dentine, problems related to the number, size and shape of teeth, and craniofacial birth defects such as cleft lip and/or palate are most important [39].

8. Basic principles of prevention of oral diseases in children

WHO Global Oral Health Programme for public health has set down basic principle approaches underlying effective oral disease prevention namely; acting on socio-determinants of health, working as one through the common risk factor approach and implementation of multiple strategies of prevention in different settings.

Socio-determinants of health: It is now apparent that individual behaviours such as oral hygiene practices, dietary patterns and attendance for dental care, which are the bases for prevention of oral diseases and conditions are largely influenced by family, social and community factors, as well as political and economical measures [40]. Therefore, WHO recommends that oral disease prevention strategies (public health strategies) need to be directed at underlying socio-determinants of health. They include; socioeconomic and political context, social position and health care system [41].

Thecommon risk factors approach as one of the underlying strategies for public health approach recognizes that chronic non-communicable diseases such as obesity, cancers, diabetes and oral diseases share a set of common risk conditions and factors. Hence providing a rationale for partnership in disease prevention which is particularly applicable in countries with limited numbers of oral health personnel.

The multiple strategies of prevention: The other underlying principle is the multiple strategies to be implemented in different settings. There should be a mix of complementary public health approaches that focus both on assisting individuals and communities to avoid disease and on the other hand to create supportive environments that are conducive to sustain good health. In the prevention of oral diseases, the high-risk approach has been largely dominant. Finally, the WHO now increasingly acknowledges that the best preventive strategy for public health approach is a combination of the high-risk and directed population approaches, [42].

9. Available prevention approaches for specific oral diseases and their effectiveness

Evidence base of oral health interventions from systematic reviews and effectiveness studies conducted between 1994 to 2005 reveal that there are several approaches for diseases prevention [43]. Water fluoridation and use of topical flourides as toothpaste, mouthrinses and varnishes were effective in reducing caries prevalence of 14 to 46% respectively. Whereas fissure sealants are reported to have caries reduction of up to 86% in 12 months and 57% in 48 months time. Dental health education provided a short term improvement in oral health knoweledge and had limited effects on oral health behaviours. While the effectivenes of dieatary control on reducing caries was not revealed. Table 2 below, summarizes the prevention approaches for specific oral diseases and their effectiveness.

Oral Diseases/Conditions prevention approach	Effectiveness in oral disease prevention
Dental health education	• Short term improvement in oral health knowledge
	• Limited effect on oral health related behaviour
	• Not effective for caries reduction
	• Short-term effect on plaque control and gingival bleeding
Topical fluorides	Caries reduction when fluoridated:
	• Toothpaste 24%
	• Mouthwashes 26%
	• Gels 28%
	• Varnishes 46%
Fissure sealants	Caries reduction ranging from 86-57% in a year or two.
Water fluoridation	Caries reduction by 14%
Dietary approach	Not effective in reducing caries.

Table 2. Available prevention approaches for specific oral diseases and their effectiveness, modified from Watt, R. G. [40]

10. Different stakeholders responsible for children's oral health

There are diverse stakeholders for children's oral health who vary in accordance to the child's age or place where the child is located on a specified period of time. Another category is the overall universal stakeholder.

The stakeholders in accordance to the child's age are presented for three age groups namely; birth to three years, four to seven years and eight to twelve years.

10.1. From birth to three years

At birth children do not have teeth. Usually the mothers are the fundamental persons in charge of the children's oral health. Under special circumstances, for example a very sick mother or a mother who pass away after delivery, caretakers may become principally accountable. Whether the mother is available or not, more carers come in as the child grows to one year and further to three years. They include; fathers, siblings, helpers and other family members. Other important responsible groups for prevention of oral diseases in young children are the professionals that is; Medical personnel (Medical doctors and nurses) and Dental personnel (Dentists, Dental Hygienists, Dental Nurses).

10.2. Four to seven years

As children grow they also assume responsibility on their health issues. Thus the stakeholders for children aged four to seven years are the mothers, fathers, children themselves, siblings, helpers, other family members and nursery/school teachers. The Medical personnel (Medical doctors and nurses) and Dental personnel (Dentists, Dental Hygienists, Dental Nurses) are accountable in prevention of oral diseases in this age group.

10.3. Eight to twelve years

The primary responsible persons for the oral health of eight to twelve years old children are the children themselves. These are supported by mothers, fathers, siblings, helpers, other family members and school teachers. The Medical personnel (Medical doctors and nurses) and Dental personnel (Dentists, Dental Laboratory Technologists, Dental Hygienists, Dental Nurses) have a big role to play in prevention of oral diseases in this age group.

The stakeholders can also be looked at in terms of location. The various locations of interest are the homes, school, health facilities and institutions for children with special health care needs.

10.4. Responsible stakeholders for children's oral health at homes

At homes the stakeholders responsible for children's oral health are Parents and guardians, children themselves and other children carers (siblings, relatives or helpers).

10.5. Responsible stakeholders for children's oral health at school

The stakeholders responsible for children's oral health at schools are teachers, children themselves and other children carers depending on the school system.

10.6. Responsible stakeholders for children's oral health at health facilities

At Health facilities responsible stakeholders for children's oral health include Medical personnel (Medical doctors and nurses), Dental personnel (Dentists, Dental Laboratory Technologists, Dental Hygienists and Dental Nurses).

10.7. Responsible stakeholders for children's oral health at Institutions for children with special health care needs

The oral health of children living at institutions is a responsibility of children carers, parents/guardians and children themselves depending on their level of dependency.

10.8. Universal stakeholders

In this chapter, governments, professional associations, Dental products manufacturers, the media and NGOs are considered universal stakeholders because their responsibilities cut across ages and locations. The governments are responsible for policies and governance of all issues pertaining to health. Whereas, professional associations' responsibilities are to safeguard the health of the people they serve. The dental products manufacturers are responsible to supply products required at all levels of prevention regardless of age or place. The NGOs can at any age and location play any role that falls within the organisation's governing regulations.

11. Assorted errands

The different tasks of various stakeholders in the prevention of oral diseases among children are presented with the centre of attention being the four levels of prevention.

11.1. Tasks of various stakeholders in executing primordial prevention of oral diseases among children

Under primordial prevention the task is to give education before the risk factor for oral diseases has occurred. The target group is the community without the risk factors.

The responsible individuals and their responsibilities are presented below;

11.2. Oral health personnel

Dentists, Dental Therapists, Dental Hygienists, Dental Nurses and Community Dental Workers or any other oral health workers are primarily responsible to give oral health education (OHE). That is; to inform the community on the common oral diseases and conditions that affect children, their causes and measures to prevent them. Important messages for the community comprise proper and timely tooth brushing of children's teeth, sensible use of sugary containing food staffs including avoiding leaving a nipple in the child's mouth at night. Other messages include maintenance of playgrounds, blunting sharp edges, securing windows and stairs as well as shunning slippery floors to protect young children against injuries, regular visit to a dentist for check-up and discouraging misconceptions, beliefs and practices harmful to children's oral health. As Narksawat et al. [44] put it that parents must be motivated to consistently spend the time required to take care of the primary dentition of their children by regular cleaning and controlling the snacking behavior of their children. Emphasis should be directed to parents of children with special health care needs, motivating and empowering them to realize these preventive strategies. In order to execute primordial prevention, the oral health personnel ought to target the community because this stage is done to a community who do not have the risk factors.

11.3. Community

The obligation of the community that is; parents, school teachers, children and other family members is to receive OHE and make use of the received information in order to avoid the risk factors. Parents of children with special health care needs, require endurance in looking after their children's oral health.

11.4. School teachers

School teachers are responsible to supervise children's playing activities, maintenance of playgrounds and controlling availability of sugary foods within school premises.

11.5. Universal stakeholders

In order for the primordial prevention to succeed, support is required from universal stakeholders, that is; Governments, Professional Associations, the Media and NGOs. The support expected is through formulation and enforcement of policies on OHE, provision of funds and personnel to take part in OHE activities as well as support to the profession to air Oral Health Education messages/campaigns through various media.

11.6. Tasks of various stakeholders in executing primary prevention of oral diseases among children

Primary prevention targets the community and the children in particular. The goal is to prevent personal exposure to risk factors.

11.6.1. Governments

Governments are in charge of policy formulation and implementation. The governm520ents therefore are liable to have in place policies supporting primary prevention of oral diseases in children such as those governing school oral health programmes including those directed to children with special health care needs, where required fluoridation of public water and fostering availability of fluoride tablets. They should provide conducive working environment, avail funds and give any other support to preventive programmes.

11.6.2. Oral health personnel

Primary prevention requires oral health personnel (Dentists, Dental Therapists, Dental Hygienists, Dental Nurses, Community Dental Workers or any other oral health workers) collectively or individually to do oral evaluation, regular dental examinations, dental prophylaxis, fissure sealants and health education with emphasis on plaque control and use of fluoridated tooth paste twice per day in the morning and evening before retiring to bed. They are also responsible to correct oral habits, and monitor occlusal development so as to prevent malocclusions. These procedures can be done at the chair side but also in communities such as primary schools or reproductive and child health clinics. Moreover, oral health care workers need to devise special primary preventive programmes for children with special health care needs bearing in mind the challenges encountered during dental treatment to these children. It may require outreach programmes to visit children at their schools where tailor-made information and instructions are given to the children.

11.6.3. Medical personnel (Medical doctors and nurses)

The medical personnel who see children for various ailments should join oral health personnel by mentioning prevention of oral diseases when they talk about prevention of other diseases particularly those sharing common risk factors such as diabetes, heart diseases, hypertension and cancers. The medical personnel attending children with special health care needs are liable to emphasise prevention of oral diseases.

11.6.4. Parents and community at large

The responsibility of parents and other community members is to advocate the use of Fluoride as a caries preventive agent and plaque control for prevention of gum diseases. Fluoride tooth paste used during tooth brushing twice a day in the morning and before retiring to be bed is universally accepted to prevent dental caries. Therefore, parents are responsible to brush their children's teeth from the eruption of the first tooth to six years of age. From age seven to 10 years, parents should supervise children's tooth brushing. In older children, parents should supervise flossing, use of dental rinses and medicinal mouthwashes. Furthermore, parents are responsible to facilitate the use of Xylitol and mouth guards if indicated. Parents should take their children for regular dental visits so that children's oral health can be monitored. Supervision and facilitation of using dental rinses and medicinal mouthwashes is another parents' task. Parents of children with special health care needs should pay special attention to prevent oral diseases for their children. This is particularly important given the hassles encountered in the dental settings by parents and oral health workers during dental treatment of children with special health care needs.

11.6.5. School and sports teachers

School children spend most of their day time at schools and therefore in contact with school teachers. The teachers are obliged to facilitate preventive actions against oral and other diseases. They can supervise tooth brushing or mouth rinse activities. They can support other programmes like Fluoride application or fissure sealing.

11.6.6. NGOs

Various national and international NGOs have funds and volunteers to support preventive programmes. They can arrange and participate in community services such as oral health screening, Fluoride application or fissure sealing programmes by giving funds and organising for personnel to take part in various programmes.

11.6.7. Dental products manufacturers

The dental product manufactures supply a wide range of products that are used to realize primary prevention of oral diseases among children. They are responsible to avail good quality products at affordable prices the dental products for prevention of diseases; tooth brushes, tooth paste, mouthwashes, fissure sealants, fluorides, dental floss, mouth mirrors as well as dental supplies including gloves, antiseptics etc.

11.7. Tasks of various stakeholders in executing secondary prevention of oral diseases among children

Secondary prevention involves actions which halt the progress of a disease at its incipient stage and prevents complications.

11.7.1. Governments

In order to facilitate provision of services to children at early stages of oral diseases so as to halt their progress and prevent complications, governments are required to provide conducive dental clinic working environments, avail funds, have in place and enforce policies on dental supplies. Governments are also responsible to oversee activities related to prevention of oral diseases in children in public sectors, private sectors and insurance companies.

11.7.2. Oral health personnel (Dentists, dental therapists, dental hygienists, dental nurses, community dental workers or any other oral health workers)

The Oral health personnel working in public or private sectors are responsible to provide or take part in treatment of various oral diseases and conditions. They should use Fluoride [45] on incipient caries, restore decayed teeth or perform root canal treatments where necessary, professional tooth cleaning and if indicated periodontal debridement. They should keep abreast with new knowledge, procedures, techniques and materials to facilitate them offer quality treatment of oral diseases at their early stages. Oral health care workers providing dental treatment to children with special health care needs should equip themselves with techniques to address the challenges encountered during dental treatment to these children.

11.7.3. Medical personnel (Medical doctors and nurses)

The medical personnel who see children for various ailments are liable to do early diagnosis of oral diseases and make prompt referral. Whereas Rozier et al. [46] demonstrated that non-dental professionals can integrate preventive dental services into their practices, the American Academy of Pediatrics recommends physician interventions in addressing dental caries to include oral health screening and referral when indicated, provision of oral hygiene instructions, dietary information, and anticipatory guidance to parents, as well as prescription of fluoride supplements. In so doing they will facilitate early identification of oral diseases, promote their readily treatment and prevention of adverse sequelae.

11.7.4. Parents

Parents have a significant role to play to aid the oral health personnel in executing secondary prevention of oral diseases among children. They have to take their children for dental consultation at early stages of the disease. For the parents to achieve this task they have to develop a practice of looking into their children's mouths and consult dentists for any abnormal development principally so for children with special health care needs. After consulting the dentists they need to comply with appointments and instructions given by professionals.

11.7.5. Dental products manufacturers

A diverse list of materials and supplies is needed to support oral health personnel in delivering secondary prevention of oral diseases among children. The dental products manufacturers are responsible to avail required materials and supplies at affordable prices and of good quality. The requirements range from instruments, dental materials and dental supplies to dental equipment.

11.7.6. School teachers

Since school teachers spend most of their working time with children, their role in secondary prevention of oral diseases among children is to remind and motivate parents as well as children to consult dentists as per professional recommendations.

11.7.7. NGOs

The NGOs can support treatment programmes through volunteer services and provision of funds to buy required instruments, dental materials, dental supplies or dental equipment depending on the NGO's capacity.

11.8. Tasks of various stakeholders in executing tertiary prevention of oral diseases among children

There are a few actions at the level of tertiary prevention of oral diseases among children:

11.8.1. Governments

As for other levels of prevention, governments are responsible to provide conducive working environment, avail dental supplies and funds to allow provision of tertiary level prevention to those children who need such services. The governments should have policies to govern provision of tertiary level oral health care.

11.8.2. Oral health personnel (Dentists, dental therapists, dental hygienists, dental nurses, dental laboratory technologists or any other oral health workers)

It is the responsibility of oral health personnel to provide or take part in provision of tertiary level oral health care. This level is provided at health facilities. The oral health personnel should bear in mind that tertiary prevention in children at times implies primary prevention of oral problems in adult life.

11.8.3. Parents

The tertiary level care in children is important for future oral health of adults. Parents are therefore required to consult dentists for this care as will be advised by dentists and to comply with appointments and instructions given by professionals.

11.8.4. Dental products manufacturers

The dental products manufacturers should avail required materials and supplies for the preparation of children's tertiary level care because they are important for future oral health of adults. Tertiary prevention in children should not to considered as cosmetic therefore the required instruments, materials and other supplies should be availed at a reasonable cost.

11.8.5. NGOs

The NGOs should support treatment programmes as per individual organisation policy and capability.

Basically, oral disease prevention is difficult to attain but it is a responsibility that has to be fulfilled. It is worth to direct efforts of disease prevention to children because they are young, easy to learn and usually what they learn at early age is retained for life thus children are likely to adopt preventive measures and maintain good oral health throughout adulthood.

12. Conclusion

Diverse groups of people are responsible to execute prevention of oral diseases in children. If they work as a team and accountable on each individual errand, oral diseases in children can be minimized or controlled thus enable children to eat well and ultimately grow well which contribute to improved children's social development, learning capacity and thus good quality of life.

13. Recommendations

The different errands should be publicized and motivate all responsible groups or individuals to be accountable with their roles in order to realize prevention of oral diseases in children.

Author details

H.S. Mbawala, F.M. Machibya and F.K. Kahabuka[*]

*Address all correspondence to: kokukahabuka@yahoo.com

Department of Orthodontics, Paedodontics and Preventive Dentistry, School of Dentistry, Muhimbili University of Health and Allied Sciences, Dar es Salaam

References

[1] Leavell, Hugh R. Clark, E.G. (1958). Preventive Medicine for the doctor in his community: epidemilogic approach. New York: McGraw-Hill.

[2] World Health Organization (WHO 2002). Global Oral Health Data Base. Geneva: World Health Organization.

[3] Petersen, P. E. (2003). The World Oral Health Report 2003: continuous improvement of oral health in the 21st century–the approach of the WHO Global Oral Health Programme. *Community Dentistry and Oral Epidemiology*, 3-24.

[4] United States Department of Health and Human Services (USDHHS). (2000) Oral Health in America: A Report of the Surgeon General. National Institute of Health. http://www.nidcr.nih.gov/datastatistics/surgeongeneral/report/executivesummary.htm

[5] Yee R, Sheiham A. (2002). The burden of restorative dental treatment for children in third world countries. *International Dental Journal* 52:1-9.

[6] Slade, G. D., Spencer, A. J., Davies, M. J., & Burrow, D. (1996). Intra-oral distribution and impact of caries experience among South Australian school children. *Australian dental journal*, 41(5), 343-350.

[7] Shepherd, M. A., Nadanovsky, P., & Sheiham, A. (1999). Dental public health: the prevalence and impact of dental pain in 8-year-old school children in Harrow, England. *British dental journal, 187*(1), 38-41.

[8] Mashoto, K. O., Astrom, A. N., David, J., & Masalu, J. R. (2009). Dental pain, oral impacts and perceived need for dental treatment in Tanzanian school students: a cross-sectional study. *Health Qual Life Outcomes, 7,* 73.

[9] Nomura, L. H., Bastos, J. L. D., & Peres, M. A. (2004). Dental pain prevalence and association with dental caries and socioeconomic status in schoolchildren, Southern Brazil, 2002. *Brazilian oral research, 18*(2), 134-140.

[10] Kiwanuka, S. N., & Åstrøm, A. N. (2005). Self-reported dental pain and associated factors in Ugandan schoolchildren. *Norsk epidemiologi, 15*(2)

[11] Gherunpong, S., Tsakos, G., & Sheiham, A. (2004). The prevalence and severity of oral impacts on daily performances in Thai primary school children. *Health Qual Life Outcomes, 2*(1), 57.

[12] David, J., Åstrøm, A. N., & Wang, N. J. (2006). Prevalence and correlates of self-reported state of teeth among schoolchildren in Kerala, India. *BMC Oral Health, 6*(1), 10.

[13] Sheiham A. Dental caries affects body weight, growth and quality of life in preschool children British Dental Journal 2006; 201: 625-626

[14] World Federation of Public Health Associations (WFPHA) (2013). Oral Health for Children www.wfpha.org/tl_files/doc/about/.../OHWG_Child%20Declaration.pdf

[15] Porta M. A Dictionary of Epidemiology (2008). Fifth Edition, *Oxforn University Press Amazon.com*

[16] Petersen PE, Bourgeois D, Ogawa H, Estupinan-Day S, Ndiaye C. (2005). The global burden of oral diseases and risks to oral health. *Bulletin of the World Health Organization* 83:661-669.

[17] Griffin SO, Jones K, Tomar SL. (2001). An economic evaluation of community water fluoridation. *Journal of Public Health Dentistry* 61:78-86.

[18] Wang NJ, Källestaal C, Petersen PE, Arnadottir IB. (1998). Caries preventive services for children and adolescents in Denmark, Iceland, Norway and Sweden: strategies and resource allocation. *Community Dentistry and Oral Epidemiology* 26:263-71.

[19] Franceschi S, Talamini R, Barra S, Baron AE, Negri E, et al. (1990). Smoking and drinking in relation to cancers of the oral cavity, pharynx, larynx, and esophagus in northern Italy. *Cancer research 50*(20):6502-6507.

[20] Giovannucci E, Colditz GA, Stampfer MJ, Willett WC (1996). Physical activity, obesity, and risk of colorectal adenoma in women (United States). *Cancer Causes & Control* 7(2):253-263.

[21]   Sanders TA (2004). Diet and general health: dietary counselling. *Caries Res* 38:3-8.

[22]   Saito T, Shimazaki Y, Kiyohara Y, Kato I, Kubo M, et al. (2005). Relationship between obesity, glucose tolerance, and periodontal disease in Japanese women: the Hisayama study. *Journal of Periodontal Research* 40(4):346-353.

[23]   Liang J, Matheson BE, Kaye WH, Boutelle KN (2013). Neurocognitive correlates of obesity and obesity-related behaviors in children and adolescents. *Int J Obes* doi: 10.1038/ijo.2013.142. [Epub ahead of print]

[24]   Kornman KS, Page RC, Tonetti MS. (1997). The host response to the microbial challenge in periodontitis: assembling the players. *Periodontol.* 14:33–53.

[25]   Hart TC, Hart PS, Bowden DW, et al. (1999). Mutations gene of the cathepsin C are responsible for Papillon-Lefevre syndrome. *J Med Genet* 36: 881–87.

[26]   Toomes, C., James, J., Wood, A. J., Wu, C. L., McCormick, D., Lench, N.,... & Thakker, N. S. (1999). Loss-of-function mutations in the cathepsin C gene result in periodontal disease and palmoplantar keratosis. *Nature genetics*, 23(4), 421-424.

[27]   Tezal M, Grossi SG, Ho AW, Genco R.J. (2004). Alcohol consumption and periodontal disease. The Third National Health and Nutrition Examination Survey. *J Clin Periodontol* 31: 484–88.

[28]   Taylor GW. (2001). Bidirectional interrelationships between diabetes and periodontal diseases: an epidemiologic perspective. *Ann Periodontol* 6: 99–112.

[29]   LeResche L, Dworkin SF. (2000). The role of stress in inflammatory disease, including periodontal disease: review of concepts and current findings. *Periodontol.* 30:2002; 91–103.)

[30]   Glendor U. (2008). Epidemiology of traumatic dental injuries –a 12 year review of the literature. *Dental Traumatol* 24: 603–611

[31]   Kania MJ, Keeling SD, McGorray SP, Wheeler TT, King GJK. (1996). Risk factors associated with incisor injury in elementary school children. *Angle Orthod* 66:423-432.

[32]   Baldava P. and Anup N. Risk factors for traumatic dental injuries in an adolescent male population in India.*J Contemp Dent Pract* 2007; 8.6: 35-42.

[33]   Harrison L. (2014). Dental trauma: guidelines for pediatricians updated. Medscape Medical News. January 27, 2014. Available at http://www.medscape.com/viewarticle/819755.

[34]   Keels MA. (2014). Management of dental trauma in a primary care setting. *Pediatrics.* 133(2):e466-76.

[35]   Carvalho JC, Vinker F, Declerck D. (1998). Malocclusion, dental injuries and dental anomalies in the primary dentition of Belgian children. *Int J Paediatr Dent.* 8(2): 137-41.

[36] McNair A and Morris D. (2008). Managing the Developing Occlusion: A guide for dental practitioners. 3rd Ed. British Orthodontic Society.

[37] Bokor-brati M. (2000). The prevalence of precancerous oral lesions. Oral leukoplakia. *Archive of Oncology* 8(4):169-70.

[38] Arendorf TM, Bredekamp B, Cloete CA, Sauer G. (1998). Oral manifestations of HIV infection in 600 South African patients. *Journal of oral pathology & medicine.* 27:176-9.

[39] Lidral AC, Murray JC, Buetow KH, Basart AM, Schearer H, Schiang R, Naval A, Layda E, Magee K, Magee W. (1997). Studies of the candidate genes *TGFB2,MSX1, TGFA,* and *TGFB3* in the etiology of cleft lip and palate in the Philippines. *Cleft Palate Craniofac J* 34(1):1-6.

[40] Newton J.T, Bower E.J. (2005). The social determinants of oral health: new approaches to conceptualising and researching complex causal networks. *Community Dentistry and Oral Epidemiology.* 33:25-34

[41] Watt, R. G. (2005). Strategies and approaches in oral disease prevention and health promotion. *Bulletin of the World Health Organization, 83*(9), 711-718

[42] World Health Organization (WHO 2000). Global strategy for the prevention and control of non-communicable diseases. Geneva

[43] Marinho, V. C., Higgins, J. P., Sheiham, A., & Logan, S. (2004). Combinations of topical fluoride (toothpastes, mouthrinses, gels, varnishes) versus single topical fluoride for preventing dental caries in children and adolescents. *Cochrane Database Syst Rev,* 1.

[44] Narksawat K, Boonthum A, Tonmukayakul U. (2011). Roles of parents in preventing dental caries in the primary dentition among preschool children in Thailand. *Asia Pac J Public Health.* 23(2):209-16. doi: 10.1177/1010539509340045. Epub 2009 Jul 2.

[45] American Academy of Pediatrics. Practice guideline endorsement. Recommendations for Using Fluoride to Prevent and Control Dental Caries in the United States. Available at: http://www.aap.org/policy/fluoride.html. (Accessed September 2014)

[46] Rozier R. G., Bawden, J. W., Slade, G. D. (2003) Prevention of Early Childhood Caries in North Carolina Medical Practices: Implications for Research and Practice. *Journal of Dental Education* 67:876-885

[47] Donovan D., McDowell I., Hunter D. (2008). AFMC Primer on Population Health A virtual textbook on Public Health concepts for clinicians. Association of Faculties of Medicine of Canada - AFMC http://phprimer.afmc.ca/inner/primer_contents

[48] Fendrychová J. Preventive Dentistry In Dostálová T, Seydlová. (2010). Dentistry and Oral Diseases for medical students. Chapter 12 Pg 191- 198. *Grada Publishing*

[49] Pine C. M., Harris R. (2007) Community Oral Health. 2nd edition Quintessence Pub.

[50] Vivekanand. (2004). Manual of Community Dentistry Chapter 9, pg 167 – 186 Jaypee Brothers Publishers.

Comparative School Dental Sealant Program to Alleviate Dental Caries Problem — Thai versus International Perspective

Sukanya Tianviwat

1. Introduction

The application of dental sealant has been recommended for caries prevention in pit and fissure surfaces. For school dental sealant programes, the Community Preventive Services Task Force recommends the implementation of school dental sealant delivery programs based on strong evidence of their effectiveness in preventing dental caries among children [1]. In the United States, school-based dental sealant programs have been implemented successfully around the country, and the American Association for Community Dental Programs and the National Maternal and Child Oral Health Resource Center have published the guideline of "Seal America" to promote the implementation of this program [2]. School dental sealant program offer several advantages over other approaches [2, 3]: increasing access to dental service among deprived children, strengthening the relationship between schools and health care institutions, and establishing the follow-up and maintenance system of the dental sealant program.

The implementation of school dental sealant programs differs from country to country. Most of the evidence of effectiveness of these programs are found in well-equipped studies conducted in developed countries. This chapter will present more than fifteen years of scientific experience of the program operating among rural primary school children in Thailand and make comparisons with scientific data published in international journals. The scope of this chapter will include several topics related to school dental sealant programs: their effectiveness, factors related to effectiveness, critical findings and most common failures, and the impact of the program on oral health status.

2. Background

In Thailand, the dental sealant program was initiated in 1996 and has been delivered to children on either a "school-based" or a "school-linked" pattern [3, 4]. In the school-based pattern, dental equipment is carried out by the dental health section of the community hospital, which visits all schools in the area under its responsibility at least once a year. Each school visit lasts 1-2 days. The mobile dental clinic, with portable field equipment, is transported from the hospital to schools by van. The equipment includes a patient chair, a portable artificial light, an operator stool, a master unit with slow-speed and high-speed handpieces with a triple syringe, a portable suction and a light polymerization unit. A temporary clinic is usually set up in an available area at each school (Figures 1 and 2). In the school-linked or hospital-based pattern, by contrast, the children receive dental sealant at the district or sub-district hospital (Figure 3). Children are screened by dentists or dental nurses at school and the parents requested to bring their children to the hospital to receive sealant. Some hospitals, however, request school teachers to bring the group of children whose parents have given permission for the child to receive dental sealant to the hospital. Some hospitals combine the two patterns of dental sealant delivery program – a school-based pattern for children in areas remote from a hospital and a school-linked pattern for children who live nearby.

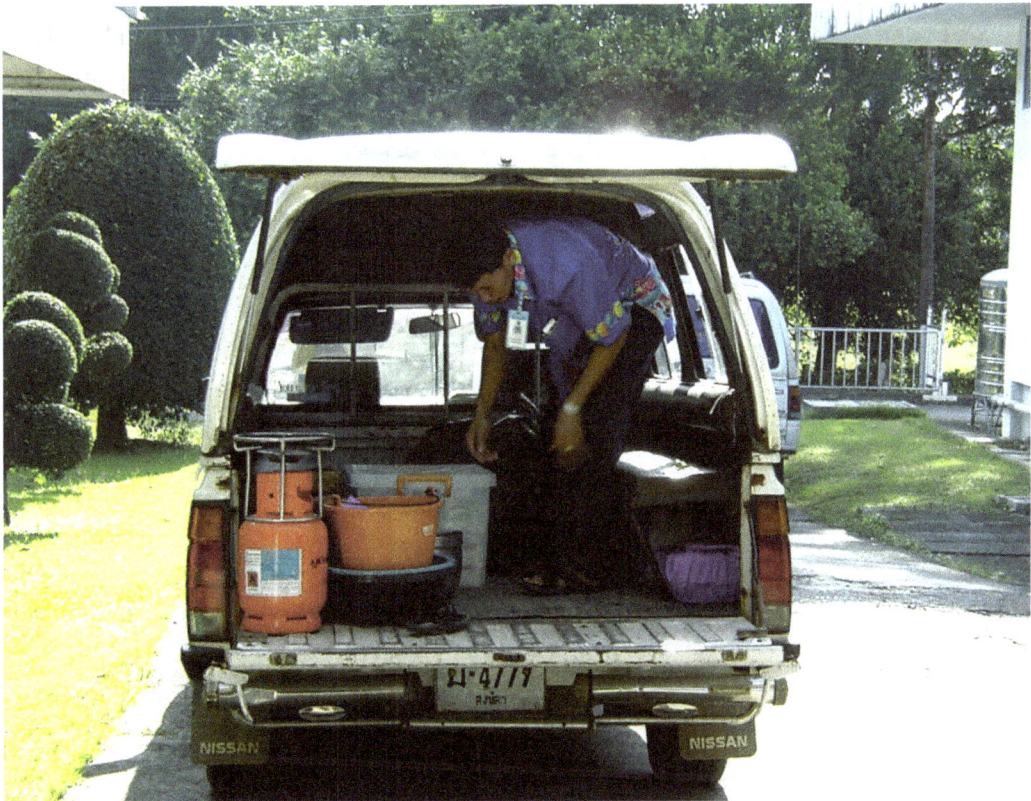

Figure 1. Mobile dental equipment delivered to school by van.

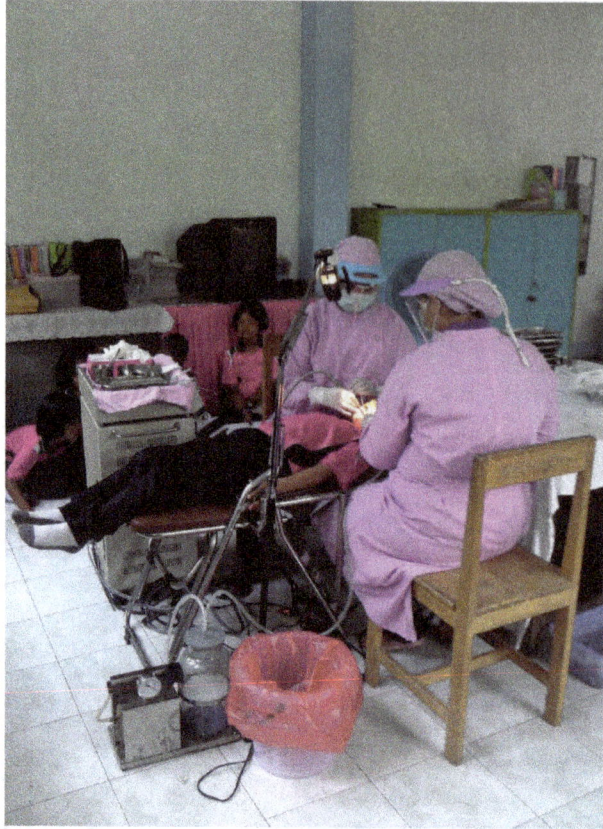

Figure 2. Mobile dental equipment set up in an available area at a school where dental services are delivered.

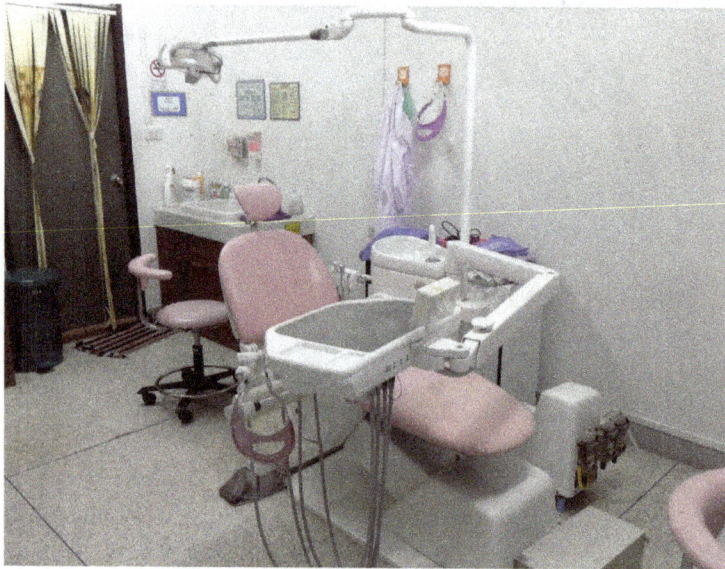

Figure 3. Dental equipment at a district or a sub-district hospital

In 2005, the Dental Health Division, Ministry of Public Health, Thailand, initiated the Oral Health Promotion and Prevention in School Children Project under the National Health Security with the slogan "Yim Sodsai Dek Thai Fun Dee" project, which can be translated as "Bright Smile and Healthy Teeth in Thai Children" [5]. One of the objectives of this project is to achieve 50% of the first grade children with an average 2.5 teeth that have received dental sealant, especially the first permanent molars. Due to this universal coverage project the number of 12-year-old children whose teeth were sealed increased from 12.7% in the year 2007 [6] to 35.2% in the year 2012 [7].

In the following text, the phrase "school dental sealant program" is used to refer to both "school-based and school-linked dental sealant programs". The content of this chapter is based mainly on reports of the sealant program implementation published since 1996, which was the year of that marked the beginning of the school dental sealant program. Experimental studies, such as those concerned with sealant materials or properties, are not included. The main content is based on resin sealant, which is in widespread use in the school programs.

3. Effectiveness of the school dental sealant program

Evaluation of the effectiveness of school dental sealant programs has been evaluated mostly on the basis of the percentage of full retention sealant and/or percentage of caries on sealed surfaces. Tables 1 and 2 compare such rates between Thailand [8-17, 25] and other countries [18-24]. Because of differences in the pattern of dental sealant delivery, in the summary of the setting, the terms "hospital" or "clinical setting" are used to represent the use of stationery dental equipment and "mobile clinic" to represent the use of mobile van or mobile dental equipment.

Major differences in sealant effectiveness between Thailand and other countries are evident. International publications report high percentages of full sealant retention within 1 to 5 years; 52.7-91.0 % [18-20, 22, 24], 74.7-85.0 % [20, 22, 24], 61.7-81.0 % [22, 24], 76 % [22] and 69% [22]. Very high long-term sealant retention at 15 and 20 years of 65% has also been reported [21]. In that study, the children had continuous access to comprehensive dental services. Moreover, the caries rate on sealed surfaces was generally low: 0.8-10.7% of the sealed teeth at one year [18-20]. Within 2 years, 0.9% of sealed surfaces had caries [20] and at 5 years 8% [22]. Very low long-term caries rate has also been reported 5.0 and 13.0% at 15 and 20 years respectively [21]. Results from Australia [23] are difficult to compare because of variation in follow-up time for evaluation of sealant retention in the study.

In Thailand, school dental sealant programs present a major difference from international results. Full sealant retention at one year in Thailand has varied between 19.6 and 67.7% [8, 9, 12, 13, 16] and that at 2 and 3 years from 8.9 to 41.8% [11, 14 - 17] and from 0 to 52.1% [9, 10, 12, 17], respectively. Moreover, higher rates of caries on sealed teeth in Thailand have been reported. At one year, the caries rate on sealed surfaces was 24% [16] and at two years 14.5-32.6% [11, 13-17]. In 2014, the 5-year caries on sealed surface rate was reported to be 13.4% [25].

In a follow-up study of sealant effectiveness in Thailand based on the Markov model [12], in which sealant was evaluated every 6 months for 30 months, the rate of sealant loss decreased with time. The first six months after application was the most vulnerable period of sealant retention, with a loss of 32.8% of teeth while caries incidence surged in the first year and also in the subsequent six months, the caries rates on sealed teeth were 10.2 % and 16.9 % in 1 and 1.5 years.

These data from the Markov model are in concordance with data presented in Tables 1 and 2, which show that school dental sealant in Thailand had relatively short-term retention and most of the caries on sealed teeth develops within 1-1.5 years after application.

4. Factors related to the school dental sealant effectiveness

Sealant retention depends on the time since application. For short-term retention, loss of sealant is related to application technique and saliva contamination. Long-term retention, on the other hand, is related to masticatory function and wear. However, a recent report of the strategy adopted to improve sealant effectiveness indicated that sealant policy also had an effect on sealant effectiveness [26]. Since, in Thailand, most of the studies have examined sealant effectiveness over the short term and have shown rather poor effectiveness, the related factors have included those dealing with basic techniques, sealant delivery conditions and strategies to improve dental sealant performance comprising attitude of the provider and sealant policy [8, 9, 26]. By contrast, international studies have dealt with more advance techniques and policy to increase coverage or access to sealant [27-32].

As mentioned above, loss of sealant in Thailand occurs within 6-12 months; such loss is related with techniques and factors of moisture control. In a study of factors related to short-term sealant retention in Thailand [8], the researcher controlled for sealant type, oral hygiene, child's cooperation and position of the teeth. After reviewing sealant procedure according to manufacturer's instruction, sealant was performed within the routine program, and after sealing for 6 months the sealant retention was examined. It was found that the checking procedure and the presence of an assistant were significant factors influencing full sealant retention. The odds of full sealant retention increased significantly, 2.8 times, when the providers checked for both occlusion and sealant retention compared with checking for sealant retention alone. The presence of an assistant increased the odds of full retention 2.3 times when compared to not having an assistant present. The shortage of dental assistants was also found to be a limitation in optimizing the mix of basic dental services (sealing, filling and extraction) for southern Thai schoolchildren [33]. This study identified the limited number of dental assistants as the crucial constraint for school dental service delivery.

The setting of the Thai school sealant program, i.e., school-based or mobile dental clinic and school-link or hospital-based dental clinic, has also been investigated as a potential factor in sealant effectiveness [9, 26], but with conflicting results. One study reported that the application of sealant in a school-based or mobile setting significantly increased the rate of sealant loss compared to that done in a hospital-based setting [26]. The other study reported a higher percentage of full sealant retention in school or mobile dental clinics than in hospital-based dental clinics [9]. However, the mobile dental conditions of two studies were different. The latter study employed a split mouth design with high power suction and the presence of a dental assistant. In each child, a dentist provided sealant on the two lower first permanent molars and restricted the number of children to be sealed in order to reduce the providers' stress from working. In this study, the percentage of full sealant retention was the highest among the studies of sealant effectiveness in Thailand (please see Table 1). On the other hand, the former study conducted in an actual situation, employing a mobile dental clinic with saliva ejector, and with no restriction on number of children or number of teeth to be sealed. Therefore, either hospital-based or school-based dental clinic could provide good results if optimal conditions for sealant – good moisture control and no tension of provider – are fulfilled. Moreover, the researcher [9] discussed that children felt more comfortable in school setting than hospital-based setting.

A recent study on strategies to improve sealant performance yielded an interesting result regarding providers' attitude and sealant policy [26]. The study examined whether audit and feedback could improve the quality of application of dental sealant in rural Thai school children. The design was a single-blind, cluster-randomized controlled trial. Sealant qualities (retention and caries), were examined prior to and after the intervention. The intervention consisted of confidential feedback of data and tailor-made problem-solving workshops. After the audit and feedback, focus group discussions (FGD) were conducted in 6 intervention clusters, including 22 dental nurses. The participating dental nurses were asked how they felt about the results from the audit and feedback and what they did when they received feedback indicating poor sealant quality. It became apparent that the participants had two distinct reactions to such feedback. The impression emerging from their direct statements was of a conflict between the quantity of children treated and the quality of service they received. On the other hand, their indirect statements indicated their wish to identify problems and to find ways of solving the problems identified by the data in the feedback. The dental nurses in all the clusters complained that the policy, which aims to maximize the number of cases in whom sealant is applied, has resulted in poor service quality because the goal of the policy does not take account of the actual situation in terms of the available manpower, overall workload, number of children needing to be treated and the condition of their teeth.

In the international perspective, more studies than in Thailand have been conducted on techniques to improve sealant effectiveness. Such studies have examined surface preparation before sealing [28, 29], four-handed sealant condition [30] and type of operator [22].

Gray et al. (2009) [28] conducted a study to review manufacturers' instructions for surface preparation in sealant use. Ten sealant products from five manufacturers which were commonly used in school sealant programs were included. The use of pumice, prophylaxis paste or prophylaxis brush was included in five products, implying handpiece use. The other five products were nonspecific. Seven products indicated that the use of fluoride-containing or oil-containing pastes should be avoided. None of the products mentioned that the operator should perform enameloplasty, fissureotomy, air abrasion or air polishing to clean the tooth surface before placing the sealant. However, one product directed the operator to remove minimal caries with a small round bur in a slow-speed handpiece after surface cleaning. In the same study, the authors conducted a review of studies comparing sealant effectiveness between mechanical preparation with pumice and using an air-water spray with sharp probe and found two studies of clinical design. Both studies reported retention rates greater than 96% at one year after sealing. Various modes of fissure preparation in combination with two filling levels were studied by Geiger (2000) [29]. In this *in vitro* study, fissure preparation was divided into three groups; no mechanical preparation, mechanical preparation with a round carbide bur, and mechanical preparation with a tapered fissure diamond bur. Then, sealant filling level in each preparation group was subdivided into minimal filling (just to the border of pit and fissure) or overfilled. The result showed that sealant penetration and retention were significantly improved in mechanically prepared compared to non-prepared fissures and preparation with a tapered fissure diamond bur was superior to that with a round carbide bur. Overfilled fissures caused significantly higher levels of micro leakage. However, nowadays, the sealant placement recommendation developed by an expert working group supported by the Centers for Disease Control and Prevention (CDC) does not recommended additional surface preparation methods, such as air abrasion or enameloplasty [27].

The effect of having a dental assistant or four-handed delivery for sealant application was reviewed after controlling for various factors, namely years since placement, tooth-surface cleaning method, isolation technique, and type of primary operator [30]. The review included 11 studies; eight studies using four-handed delivery and the other three using two-handed delivery. Summary retention rates in studies using four-handed delivery were higher than those in studies using two-handed delivery at 1, 2 and 3 years; 89.8% vs 84.8%, 83.0 % vs 72.4% and 83.0% vs 67.9%, respectively. Multivariate analysis indicated that four-handed delivery increased sealant retention by about 9 percentage points compared with two-handed delivery.

Most school dental sealant application in Thailand is implemented by dental nurses. From Tables 1 and 2, the sealant effectiveness does not obviously differ between dentists and dental nurses. In other countries sealant application in school programs is mostly done by dentists (Table 1 and 2). There was the review to identify the effect of operator and sealant effectiveness [30]. This review showed unexpected finding of the association between having a dentist as the primary operator and lower sealant retention rates. The authors suggested two possible reasons for unexpected results. First, many dentists likely had limited experience with sealant materials and/or placement techniques. And the studies in which dentists were the primary operators may have been less likely to provide training in sealant placement than the studies in which the primary operators were non dentists.

There has been an effort to distribute the simple task of sealant application to other dental personnel, i.e., dental assistants [22] or dental therapists [23]. Very high sealant was achieved when sealing was performed by a dental assistant [22]. In another study, conducted in Australia [23], it was difficult to evaluate the performance of dental therapists owing to variation of follow-up time of the sealant. It seems, therefore, that type of operator is not a critical factor influencing sealant effectiveness.

Table 1. Full sealant retention rates in Thailand and other countries by period of follow-up

First author, year	Age, tooth	Number of children, teeth at baseline	Setting, Provider	Material	Full sealant retention rate (% of teeth) — Period of follow-up (years)							
					1	2	3	4	5	10	15	20
Thailand												
Tianviwat, 2011 [8]	Grade 1§, M1	206, 347	M, DN with or without DA	Light-cured resin	67.7†							
Choomphupan, 2011 [9]	6-9, M1	212, 848	M, D / H, D	Light-cured Helioseal F	62.7 / 42.5		35.9 / 24.6					
Charnvanishporn, 2009 [10]	Grade 1§, M1	175, 355	M, NA	NA			52.1					
Thamtadawiwat, 2008 [11]	6-8, M1	183, 349	H, DN	Light-cured Prevocare		41.8						
Tianviwat, 2008 [12]	Grade 1§, M1	184, 332	M and H, DN	Light-cured resin	54.8		30.7†					
Obsuwan, 2008 [13]	6-8, M1	500, 2000	H, NA	NA	45.6*							
Kongtawelert, 2008 [14]	6-8, M1	865, 2193	H, DN without DA	Light-cured resin		36.0						
Kantamaturapoj, 2008 [15]	6-8, M1	320, 1280	H, NA	Resin (not specific)		33.2**						
Thipsoonthornchai, 2003 [16]	6-7, M1	107, 107	M, NA	Light-cured resin	19.6	8.9						
Tianviwat, 2001 [17]	6-7, M1	102, 260 / 20-21 months: 86 teeth / 32-33 months: 174 teeth	M, DN	NA		18.6**	0***					
Other countries												
Hsieh, 2014 Taiwan [18]	6-9, M1	122, 229	M, 1D:1DA	Light-cured 3M ESPE	86.0							
Muller-Bolla, 2013 France [19]	6-7, M1	253, 421	H, 1D:1DA	Light-cured Delton	52.7							
Francis, 2008 Kuwait [20]	6-8, M1	452, 1372	H, D	Light-cured Delton plus	79.8	75.0						
Wendt, 2001 Sweden [21]	NA, M1 / NA, M2	45, 153 / 45, 161	H, D / H, D	Self-cured Delton							65.0	65.0
Holst, 1998 Sweden [22]	6-10, M1 11-14, M2	976, 3218	H, DA	Light-cured Delton	91.0	85.0	81.0	76.0	69.0			
Messer, 1997 Australia [23]	6-12, All	774, 2875	H, 2DT: 1DA	NA Conseal	56.0 (1-48 months)							
Bravo, 1996 Spain [24]	6-8, M1	104, 416	M, 1D:1DA	Light-cured Delton	87.3	74.7	61.7					

§average 6-8 years old; * follow-up at 6 months; †follow-up at 20-21 months at 30 months; ** follow-up at 20-21 months; *** follow-up at 32-33 months
M1 = first permanent molar; M2 = second permanent molar; All = permanent premolar and molar; NA = not available
M = mobile dental equipment or van; H = hospital or clinical dental equipment; DN = dental nurses; D = dentist; DT = dental therapist; DA= dental assistant

First author, year	Age, tooth	Number of children, teeth at baseline	Setting, Provider	Material	Caries rate on sealed surfaces (% of teeth) Period of follow-up (years)							
					1	2	3	4	5	10	15	20
Thailand												
Plengsringam, 2014 [25]	Grade 1§, M1	473, 1795	NA, NA	NA								
Charnvanishporn, 2009 [10]	Grade 1§, M1	175, 355	M, NA	NA			21.5		13.4			
Thamtadawiwat, 2008 [11]	6-8, M1	183, 349	H, DN	Light-cured Prevocare		16.3						
Tianviwat, 2008 [12]	Grade 1§, M1	184, 332	M and H DN	Light-cured resin			26.1#					
Obsuwan, 2008 [13]	6-8, M1	500, 2000	H, NA	NA		32.6						
Kongtawelert, 2008 [14]	6-8, M1	865, 2193	H, DN without DA	Light-cured resin		14.5						
Kantamaturapoj, 2008 [15]	6-8, M1	320, 1280	H, NA	Resin (not specific)		29.7*						
Thipsoonthornchai, 2003 [16]	6-7, M1	107, 107	M, NA	Light-cured resin	24	25						
Tianviwat, 2001 [17]	6-7, M1	20-21 months: 86 teeth; 32-33 months: 174 teeth	M, DN	NA		22.1*	21.9**					
Other countries												
Hsieh, 2014 Taiwan [18]	6-9, M1	122, 229	M, 1D:1DA	Light-cured 3M ESPE	6.1							
Muller-Bolla, 2013 France [19]	6-7, M1	253, 421	H, 1D:1DA	Light-cured Delton	10.7							
Francis, 2008 Kuwait [20]	6-8, M1	452, 1372	H, D	Light-cured Delton plus	0.8	0.9						
Wendt, 2001 Sweden [21]	NA, M1 / NA, M2	45, 153 / 45, 161	H, D / H, D	Self-cured Delton							5.0	13.0
Holst, 1998 Sweden [22]	6-10, M1 / 11-14, M2	976, 3218	H, DA	Light-cured Delton					8			

§ average 6-8 years old; † follow-up at 30 months; * follow-up at 20-21 months; ** follow-up at 32-33 months
M1 = first permanent molar; M2 = second permanent molar; All = permanent premolar and molar; NA = not available
M = mobile dental equipment or van; H = hospital or clinical dental equipment; DN = dental nurses; D = dentist; DT= dental therapist; DA= dental assistant

Table 2. Caries rates on sealed surfaces in Thailand and other countries by period of follow-up

5. Critical findings and most common failures

Most studies of sealant effectiveness have reported sealant retention as full, partial or total loss, and reported caries or no caries on sealed surfaces. However, among these sealant failures, there were a few common or typical types of sealant loss, and these reflect the cause of failures and could suggest how to improve school dental sealant effectiveness [26]. The most common failure scenarios in the Thai context are presented below with illustrations. In each picture, a combination of failures might be seen; however, for explanation purposes the major failure is demonstrated. The causes of failure which were summarized from a problem-solving work-shop in the audit and feedback study [26] are also discussed.

5.1. Partial retention with ledge and caries present

The common characteristics of this type of loss are loss of some sealant and a pit/fissure with ledge exposed when exploring with a sharp probe. Caries is present with loss of tissue beyond the boundaries of the pits and fissures on occlusal surfaces and lesions contain demineralized dentine, usually light brown, and have a soft texture when explored with a blunt probe using gentle pressure (Figure 4). This common failure was present in 67.6% of the total caries on sealed surfaces at 6 months follow-up after a single sealant application [26] (data available from author). The same result was found in a long-term follow-up study in the context of high caries risk children in an inefficient school dental sealant program [12]. The effect of partial sealant retention with ledge present is to increase the risk of caries 3.1 times compared with total sealant loss [12]. A study in Scotland [34] confirmed the result: teeth with partially retained sealant at baseline were found to have a significantly higher percentage of caries (22.9%) than teeth with complete sealing (14.4%).

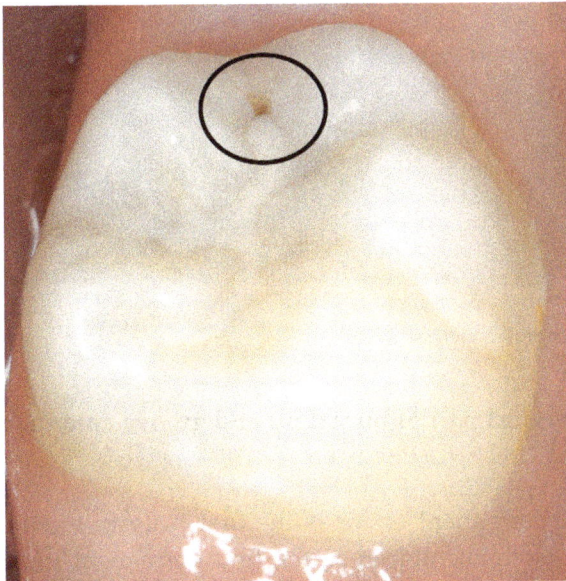

Figure 4. Partial retention with ledge and caries present

One review has addressed the controversy over the caries risk in formerly sealed teeth [35]. The authors examined the risk of caries development in teeth with partially or fully lost sealant relative to the risk in teeth that had never received sealants and concluded that teeth with fully or partially lost sealant were not at a higher risk of developing caries than teeth that had never been sealed. The studies included in the review were conducted in developed countries, where the risk of caries is quite low, the services are provided in well-equipped clinics and the sealant effectiveness is high.

It is obviously important that follow-up and repair of sealant loss should be promoted to increase the effectiveness of any school dental sealant program.

5.2. Loss of sealant at poor oral hygiene surfaces

From observational study, this type of loss accounts for approximately 60.7% of all failures of dental sealant [26]. Poor oral hygiene gauged by the presentation of soft debris covering more than 2/3 of the exposed tooth surface (Figure 5) based on the Debris index of Simplified Oral Hygiene Index [36]. The characteristics are partial or total loss of sealant and the presence of poor oral hygiene. This recent finding indicates a significant effect of poor oral hygiene on failure of sealant retention.

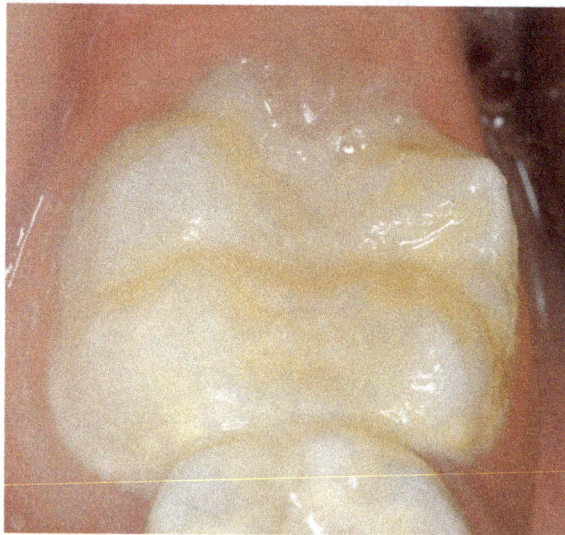

Figure 5. Loss of sealant at poor oral hygiene surfaces

5.3. Loss of sealant at cervical part of buccal pit and groove among lower first permanent molars.

In Thailand, lower first permanent molar is the first priority for the school dental sealant program among grade 1 schoolchildren as the first permanent molars present the highest percentage of caries: 51.4% in 12-year-old children [37]. Among all children, the lower first permanent molars comprised 36.4% and the upper first permanent molars 17.5% of all carious teeth [5]. The ratio of sealant service between lower teeth and upper teeth varied between 1.4:1 and 2.2:1 [8, 26]. This failure is characterized by a lack of sealant remaining at the lower end of the the buccal pit and groove (Figure 6) and was found in approximately 31.9% of sealed lower permanent molars. The significant concern of the scenario is the frequent presentation of caries development. The causes are related to tooth eruption and policy. Findings from focus group discussion in the sealant study [26] revealed that the policy of achieving 50% of first grade children being sealed placed a considerable burden on providers and had a negative impact on the quality of the program. A study of the eruption pattern in American children [38] found that only 57 % of first graders had all first permanent molars sufficiently erupted for sealing. In Taiwan [18], children aged 6-9 years presented only 46.9% (229 teeth among 488 teeth) of first permanent molars had erupted without decay, and eruption with decay or filling was present in 23.8% (116 teeth among 488 teeth). The loss of buccal surface was higher than that of occlusal surface among lower first permanent molars [23].

A study of eruption pattern of first permanent molar among Thai kindergarten level 2 and grade 1 and grade 2 schoolchildren [39] found that the percentages of at least one first permanent molar eruption were 6.0%, 75.1% and 98.5%, respectively. Among grade-1 children, who are the target group of the school dental sealant program in Thailand, the right lower first permanent molar had erupted 65.3% and caries was found 12.1%, whereas on the left side 64.3% had erupted and caries was present 9.1%. In the context of high caries prevalence, it is likely that the provider might seal teeth that are not in a suitable condition for sealing, such as being insufficiently erupted which more than half of the buccal surface covered by gingival tissue.

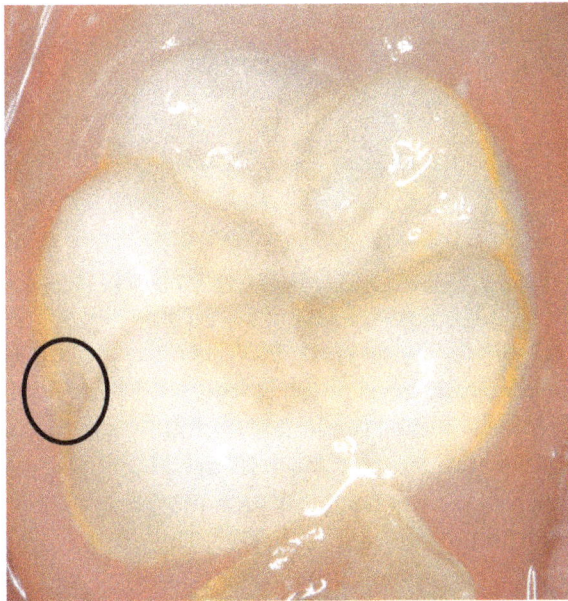

Figure 6. Loss of sealant at cervical part of buccal pit and groove among lower first permanent molars.

5.4. Loss of sealant at distal pit and groove of the occlusal surface of lower molars

The characteristics of this failure were no sealant remaining at the distal pit and groove of the occlusal surfaces of the lower molars and the presence of a ledge (Figure 7). The sealant was often was bulked or thick. This type of failure was seen in 16.3% of sealed lower permanent molars [26] (data available from author). The cause of failure, summarized from the problem-solving workshop, concerned the application technique. The provider used a brush to deliver sealant onto the tooth surface and the excess sealant flowed under gravity collecting in bulk and forming a thick layer at the distal end of the groove. When the children chewed, this area was at risk of fracture.

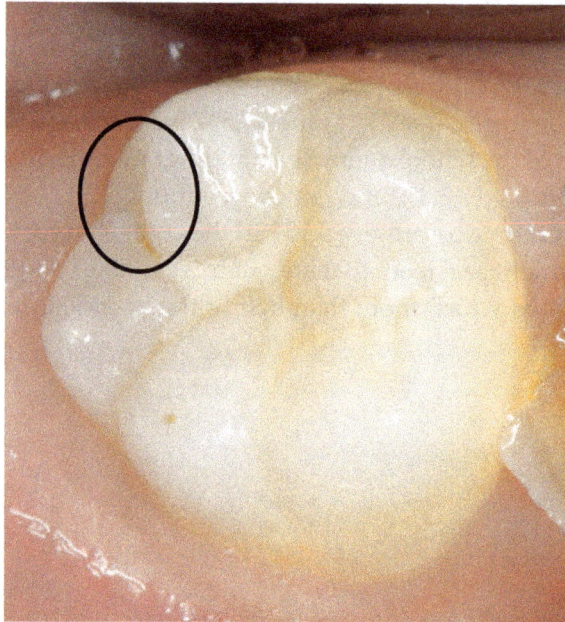

Figure 7. Loss of sealant at distal pit and groove of the occlusal surface of lower molars

There were other failures related with case selection and sealant technique; for instance, operculum covered on sealed surfaces (Figure 8), and void in sealant with or without caries (Figure 9). Most of the failures could be prevented by following the correct sealant procedure and instructions. The study of audit and feedback showed that these common failure scenarios and their own performance data as reflected in retention and caries rates could change the provider's attitude toward dental service quality [26]. The result from focus group discussion showed that they realized the poor quality of the dental service and felt they had to achieve a balance between quantity and quality of school dental sealant. They identified the means of solving their problems of service quality in terms of reallocating manpower, increasing their awareness, and improved equipment maintenance and sealant technique.

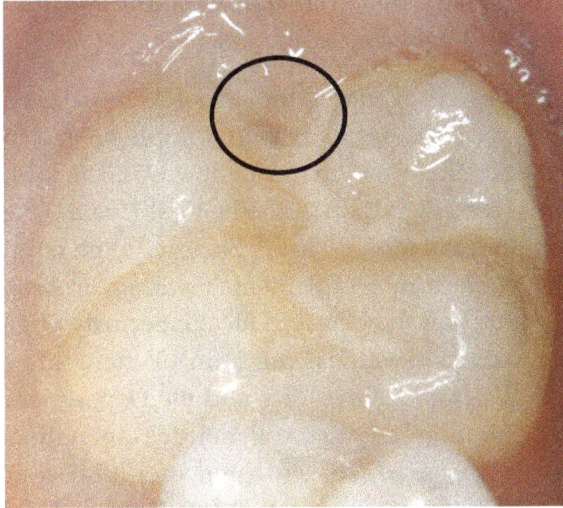

Figure 8. Operculum cover on sealed surface

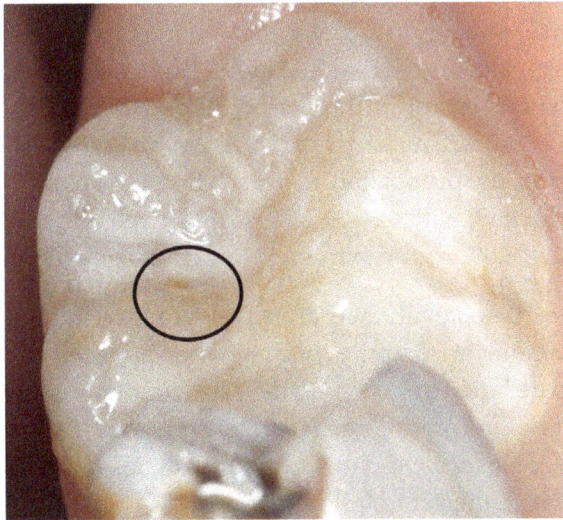

Figure 9. A void in sealant with caries

6. Impact of school dental sealant on oral health status

Evidence showing the effectiveness of dental sealant for caries prevention is drawn from several scientific papers [27, 40, 41]. Data from the evaluation of the school dental sealant program under the universal coverage of health care service in Thailand are presented. The macro scale data from Ministry of Public Health and data from each area and published in Thai journals are included. The impact of the program on the dental status of children as reflected in reports of the National Oral Health Survey before and after implementation of the school dental sealant program is also discussed.

As mentioned at the beginning of the chapter, the school As mentioned at the beginning of the chapter, the school sealant sealant program was first implemented in Thailand in 1996 on a small scale [17]. By 2001, the coverage of dental sealant was still very low; only 4.5% of 12-year-old children received dental sealant [42]. In 2005, the Oral Health Promotion and Prevention in School Children Project under National Health Security "Yim (smile) Sodsai (Bright), Dek Thai (Thai Children) Fun Dee (Health Teeth)", which was a joint project of the Dental health division, Department of health, and the National Health Security Organization was launched [5]. This project was managed as a vertical program by signing a contract between chief executive officers of the Provincial Health Office and the Department of Health. The project included prevention and promotion activities; full mouth examination of first grade and third grade students, sealant for the first grade students, and after-lunch tooth brushing for primary school children. Sealant activities of the project during 2005-2007 were evaluated based on monthly reports via a web-based system. After-lunch tooth brushing activity is an on-going activity which has been conducted since 1988 in the Oral Health Surveillance and Dental Health Promotion Program for primary school children [43].

The percentages of dental examination and sealant activities are presented in Table 3. The data were retrieved from 75 provinces in Thailand. Among first grade primary school children 35.9 – 48.8% had access to dental sealant in the period 2005-2007. In 2007, the number of sealed children was lower than in 2005-2006, partly explained by the diminished incentive for sealant service providers. However, the proportion of sealed children was still lower than that in other countries, for example, Slovenia with 62-100% (1988) [44], Ireland with 50-80% (1997) [45], and the United States with 51.1-88.0% and an extremely low coverage in one area of 41.0% (2002) [46].

The impact of the program was evaluated after two years of implementation based on the number of carious teeth among third grade children who had received sealant when they were in grade 1. Table 4 compares data between grade 3 sealed and unsealed children. Number of caries in first permanent molars among sealed children was 33.1% - much lower than that in unsealed children (66.9%). Nevertheless the number of caries in sealed group was quite high compared to other studies at the same follow-up period in Thai context (please see table 2). Evidence to support dental sealant effectiveness has been reported in several international publications. However, reports of the impact of the school dental sealant program at the macro level are few. In Slovenia, the most recent caries decline during 1987-1998; i.e. from 5.1 to 1.8 for 12-year-olds, and from 10.2 to 4.3 for 15-year-olds, was most likely due to supervised brushing with concentrated fluoride gel taking place several times a year in primary schools attended by children aged 7–15 years, improved oral hygiene, and a comprehensive program of applying fissure sealants, particularly on first molars. The Cochran database published a review of pit and fissure sealants for preventing dental decay in the permanent teeth of children and adolescents [40]. The review showed that the probability of sealed teeth remaining non-carious in patients who had received resin sealant at 24 months was 4.5 times less than that in the corresponding teeth of unsealed children (relative risk= 0.22; 95% confidence interval 0.34 to 0.22).

Activities	Educational year 2005		Educational year 2006		Educational year 2007	
	Number	Percent	Number	Percent	Number	Percent
Examination grade 1 and 3 (children)	1,299,959	81.3	1,257,486	78.6	941,968	58.9
Sealant grade 1 (children)	414,827	48.6	430,044	48.8	316,404	35.9
(teeth)	1,051,542	NA	1,212,398	NA	901,704	NA
Brushing (school)	28,647$	91.8	27,771#	94.1	27,432#	95.4
(children)	4,604,179$	87.5	4,190,561#	88.6	4,194,000#	92.5

NA = not available; $ data from 75 provinces; # data from 70 provinces

Source: Modified from Jirapongsa W, Prasertsom P. [5]

Table 3. Percentage coverage of dental examination and dental sealant in the Oral Health Promotion and Prevention in School Children Project under National Health Security

Group	Number of examined children	Percent of children who had carious in first permanent molars
Children who receive sealant	149,837	33.1
Children who did not received sealant	303,023	66.9

Source: Jirapongsa W, Prasertsom P. [5]

Table 4. Number of children and percentage of carious first permanent molars classified by sealed and unsealed grade 3 primary school children

An area-based study in Thailand found a marginally significant impact of the program regarding the proportion of children in whom caries was prevented [13]. This was a cohort study comparing sealed and unsealed groups of children. Both groups were enrolled in after-lunch tooth brushing with fluoride toothpaste. Table 5 presents the frequency of caries on first permanent molars in the two groups. A high percentage of early sealant loss was found in this study; at 6 months only 45.6% had full sealant retention – a value that is quite low compared to the data for the same period in Thailand, 54.8-67.7 % (Table 1). Therefore, in the high and early sealant loss area, the caries preventive effect was difficult to reach.

Group	Number of children	Number of children with caries (%)		Carious teeth Mean (sd)
Children who receive sealant	500	163 (32.6)	p-value	p-value < .001
Children who did not received sealant	500	159 (31.8)	0.052	

Source: Obsuwan K. [13]

Table 5. Caries on first permanent molars at 24 months between sealed and unsealed group

The percentages of sealed and unsealed surfaces having caries have been compared in several cross-sectional studies using baseline data from the web-based system and examined caries at the end of the study. Table 6 summarizes the caries data from three studies comparing children who received dental sealant with others who did not. The differences were only marginally significant (rows 1 and 3) or non-significant (row 2). The sealant retention rates in these studies were quite low (please see Table 1). In two of the studies; 42% at 2 years [11] and 33.2% at 20 months [15], although somewhat higher in the third study, 52.1% at three years [10]. Thus, under low effectiveness conditions, caries preventive effect was low.

First author	Number of sealed children at last follow up	Number and percent of caries	Number of unsealed children at last follow up	Number and percent of caries	p-value
Charnvanishporn, 2009 [10]	130	28 (21.5%)	130	54 (41.5%)	0.038
Thamtadawiwat, 2008 [11]	183	57 (16.3%)*	215	56 (13.3 %)*	0.14
Kantamaturapoj, 2008 [15]	300	85 (28.3 %)	300	108 (36.0 %)	0.044

*only carious data at teeth level are available: 57 from 349 teeth (16.3%) among sealed group and 56 from 422 teeth (13.3%) among unsealed group

Table 6. Percentage of caries in sealed and unsealed children

In Thailand, the Dental Health Division, Department of Health, has conducted a National Oral Health Survey every 5 years, the most recent one was the 7th survey conducted in 2012. The data from 4 surveys were used to reveal the impact of dental sealant on the oral health status of children (Figure 10). As the target group of the school dental sealant project was grade 1 primary-school children, aged 6-8 years, the data of 12-year-olds were used. The number of examined children and caries experience in permanent teeth of each survey are shown in Table 7. The survey data did not report caries experience in first permanent molars (only the 4th survey reported caries by tooth), therefore the total caries experience in permanent teeth is present as proxy for caries experience of first permanent molars since 51.4% of caries teeth in 12 years old children were in first permanent molars [37].

The 4th, 6th and 7th surveys were conducted in 17 provinces, 4 provinces from each region (north, south, north-east and central) and Bangkok, the capital province. The sample size of the 5th survey was very large because the Dental Health Division expanded the survey from 17 to 48 provinces and increased the size of the sample for improved representativeness at the provincial level (Table 7). The 4th survey was conducted before the small scale implementation of school dental sealant activity, therefore the data from this survey together with other dental health programs could be used as baseline data. Data from the 5th survey were used to assess the impact of the small scale school dental sealant program. The 6th and 7th survey data were used to assess the impact of the large scale program. Caries experience of 12-year-old children from the four surveys is presented in Table 7. Coverage of dental sealant is shown in Table 8. Other dental health care programs implemented during 1994 to date are summarized in Table 9.

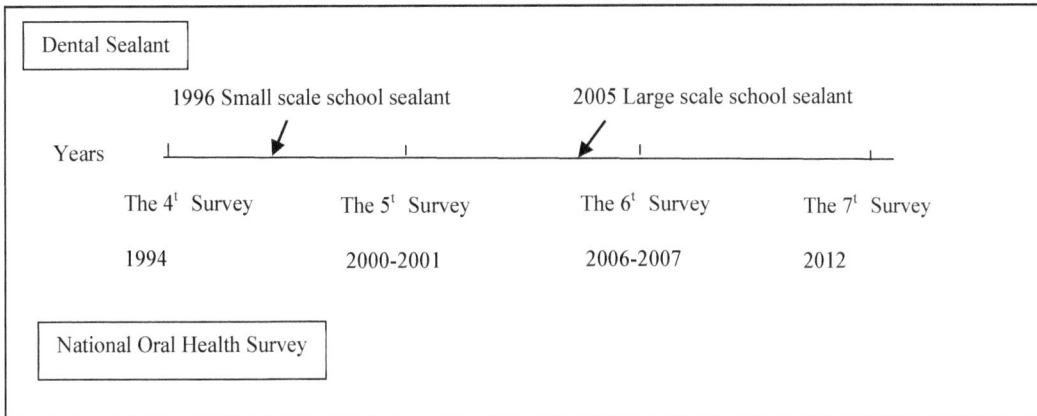

Figure 10: Summary of implementation timeline of National Oral Health Surveys and the dental sealant programme

During the period 1994 to 2000/2001 [42, 47], the percentage of children affected by caries increased but the average caries experience in permanent teeth was quite stable (Table 7). The oral health program at that time comprised school dental sealant on a small scale, ongoing after-lunch tooth brushing and oral health education (Tables 8 and 9). However, from the 5th survey, the proportion of children who enrolled every day in the after-lunch tooth brushing program was low, only 26.3%. The proportion of children who brushed their teeth every day was 86.2% in the morning and 34.6% in the evening.

Between 2000/2001 and 2006/2007 [42, 6], caries experience in terms of percentage of children affected by caries and average carious teeth per child among 12-year-olds was slightly decreased (Table 7). Sealant service was increased 2.8 times from the 5th to the 6th survey. This period included the first phase of the large scale implementation of school dental sealant and the campaign to control of sugar consumption, which emphasized the creation of networks and activities in childcare centers. However, the number of sealed children was still low (Table 8). Other dental heath activities, such as after-lunch tooth brushing and oral health education, were ongoing. The proportion of children who brushed their teeth every day at school decreased to 21.7% and that of children who did not brush increased to 57.9%. Brushing at home seemed to increase slightly (Table 8).

During the 6th and 7th surveys [6, 7], the proportion of children having caries decreased approximately five percentage points and the average number of carious teeth decreased from 1.55 to 1.3 teeth per child. The percentage of children with sealant at 12 years of age increased from 12.7% to 35.2% (Table 8). The large scale dental sealant was implemented for nearly 7 years. The percentage of tooth brushing occasion continued on the rise. However, snack consumption also increased during the same period (Table 8).

	The 4th survey [47] (1994)	The 5th survey [42] (2000-2001)	The 6th Survey [6] (2006-2007)	The 7th Survey [7] (2012)
Number of children	2,801	35,623	2,208	2,618
Percent caries	53.9	57.3	56.9	52.3
Mean DMFT and SE	1.6± 0.04	1.64*	1.55*	1.30*

*SE data are not available

Table 7. Number of children, percentage and mean caries experience of 12-year-olds from four surveys

Activities	The 4th survey [47] (1994)#	The 5th survey [42] (2000-2001)	The 6th Survey [6] (2006-2007)	The 7th Survey [7] (2012)
Dental sealant*	NA	4.5	12.7	35.2
Daily tooth brushing after-lunch	NA	26.3	21.7	17.8$
Tooth brushing occation@	NA	Morning 86.2 Evening 34.6	Every day 89.6 Mean 2.2 times a day	Morning 97.7 Evening 71.5
Use Fluoride toothpaste	NA	94.1	89.9	91.4
Eating snack everyday		NA	28.2	38.8

NA = not available

* received dental sealant and dental sealant presence at 12 years old

Data of 12 years-old were not available since oral health care behavior interviewed in 17 years and older.

$ The question was not specific to after-lunch tooth brushing program at school

@ In each survey, different questions were applied - the 5th and 7th asked whether he/she brushed every day in the morning and evening, the 6th survey asked whether he/she brushed his/her teeth every day and how often

Table 8. Percentage of 12-year-old children enrolled in the oral health prevention and promotion activities

It is difficult to draw conclusion with certainty on the reasons explaining the decline of caries [44]. In Thailand, among 12-year-old children, the important factors related to caries decline seem to be the large scale school dental sealant and frequent tooth brushing with fluoride toothpaste [7]. Since the number of children with sealants in the survey was the number of children who received dental sealant and in whom the dental sealant was still present at 12 years of age, the actual coverage should be larger than the reported figures of 12.7% and 35.2% at the 6th and 7th surveys, respectively. The percentages of children having tooth-brushing behavior with fluoride toothpaste were high. The percentage with normal gingival condition also increased from 18.0% to 29.9% from the 6th to the 7th survey. This increase could be ascribed to the tooth brushing behavior [7]. However, the eating habit is a major problem that remains to be solved.

Period	Program	Brief activities
1988	Oral Health Surveillance and Dental Health Promotion Programme for primary school Children	Dental examination by school teachers After-lunch tooth brushing program Oral health education
1996	Small scale school dental sealant	Sealant in grade 1
1999	Health Promoting School (Oral health integrated in health promotion)	Key indicators for oral health; dental examination, no caries on permanent teeth (fillings are acceptable), no gingivitis After-lunch tooth brushing with fluoride toothpaste Healthy food in school
2003	Sweet enough project	Creating network and campaign to reduce sugar consumption
2005	Oral Health Promotion and Prevention in School Children Project under National Health Security (Large scale school dental sealant)	Full mouth examination grade 1 and 3 children Sealant grade 1 children After-lunch tooth brushing in primary school

Table 9. Dental health care programs implemented for school children in Thailand

7. Conclusion and suggestion

Although the effectiveness of school dental sealant program in Thailand has continuously improved, there is still much room for further improvement. This chapter has presented the findings on effectiveness and on failures in context of the actual school programs, where more factors are operating than in the context of experimental research. Looking at failures may provide valuable information. In this case, the types of failure could reflect their causes, and be used to improve performance. In the Thai context, short-term retention is still a problem. Improvement in the related factors such as equipment, application technique and presence of chair-side assistant might result in increased effectiveness. Important improvement measures may include adjusting the goal or key performance indicators of the sealant program based on actual workload, adding in some indicator to reflect the quality of the program and initiating evaluation by an external evaluator. The quality indicator must not place additional pressure on providers; evaluation should be reward-based rather than punishment-based. The guideline and recommendation on sealant application should be strictly followed and emphasized to providers.

A school dental sealant program alone could not have much impact on oral health status since its effect is only on pit and fissure surfaces. Comprehensive prevention and promotion should be strengthened, inclusive of dental sealant, tooth brushing with fluoride toothpaste and eating behavior.

Acknowledgements

I would like to acknowledge the Thailand Dental Public Health Society and the Lion Corporation (Thailand) Limited for the Lion award of Oral Health for School Sealant Project, which supported the publication of this chapter. I am also grateful to my respected PhD advisor, Professor Dr. Virasakdi Chongsuvivatwong, who gave me many valuable ideas; and I especially acknowledge Associate Professor Dr. Songchai Thitasomakul, Assistant Professor Dr. Janpim Hintao and Dr. Banyen Sirisakulveroj for their long-time of friendship and great assistance. Special appreciation is expressed to Dr. Alan Geater and Mr. Sakda Pongcharoenyong for their kindness to review and edit this book chapter. I am also grateful to all the dental nurses and children who participated in the study.

Author details

Sukanya Tianviwat[1,2]

Address all correspondence to: Sukanya.ti@psu.ac.th

1 Faculty of Dentistry, Prince of Songkla University, Songkhla, Thailand

2 Common Oral Diseases and Epidemiology Research Center, Faculty of Dentistry, Prince of Songkla University, Songkhla, Thailand

References

[1] Guide to Community Preventive Services. Preventing Dental Caries: School-Based Dental Sealant Delivery Programs. www.thecommunityguide.org/oral/caries.html. (accessed 3 August 2013).

[2] Carter NL, with the American Association for Community Dental Programs and the National Maternal and Child Oral Health Resource Center. Seal America: The Prevention Invention (2nd ed., rev.). Washington DC: National Maternal and Child Oral Health Resource Center; 2011. http://www.mchoralhealth.org/seal/intro.html#school (accessed 12 May 2013).

[3]   Tianviwat s, Hoerup NJ. Evaluation of an outreach oral health service and use of mobile dental equipment in Southern Thailand. Journal of Public Health 2002; 32(3): 167-177.

[4]   Centers for Disease Control and Prevention. Infrastructure Development Tools Activity 5a: School-Based/School-Linked Dental Sealant Programs. http://www.cdc.gov/oralhealth/state_programs/infrastructure/activity5a.htm (accessed on 9 Sept 2014).

[5]   Jirapongsa W, Prasertsom P. Evaluation of Oral Health promotion and Prevention in School Children Project under National Health Security "Yim (smile) Sodsai (Bright), Dek Thai (Thai Children) Fun Dee (Health Teeth)" 2005-2007. Thailand Journal of Dental Public Health 2008; 13(5): 85-96.

[6]   Dental Division. The 6th Thailand National Oral Health Survey report 2006-2007. Bangkok: Health Department (Thailand), Ministry of Public Health; 2008.

[7]   Dental Division. The 7th Thailand National Oral Health Survey report 2012. Bangkok: Health Department (Thailand), Ministry of Public Health; 2013.

[8]   Tianviwat S, Hintao J, Chongsuvivatwong V, Thitasomakul S, Sirisakulveroj B. Factors related to short-term retention of sealant in permanent molar teeth provided in the school mobile dental clinic, Songkhla province, Southern Thailand. Journal of Public Health 2011; 41(1):50-58.

[9]   Choomphupan V. Comparison of pit and fissure sealant retention rate between mobile dental unit in school and dental unit in health center at 6, 12, and 36 months in Minburi district, Bangkok. Thailand Journal of Dental Public Health 2011; 16(2): 33-42.

[10] Charnvanishporn S. The retention of sealed teeth of the students in third grade primary school, after 3 years of mobile sealant project in Ranong provinces, 2007. Thailand Journal of Dental Public Health 2009; 13(3): 63-70.

[11] Thamtadawiwat D. The effectiveness of dental pit and fissure sealant program for the student in Prathomsueksa 1 Cha-am district, Phetchaburi province. Thailand Journal of Dental Public Health 2008; 13(1): 25-36.

[12] Tianviwat S, Chongsuvivatwong V, Sirisakulveroj B. Loss of sealant retention and subsequent caries development. Community Dental Health 2008; 25(4): 216-220.

[13] Obsuwan K. The effectiveness of the pit and fissure sealant in the "Save our six" project Chiang Rai, Thailand. Thailand Journal of Dental Public Health 2008; 13(1): 52-62.

[14] Kongtawelert P. A two-year evaluation of pit and fissure sealant of first permanent molars in school-based program (Yim Sod Sai Dek Thai Fun Dee) in Sukhothai province during 2005-2007. Thailand Journal of Dental Public Health 2008; 12(3): 86-96.

[15] Kantamaturapoj K. The effectiveness of dental pit and fissure sealant program in primary school children in Kamphaengphet province. Thailand Journal of Dental Public Health 2008; 12(2): 7-16.

[16] Thipsoonthornchai J. The comparative study on retention rate and caries prevention between glass ionomer and resin using as pit and fissure sealant in mobile dental service, Buriram province. Thailand Journal of Dental Public Health 2003; 8(1-2): 62-77.

[17] Tianviwat S, Chukadee W, Sirisakunweroj B, Leewanant R, Larsen MJ. Retention of pit and fissure sealants under field conditions after nearly 2-3 years. Journal of the Dental Association of Thailand 2001; 51(2): 115-120.

[18] Hsieh H, Huang S, Tsai C, Chiou M, Liao C. Evaluation of a sealant intervention program among Taiwanese aboriginal schoolchildren. Journal of Dental Sciences 2014; 9 (2): 178-184.

[19] Muller-Bolla M, Lupi-Pe´gurier L, Bardakjian H, Velly AM. Effectiveness of school-based dental sealant programs among children from low-income backgrounds in France: a pragmatic randomized clinical trial. Community Dentistry and Oral Epidemiology 2013; 41(3): 232–241.

[20] Francis R, Mascarenhas AK, Soparkar P, Al-Mutawaa S. Retention and effectiveness of fissure sealants in Kuwaiti school children. Community Dental Health 2008; 25(4): 211-215

[21] Wendt LK, Koch G, Birkhed D. On the retention and effectiveness of fissure sealant in permanent molars after 15-20 years: a cohort study. Community Dentistry and Oral Epidemiology 2001; 29(4): 302-307.

[22] Holst A, Braune K, Sullivan A. A five-year evaluation of fissure sealants applied by dental assistants. Swedish Dental Journal 1998; 22(5-6): 195-201.

[23] Messer LB, Calache H, Morgan MV. The retention of pit and fissure sealants placed in primary school children by Dental Health Services, Victoria. Australian Dental Journal 1997; 42(4): 233-239.

[24] Bravo M, Osorio E, García-Anllo I, Llodra JC, Baca P. The influence of dft index on sealant success: a 48-month survival analysis. Journal of Dental Research 1996; 75(2): 768-774.

[25] Plengsringam N, Tharasombat S. Effectiveness of dental sealant in preventing dental caries among students in a school dental health program of Pranangklao hospital, Nonthaburi. Journal of Health Science 2014; 23(1): 91-98.

[26] Tianviwat S. Performance improvement of dental service quality in the school dental sealant program following the implementation of an audit and feedback system. Bangkok: Thailand Research Fund. 2012-2013.

[27] Gooch B, Griffin S, Gray S, Kohn W, Rozier R, et al. Preventing Dental Caries Through School-Based Sealant Programs: Updated Recommendations and Reviews of Evidence. Journal of the American Dental Association 2009; 140(11):1356-1365.

[28] Gray SK, Griffin SO, Malvitz DM, Gooch BF. A comparison of the effects of tooth brushing and handpiece prophylaxis on retention of sealants. Journal of the American Dental Association 2009; 140(1): 38-46.

[29] Geiger SB, Gulayev S, Weiss EI. Improving fissure sealants quality: mechanical preparation and filling level. Journal of Dentistry 2000; 28(6):407-412.

[30] Griffin SO, Jones K, Gray SK, Malvitz DM, Gooch BF. Exploring four-handed delivery and retention of resin-based sealants. Journal of the American Dental Association 2008; 139(3): 281-289.

[31] Albert DA, McManus JM, Mitchell DA. Models for delivering school-based dental care. Journal of School Health 2005; 75(5): 157-161.

[32] Jackson DM, Jahnke LR, Kerber L, Nyer G, Siemens K, et al. Creating a successful school-based mobile dental program. Journal of School Health 2007; 77(1): 1-6.

[33] Tianviwat S, Chongsuvivatwong V, Birch S. Optimizing the mix of basic dental services for Southern Thai schoolchildren based on resource consumption, service needs and parental preference. Community Dentistry and Oral Epidemiology 2009; 37(4): 372-380.

[34] Chestnutt I, Schafer F, Jacobson P, Stephen K. The prevalence and effectiveness of fissure sealants in Scottish adolescents. British Dental Journal 1994; 177(4): 125-129.

[35] Griffin S, Gray S, Malvitz D, Gooch B. Caries Risk in Formerly Sealed Teeth. The Journal of the American Dental Association 2009;140(4):415-423.

[36] Green JC, Vermillion JR. The simplified oral hygiene index. The Journal of the American Dental Association 1964; 68: 7-13.

[37] Dental Division. Oral Health Promotion and Prevention in School Children Project under National Health Security. http://www.anamai.ecgates.com/news/news_detail.php?id=323. (accessed 3 May 2014).

[38] Kuthy R, Ashton J. Eruption pattern of permanent molars: Implication for school-based dental sealant program. Journal of Public Health Dentistry 1989; 49(1):7-14.

[39] Muangmuen T. Permanent First Molar Eruption and Dental Caries in Children of Banklang Subdistrict, Lomsak District, Pethchabun Province. Thailand Journal of Dental Public Health 2014; 19(1): 9-20.

[40] Ahovuo-Saloranta A, Hiiri A, Nordblad A,MäkeläM,Worthington HV. Pit and fissure sealants for preventing dental decay in the permanent teeth of children and adolescents. Cochrane Database of Systematic Reviews 2008, Issue 4. Art. No.: CD001830. DOI:10.1002/14651858.CD001830.pub3.

[41] Ahovuo-Saloranta A, Forss H, Walsh T, Hiiri A, Nordblad A, et al. Sealants for pre-venting dental decay in the permanent teeth. Cochrane Database of Systematic Reviews 2013, Issue 3. Art. No.: CD001830. DOI: 10.1002/14651858.CD001830.pub4.

[42] Dental Division. The 5th Thailand National Oral Health Survey report 2000-2001. Bangkok: Health Department (Thailand), Ministry of Public Health; 2002.

[43] Dental Division. Manual of Dental Health Surveillance Project for Primary School Children. Bangkok: The War Veterans Organization of Thailand Publishing; 1988.

[44] Vrbic V. Reasons for caries decline in Slovenia. Community Dentistry and Oral Epidemiology 2000; 28(2):126-132.

[45] O'Mullane D, Clarke D, Daly F, McDermott S, Murphy B, et al. Use of fissure sealants in the Eastern Health Board in the Republic of Ireland. 45th ORCA Congress. Caries Research 1998; 32(4):267–317 (abstract no. 42).

[46] Kumar JV, Wadhawan S. Targeting dental sealants in school-based programs: evaluation of an approach. Community Dentistry and Oral Epidemiology 2002; 30(3): 210–215.

[47] Dental Division. The 4th Thailand National Oral Health Survey report 1994. Bangkok: Health Department (Thailand), Ministry of Public Health; 1995.

Permissions

List of Contributors

Elena Preoteasa, Laura Iosif, Catalina Murariu Magureanu and Marina Imre
Department of Prosthodontics, Faculty of Dental Medicine, Carol Davila University of Medicine and Pharmacy, Bucharest, Romania

Cristina Teodora Preoteasa
Department of Oral Diagnosis, Ergonomics, Scientific Research Methodology, Faculty of Dental Medicine, Carol Davila University of Medicine and Pharmacy, Bucharest, Romania

Ana Isabel García-Kass, Juan Antonio García-Núñez and Victoriano Serrano-Cuenca
Department of Stomatology III, School of Dentistry, Complutense University of Madrid, Spain

Ticiana Sidorenko de Oliveira Capote and Marcela de Almeida Gonçalves
Dental School at Araraquara, Univ. Estadual Paulista, UNESP, Department of Morphology, Araraquara, São Paulo, Brazil

Andrea Gonçalves and Marcelo Gonçalves
Dental School at Araraquara, Univ. Estadual Paulista, UNESP, Department of Diagnostic and Surgery, Araraquara, São Paulo, Brazil

J. M. F. A. Fernandes and V. A. Menezes
Post-graduation in Pediatric Dentistry, Faculty of Dentistry, University of Pernambuco, Camaragibe, Pernambuco, Brazil

A. J. R. Albuquerque
RENORBIO, Northeast Network of Biotechnology, Federal University of Paraiba, Biotechnology Centre, Campus I, Joao Pessoa, Paraiba, Brazil

M. A. C. Oliveira and K. M. S. Meira
Post-graduation in Dentistry, Health Science Center, University of Paraíba, João Pessoa, Paraíba, Brazil

F. C. Sampaio
RENORBIO, Northeast Network of Biotechnology, Federal University of Paraiba, Biotechnology Centre, Campus I, Joao Pessoa, Paraiba, Brazil
Post-graduation in Dentistry, Health Science Center, University of Paraíba, João Pessoa, Paraíba, Brazil

R. A. Menezes Júnior
Alternative and Renewable Energy Center, Department of Renewable Energy Engineering, Federal University of Paraíba, João Pessoa, Paraíba, Brazil

Anna Maria Heikkinen, Päivi Mäntylä and Jussi Leppilahti
Institute of Dentistry, Helsinki University, Central Hospital Helsinki, Finland

Jukka Meurman
Institute of Dentistry, Helsinki University, Central Hospital Helsinki, Finland
Departments of Oral and Maxillofacial Diseases and Periodontology, Helsinki University, Central Hospital Helsinki, Finland

Timo Sorsa
Institute of Dentistry, Helsinki University, Central Hospital Helsinki, Finland
Departments of Oral and Maxillofacial Diseases and Periodontology, Helsinki University, Central Hospital Helsinki, Finland
Division of Periodontology, Department of Dental Medicine, Karolinska Institutet, Huddinge, Sweden

Nilminie Rathnayake
Division of Periodontology, Department of Dental Medicine, Karolinska Institutet, Huddinge, Sweden

Marisa Alves Nogueira Diaz and Isabela de Oliveira Carvalho
Departament of Biochemistry and Molecular Biology, Federal University of Viçosa, Viçosa, Minas Gerais, Brazil

Gaspar Diaz
Departament of Chemistry, Federal University of Minas Gerais, Belo Horizonte, Minas Gerais, Brazil

H. S. Mbawala, F. M. Machibya and F. K. Kahabuka
Department of Orthodontics, Paedodontics and Preventive Dentistry, School of Dentistry, Muhimbili University of Health and Allied Sciences, Dar es Salaam

Sukanya Tianviwat
Faculty of Dentistry, Prince of Songkla University, Songkhla, Thailand
Common Oral Diseases and Epidemiology Research Center, Faculty of Dentistry, Prince of Songkla University, Songkhla, Thailand

Index

A
Alveolar Ridge Resorption, 6, 8-10
Antimicrobials, 86, 89-94, 97, 140, 153
Arterial Calcifications, 55, 60, 63

B
Bifid Mandibular Canal, 55, 57, 59, 76-77, 79
Bifurcation, 57-58, 63-64, 66
Biofilm, 37-39, 85-90, 93, 95-100, 102, 110, 114, 139, 142, 144-146, 149, 151, 160, 169
Biofilm Growth, 85, 88
Blood Debris, 38
Bone Density, 10, 60

C
Calcified Carotid Atheroma, 64
Calcified Stylohyoid Complex, 55, 60-63, 79
Candidal Leukoplakia, 17
Cardiovascular Disease, 127
Cavitation, 34-36, 39, 41, 43, 46, 49
Cervical Arthritis, 63
Chitosan, 142, 153-154
Chlorhexidine, 15, 18, 25, 86, 90, 95, 105, 115, 118, 140, 142, 144, 146, 148, 150, 154
Combination Syndrome, 12, 14, 18, 25
Cytokine, 137

D
Dental Caries, 29, 85-86, 93, 98, 101, 110, 140, 149-150, 153, 163, 166-167, 175, 177, 180, 182, 184, 204, 206-207
Dental Restorative Material, 86
Dental Treatment, 2, 8, 163-164, 176, 179-180
Denture, 1-20, 23-32, 146, 165, 167
Denture Stomatitis, 4-6, 8, 11, 16-18, 32
Diabetes, 6, 8, 10, 16, 63-64, 66, 103, 127-128, 137, 142, 166, 168, 170, 175, 181

E
Edentulism, 1-3, 5-8, 10-12, 14, 18, 21, 28-30, 128
Elastase, 121, 123-125, 130, 132, 136-137

E
Endodontic Surgery, 47, 50
Escherichia Coli, 95, 152
Etiology, 8, 10, 14-16, 18, 21, 31-32, 60, 73, 75, 138, 182
Exostosis, 9, 11, 14

F
Fibrous Hyperplasia, 15-16

G
Gingival Hyperplasia, 4

H
Halitophobia, 104
Halitosis, 75, 103-105, 109, 112-114, 116, 118
Hinokitiol, 105, 107, 109, 116
Hyperpigmentation, 22-23
Hyperplasia, 4, 8, 15-17, 27, 31

I
Immunoglobulin, 110
Implant Overdenture, 4, 21, 26-27, 33
Inflammatory Papillary, 15-17

L
L. Reuteri, 108, 111
Lactoferrin, 105, 108, 110, 116

M
Mandibular Anterior Teeth, 12
Mandibular Edentulism, 11, 14
Mastication, 4-5, 8-9, 20, 27, 120
Mastication Deficiencies, 4, 8
Matrix Metalloproteinase, 122, 132-134, 137
Maxillary Tuberosity, 10, 12
Mikulicz Syndromes, 17
Muscular Hypotonia, 19
Mylohyoid Muscle, 12, 58
Myofacial Pain, 63

N
Neutrophil, 120, 123, 125-126, 134-136

O

Occlusal Trauma, 12

Oral Cavity, 31, 39, 85-86, 90, 97, 103-105, 128, 138, 142, 144-146, 148-149, 170, 180

Oral Health, 2, 5-8, 27, 29-32, 60, 86, 97, 99, 110, 114, 118, 122, 129, 132, 135, 141, 151, 155, 163-164, 166, 180, 182, 197-199, 205, 207-208

Oral Mucosa, 8, 11, 15-16, 18, 20, 32, 85, 106, 170

Osseous Density, 49

Ostectomy, 39, 50

P

Panoramic Radiography, 55-70, 72-75, 78, 80-81

Passive Ultrasonic Irrigation, 45-46, 54

Periodontal Disease, 2, 8-10, 13, 25, 39, 51, 56, 103, 109, 111, 120, 123, 128-136, 142, 168, 181

Periodontitis, 25, 34, 38-40, 103, 107, 111, 113, 117, 119-126, 128-138, 147, 149, 167-168, 181

Phleboliths, 55, 70-73, 82-83

Probiotic Bacteria, 105, 108, 110

Prophylaxis, 35, 40, 104, 165, 189, 207

Propolis, 141-142, 152-153

Protease, 109, 116, 125

R

Retromolar Pad, 10, 12

Rheumatoid Arthritis, 127-128, 134, 137

S

Sialolithiasis, 55, 63, 67, 70, 73, 75, 81-82

Streptococcus Pyogenes, 110, 117

Stylohyoid Complex, 55, 60-63, 79-80

Systemic Inflammation, 119-120, 127

T

Tonsillolith, 73, 83-84

Traumatic Ulcer, 6, 15

U

Ultrasonic Instrumentation, 34, 41-43, 45-46, 53

www.ingramcontent.com/pod-product-compliance
Lightning Source LLC
Chambersburg PA
CBHW061958190326
41458CB00009B/2902